Praise for *Medic, a Diary*

"It's one thing to be told these stories but another altogether to watch them. Which is exactly what Horowitz has given us—a chance to bear witness. Profane in its depiction, exquisite in its simplicity, *Medic* drags you right up next to the dead and forces you to look. The great magic trick is that in each panel he's managed to squeeze in all the humor, indifference and grace that define a life on the ambulance. This book will blow you away."

— Kevin Hazzard, award-winning writer of *No One's Coming,*
A Thousand Naked Strangers, and *American Sirens*

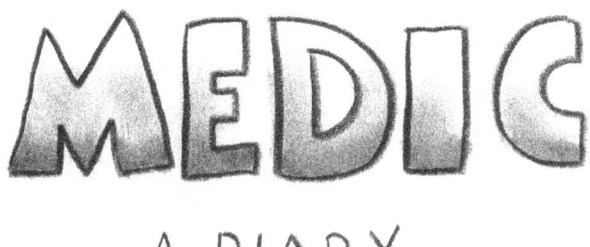

MEDIC

A DIARY

MEDIC

A DIARY

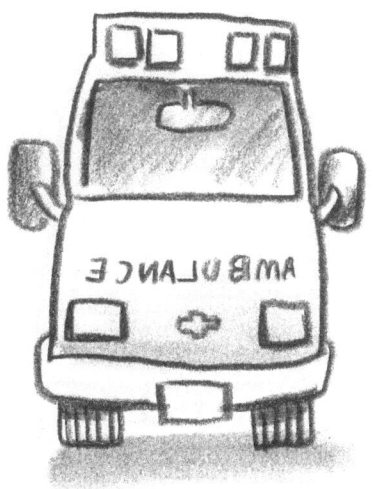

DAVE HOROWITZ

Black Pencil Press

Author's note: This book is based on my experiences working commercial EMS in New York's Hudson Valley. Many of my coworkers have graciously allowed me to use their names and likenesses in this book (they know who they are). Details and characteristics of all other people and details of events in this book have been changed or are entirely fictional. Any similarities to real people (who have not granted permission) or events in this work are purely coincidental.

The art was done with black colored pencil and charcoal on paper.

Acknowledgments: Special thanks to Scott Shortle for motivating me to keep going, page after page. Thanks to Rachel Crozier and Anissa Kapsales for copy-editing.

Thanks to all my partners, especially James "Cow" Cowperthwaite, Scott Shortle, Jen Christiansen, Ryan Lynch, Timmy Mitzel, Steve Delage, Chris Hyatt, Steve Helsley, Tim Lena, Jodie Gregory, Kim Winkler, Phil Sinagra, Joe Orr, Walanya Green, Chuck Foster, Joe Vitti, Karl Forst, Bill Drakert, Mark Caserto, Jon Edouard, Nick Violaris, Ellen Murray, Jesse Galina, Leroy Burnett, Ariel Zangla, and Kathy Hydos.

Thank you to every patient who allowed me to try to help them.

Copyright © 2025 by Dave Horowitz

All rights reserved. Published by Black Pencil Press.
blackpencilpress.com

ISBN 979-8-218-81041-2

for my wife

Introduction

I had just started medic school when I went to my first "unattended."

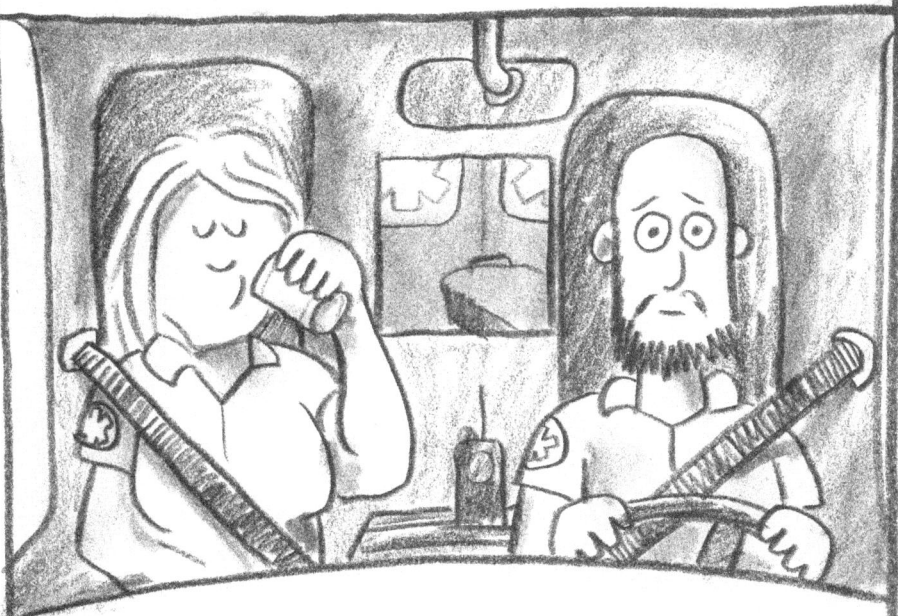

I was an EMT (emergency medical technician), and my partner, Kim, was the paramedic. Kim had many more years of training and experience. I was pretty much a noob.

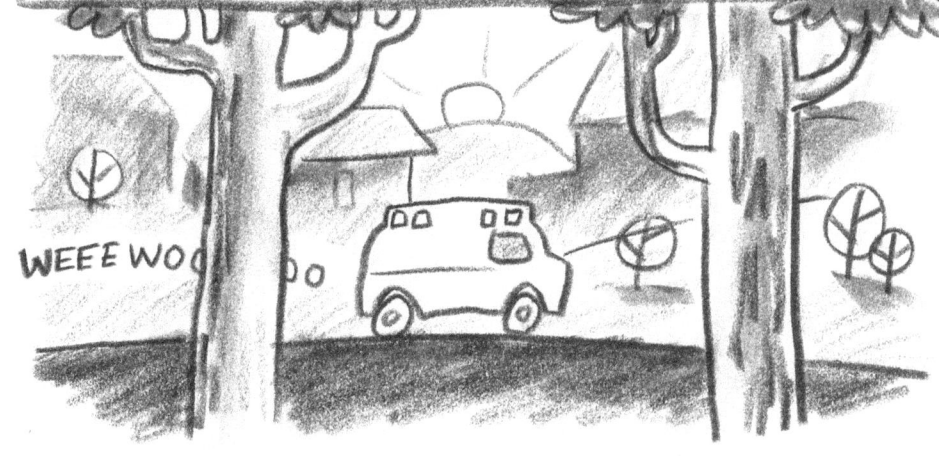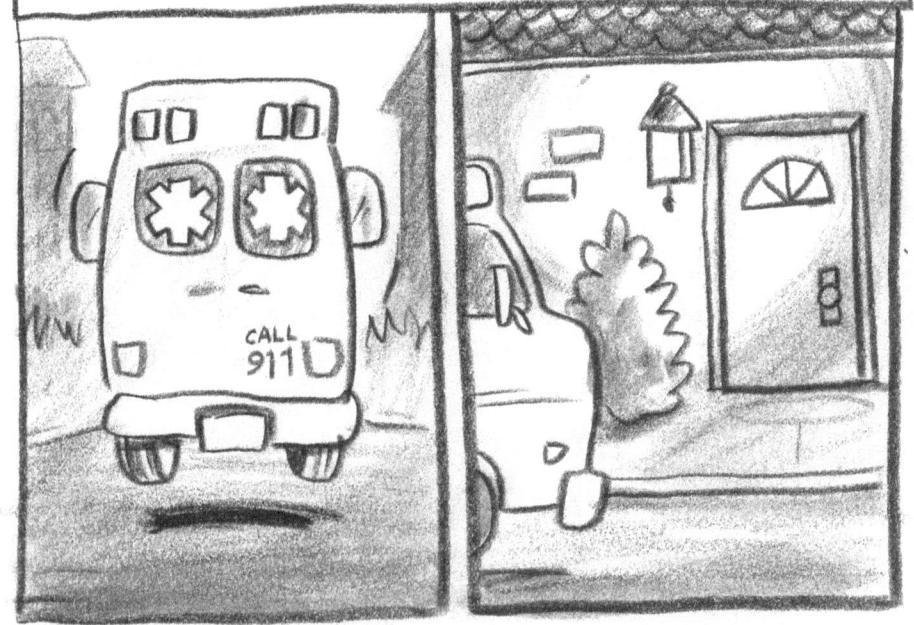

In emergency medicine, an unattended is just what it sounds like - a person died, usually alone. By the time they are found it is too late to do anything for them.

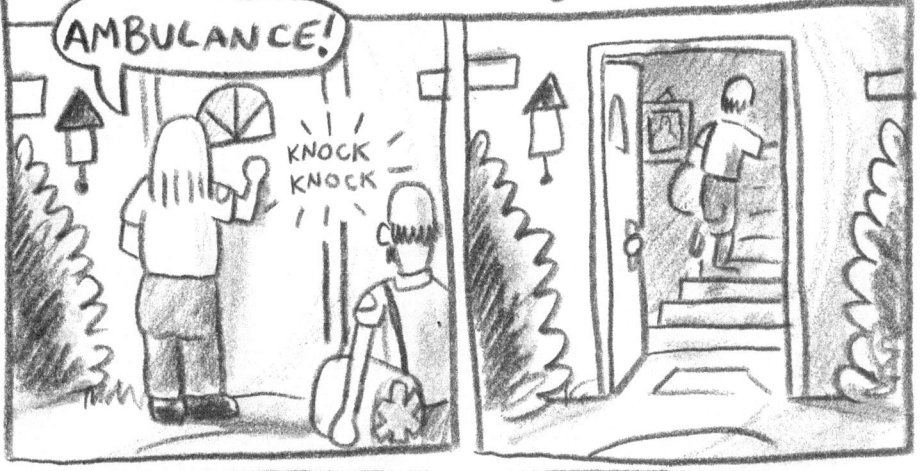

Either rigor mortis has set in, or blood has given up to gravity and made big purple welts called lividity.

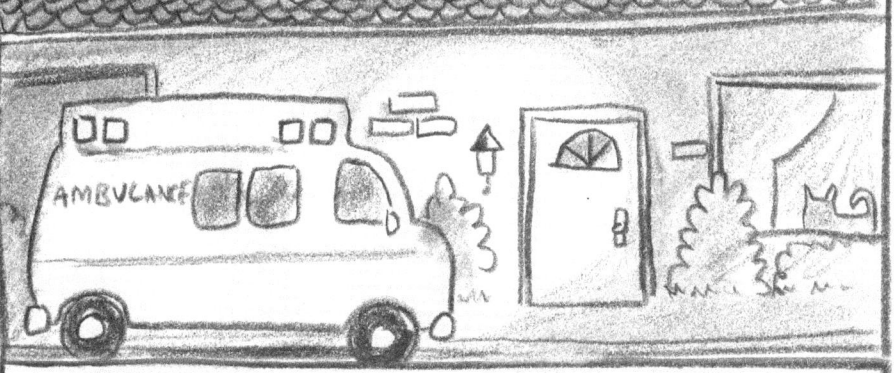

On the one hand, unattendeds are easy; there's nothing you have to do.

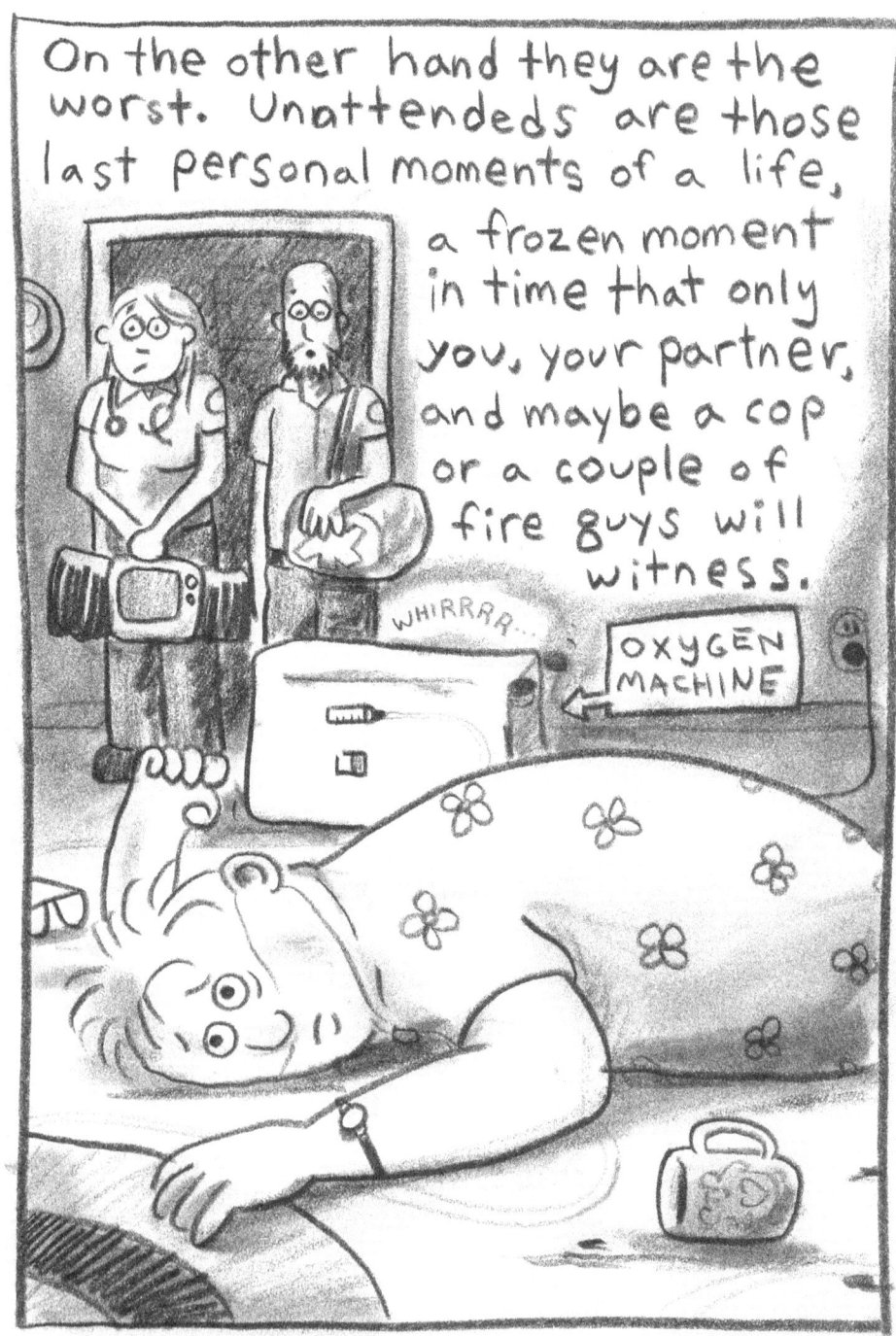

On the other hand they are the worst. Unattendeds are those last personal moments of a life, a frozen moment in time that only you, your partner, and maybe a cop or a couple of fire guys will witness.

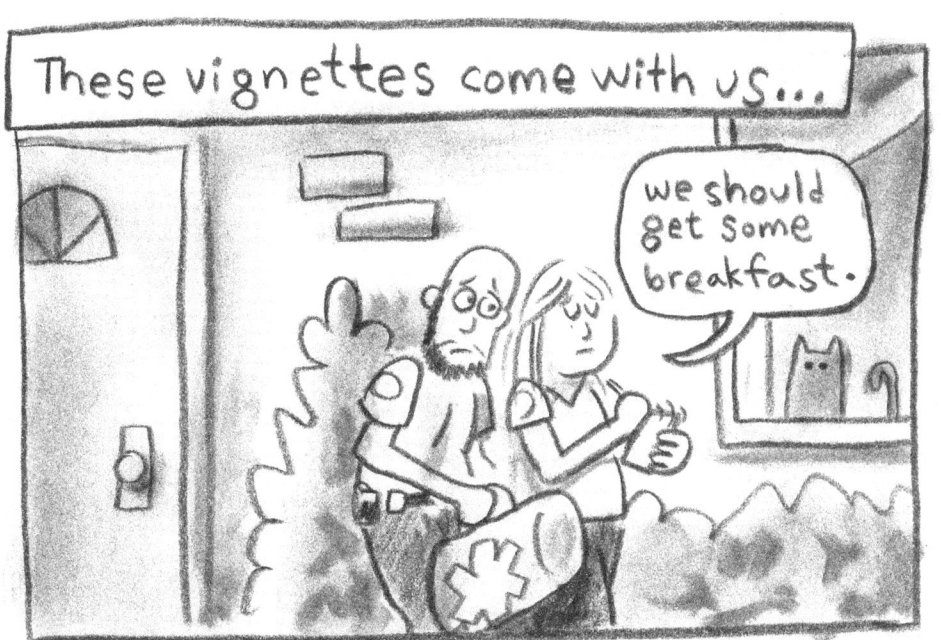

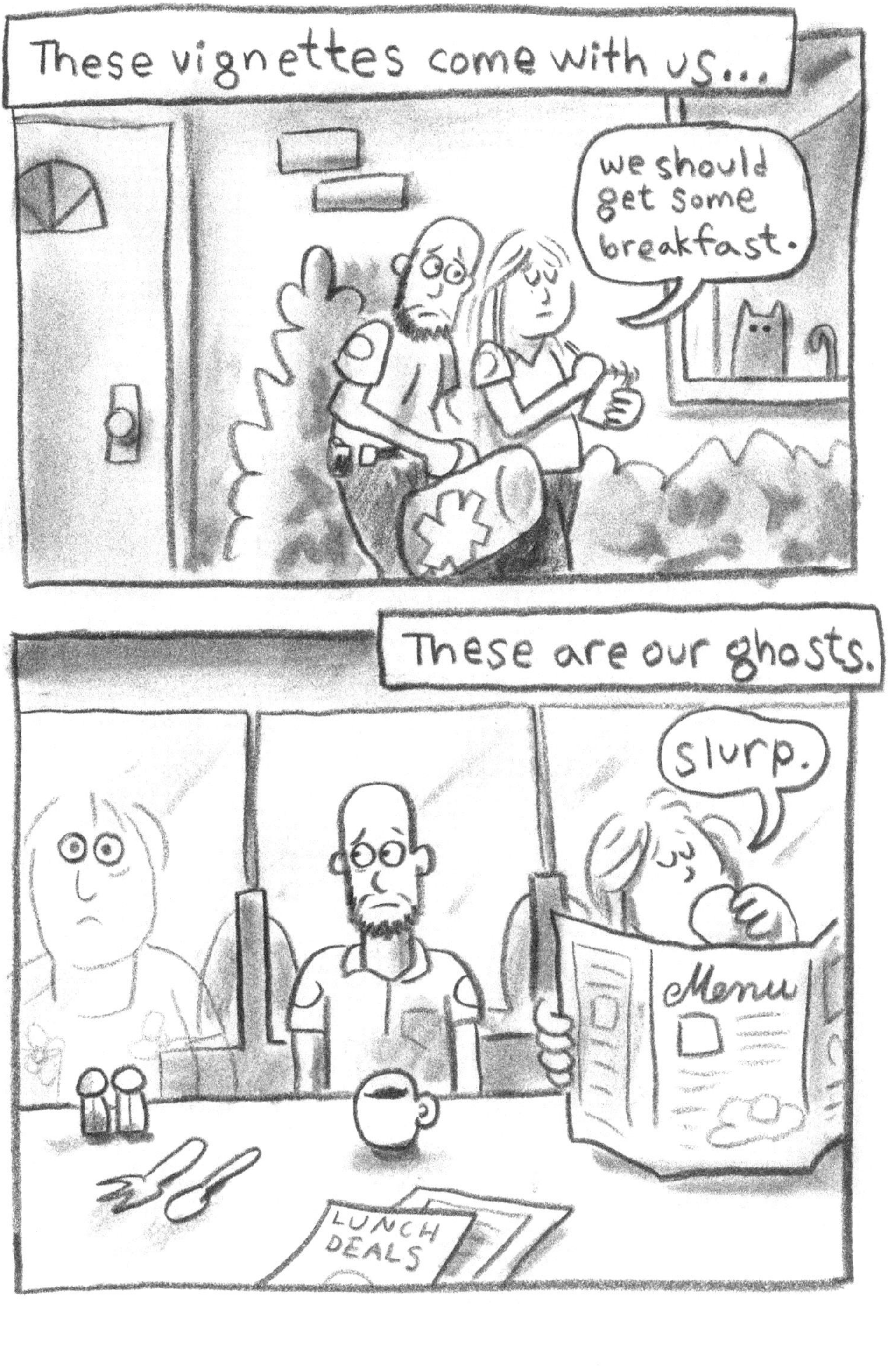

Part 1

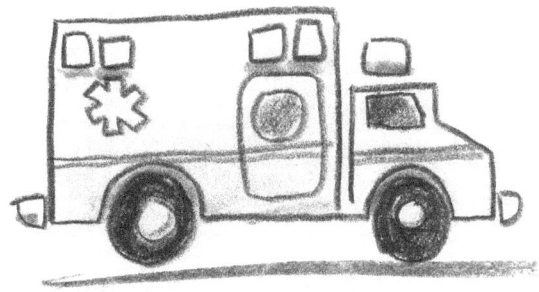

Trash Can

It was easily the worst ambulance company in the region. But they were the only one to return my calls.

TRANSCARE AM

NO PARKING

I was fresh out of EMT school, and I really needed the work.

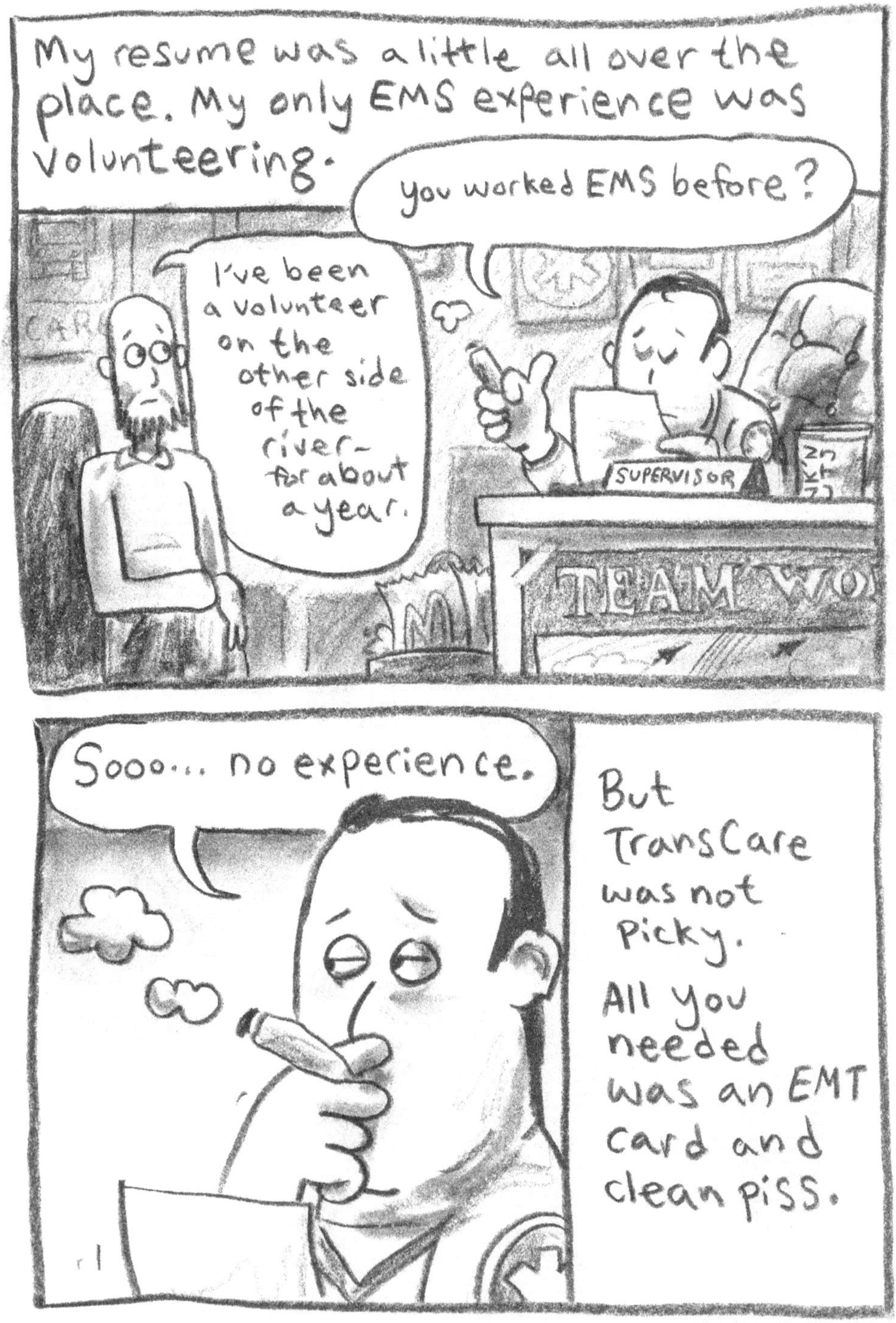

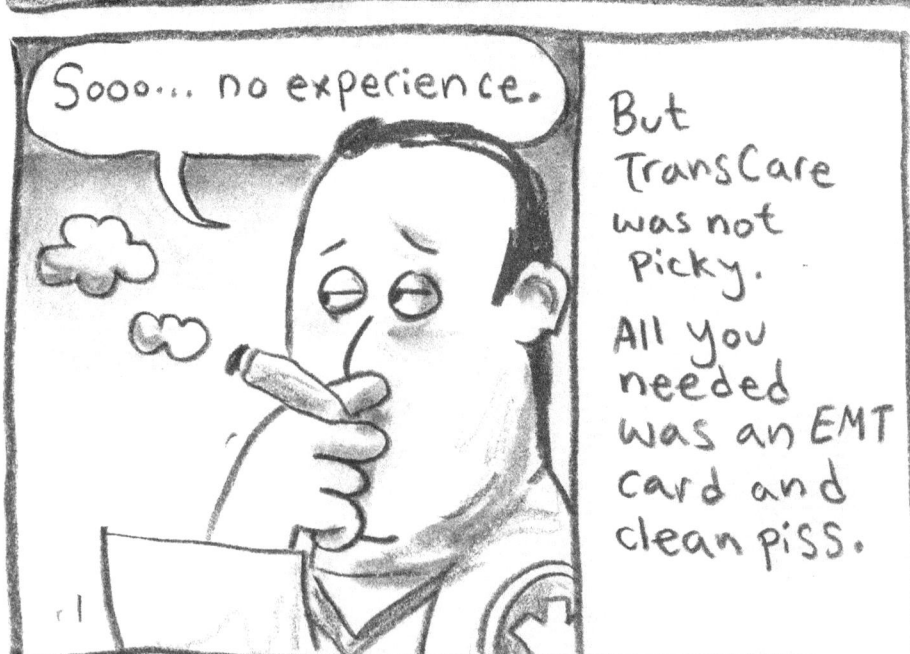

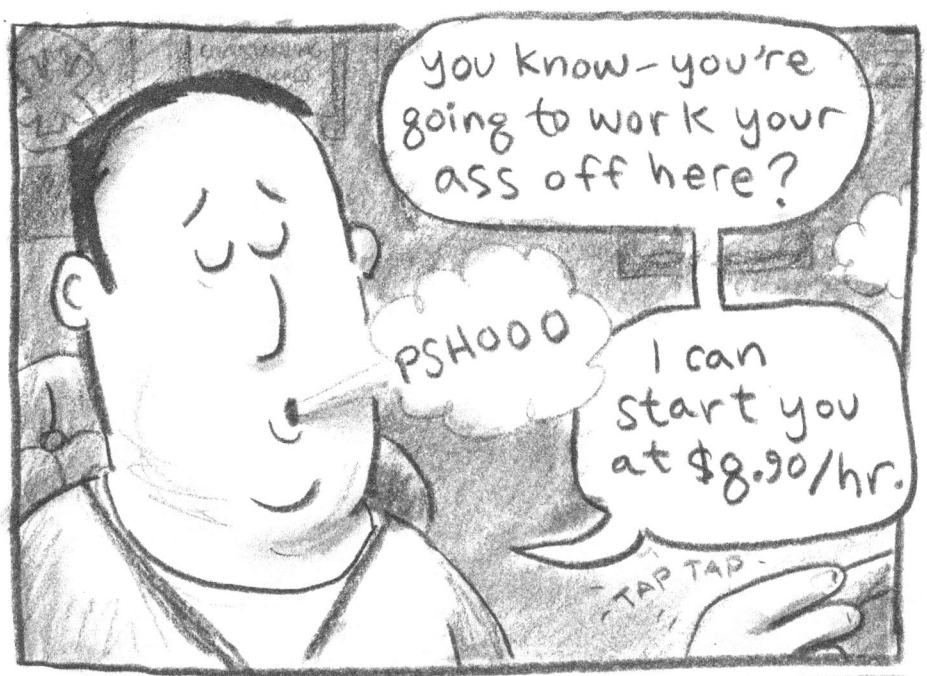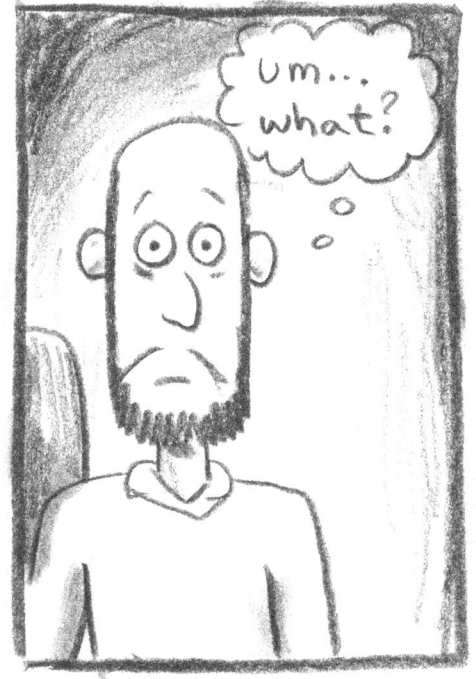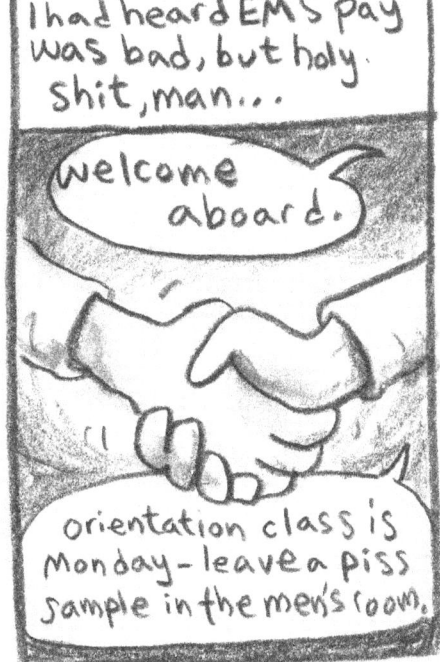

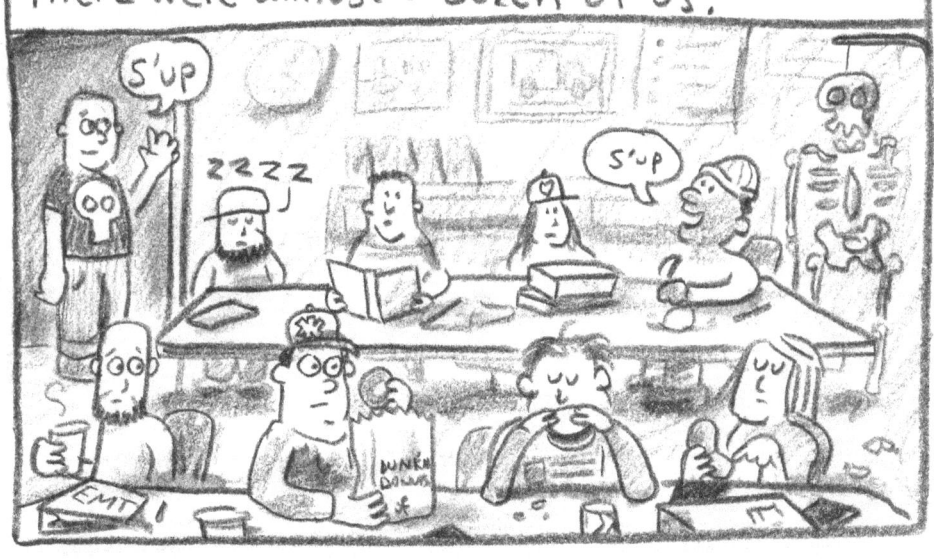
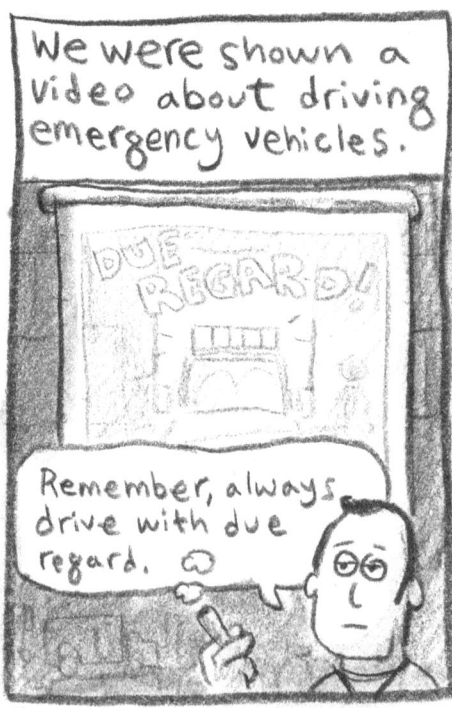
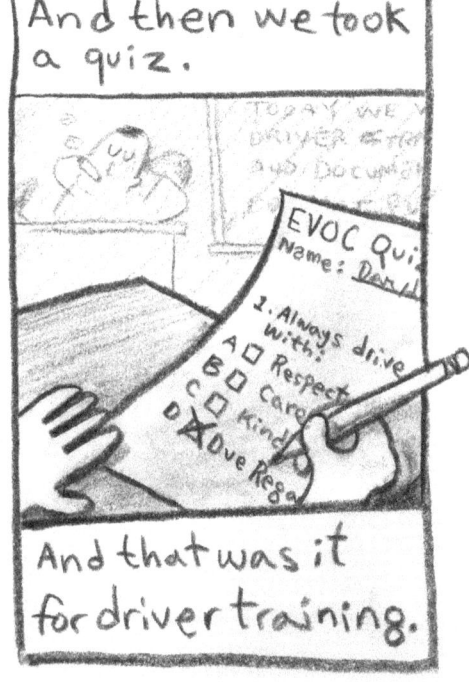

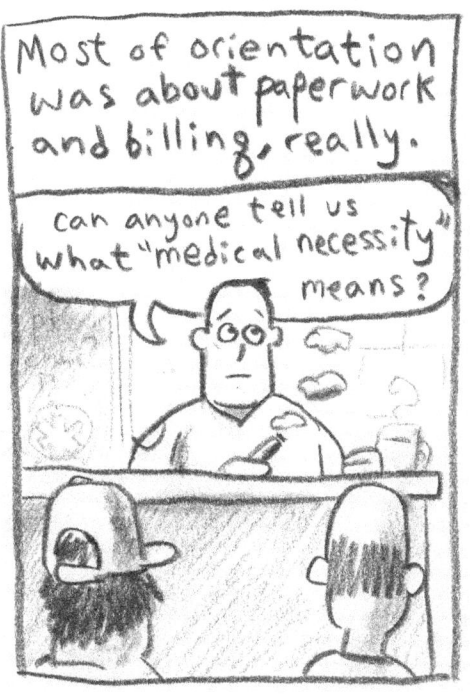
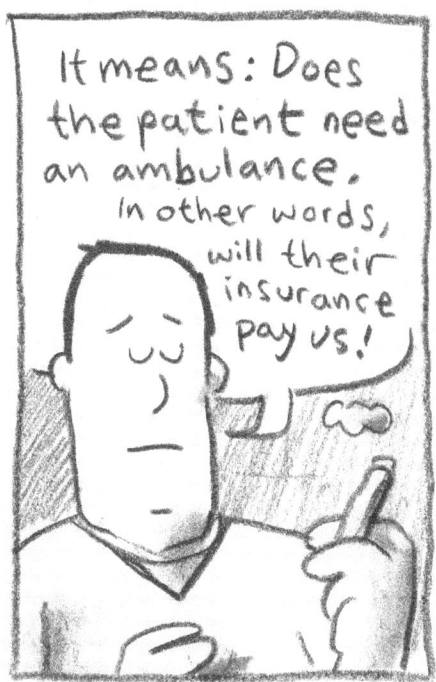
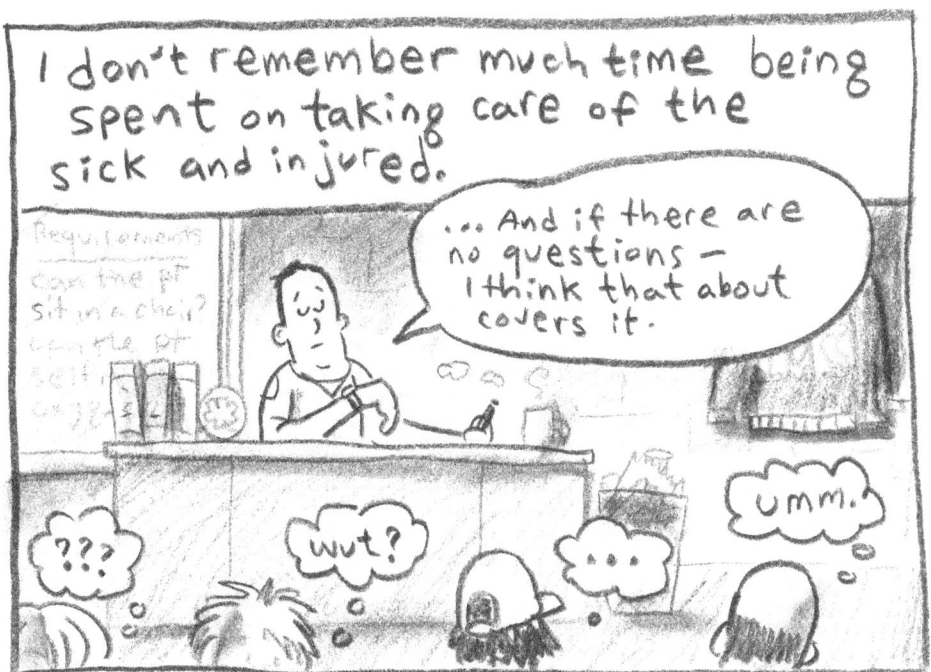

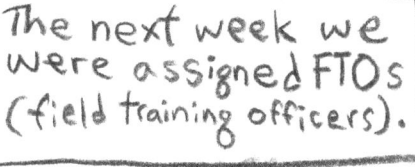
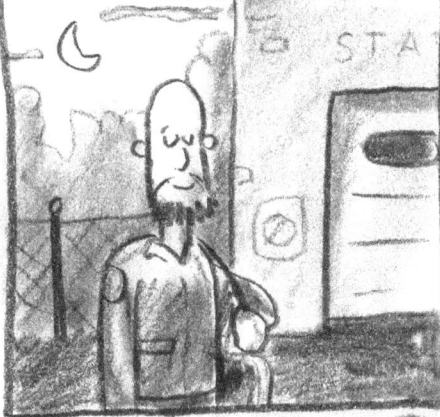
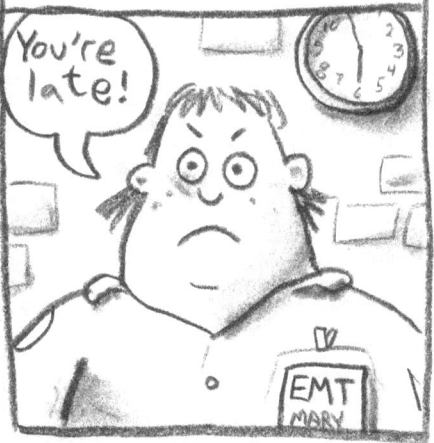
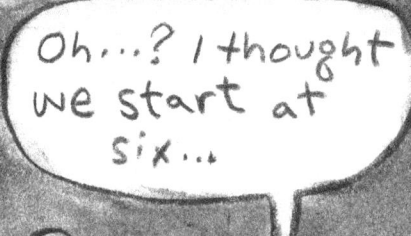
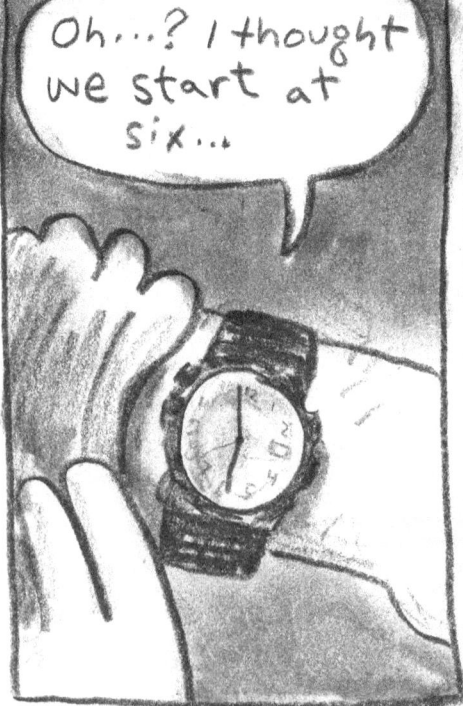
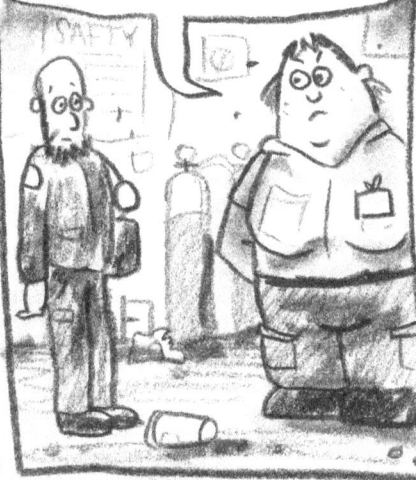

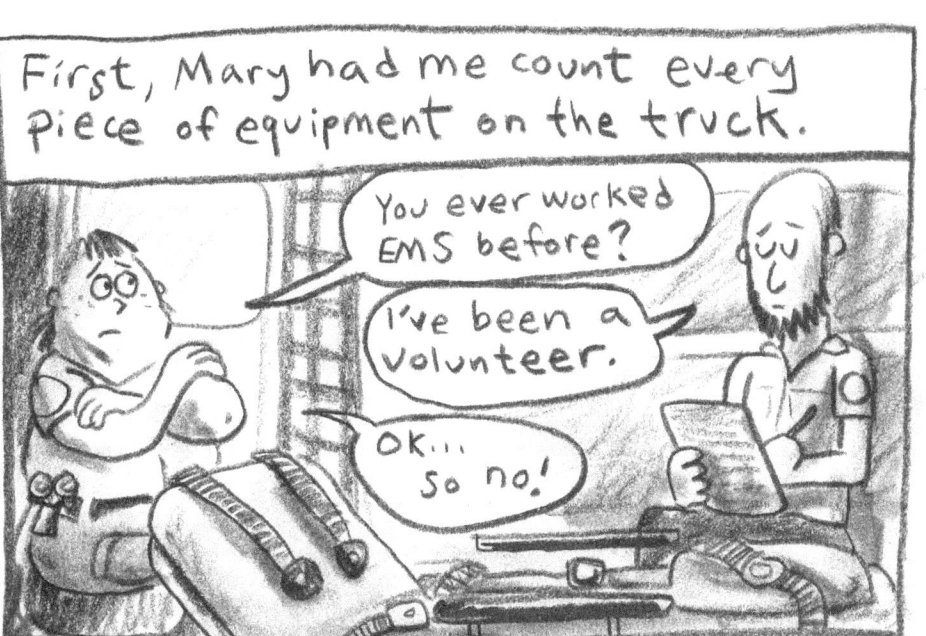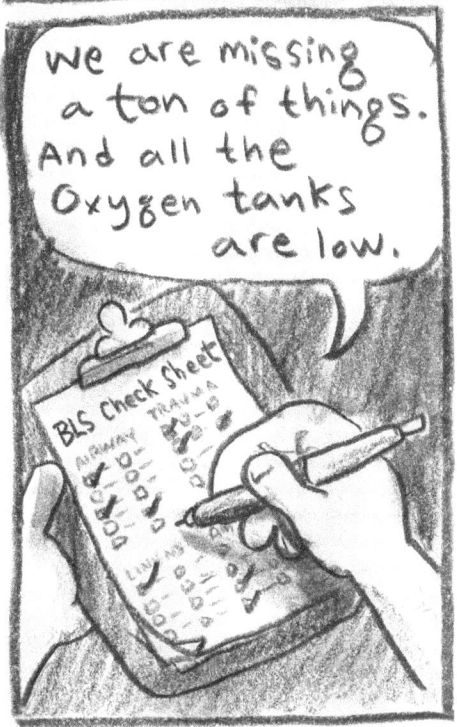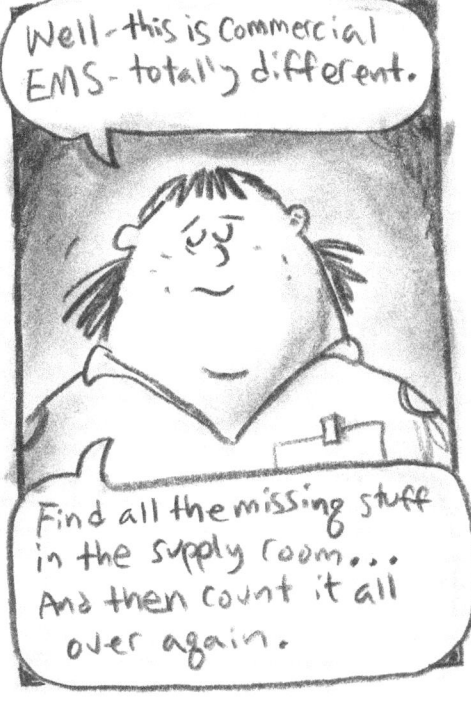

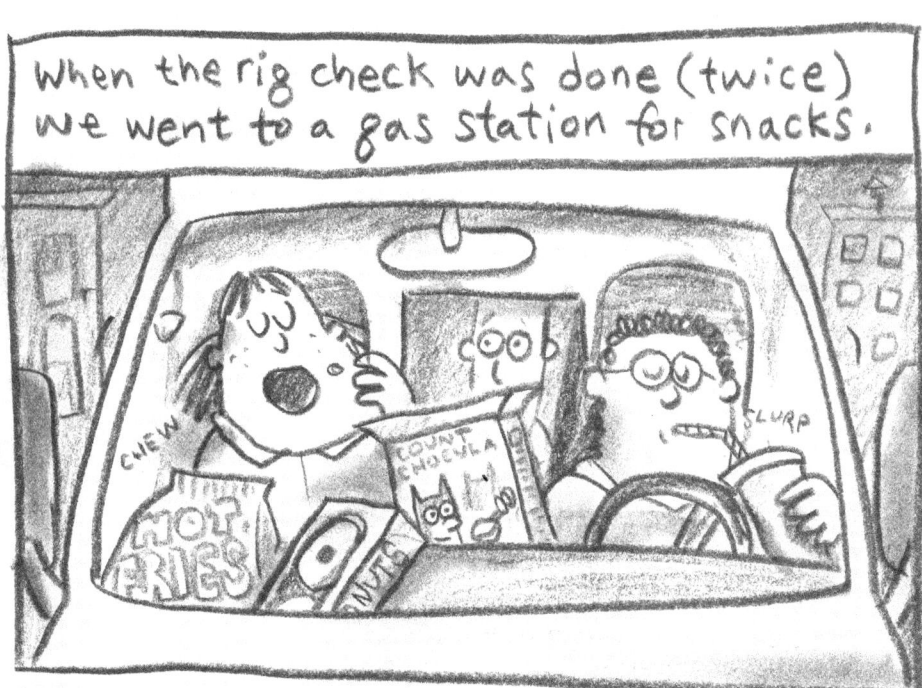

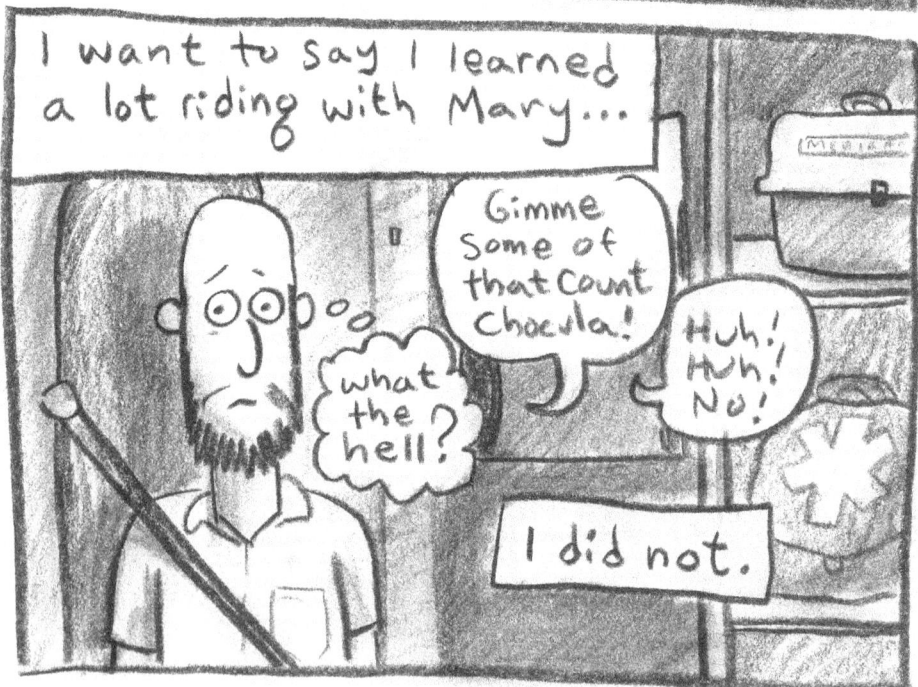

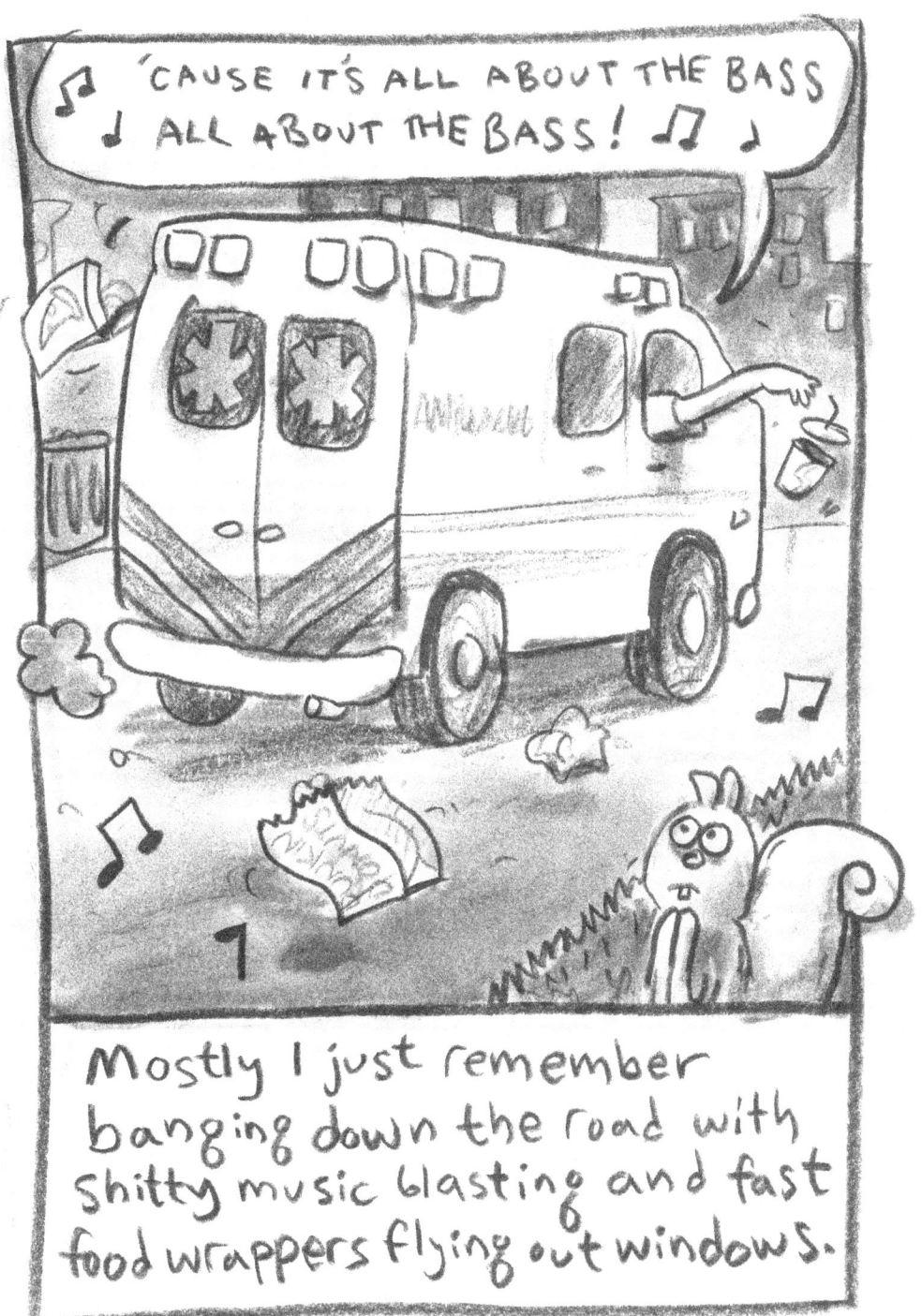

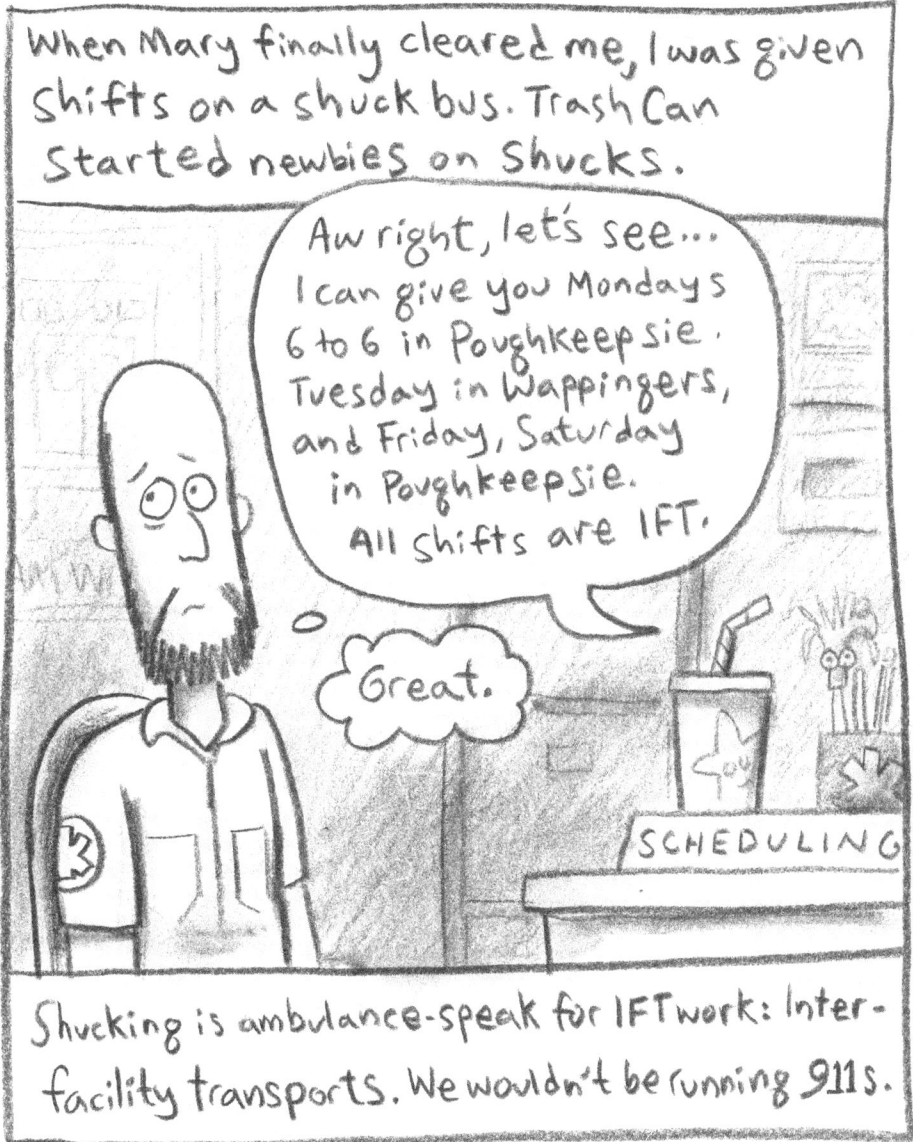

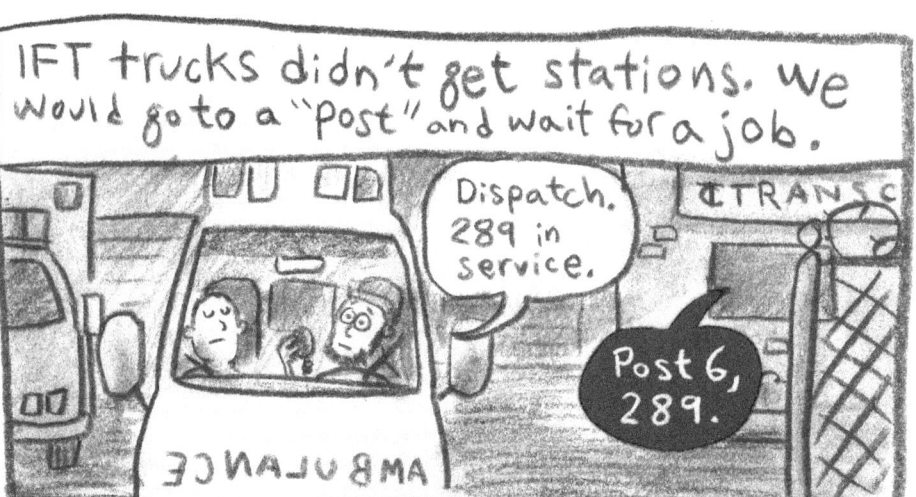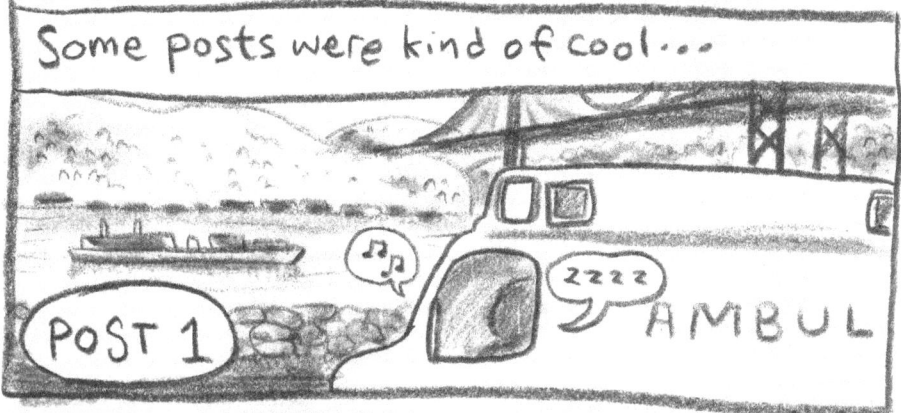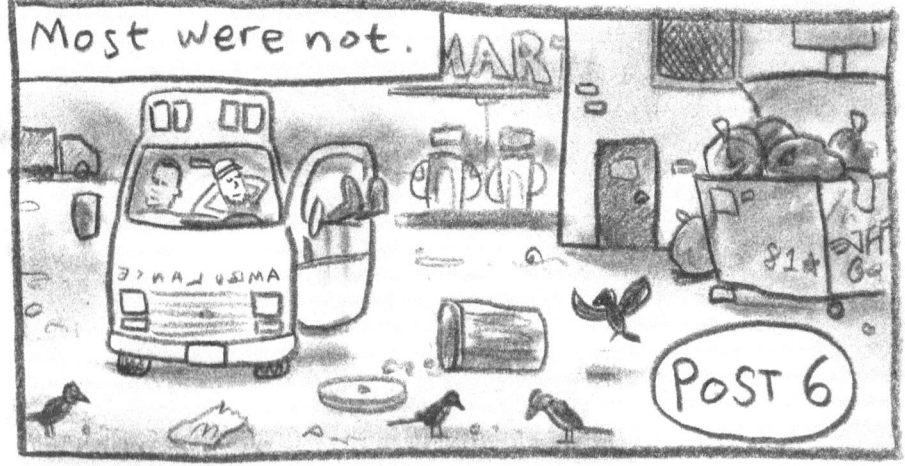

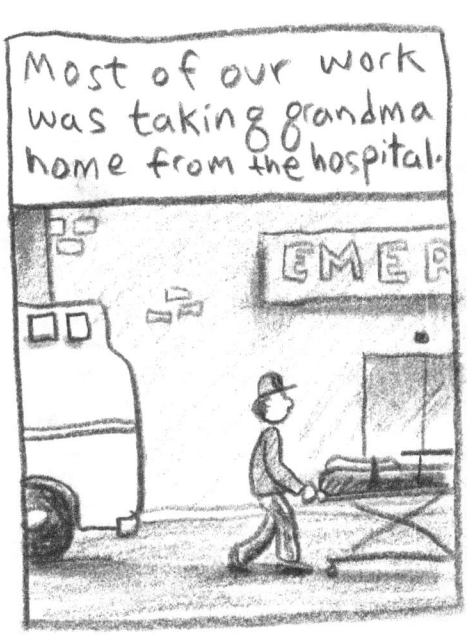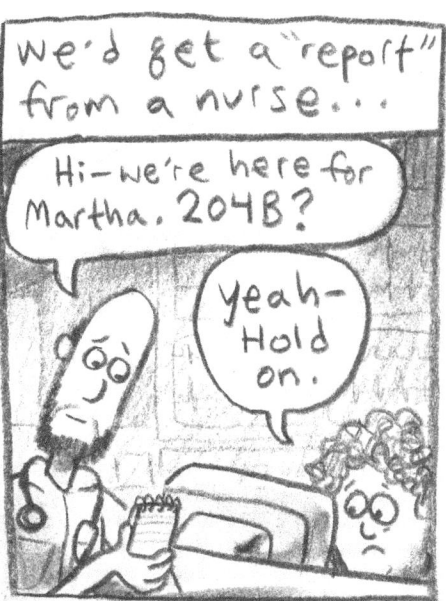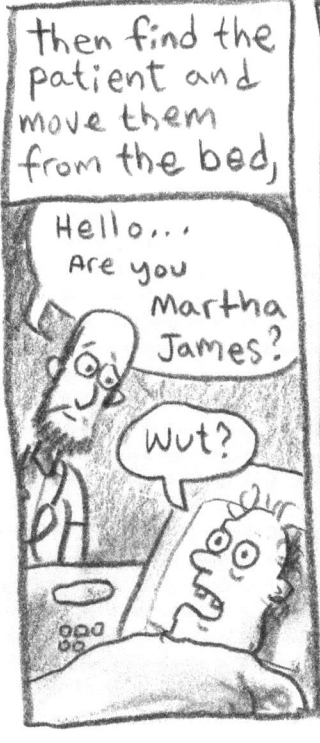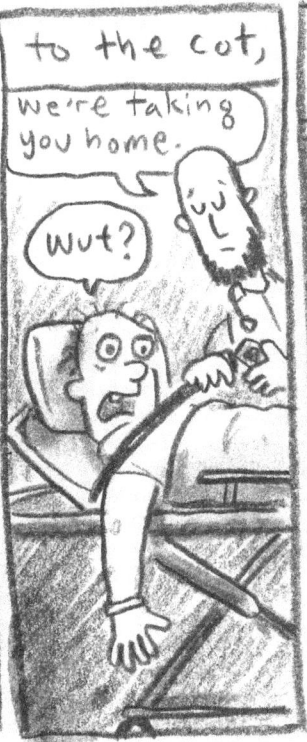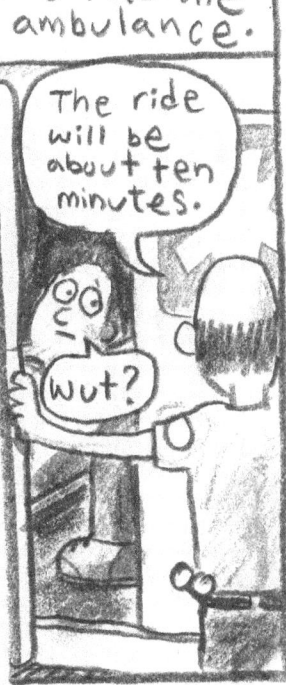

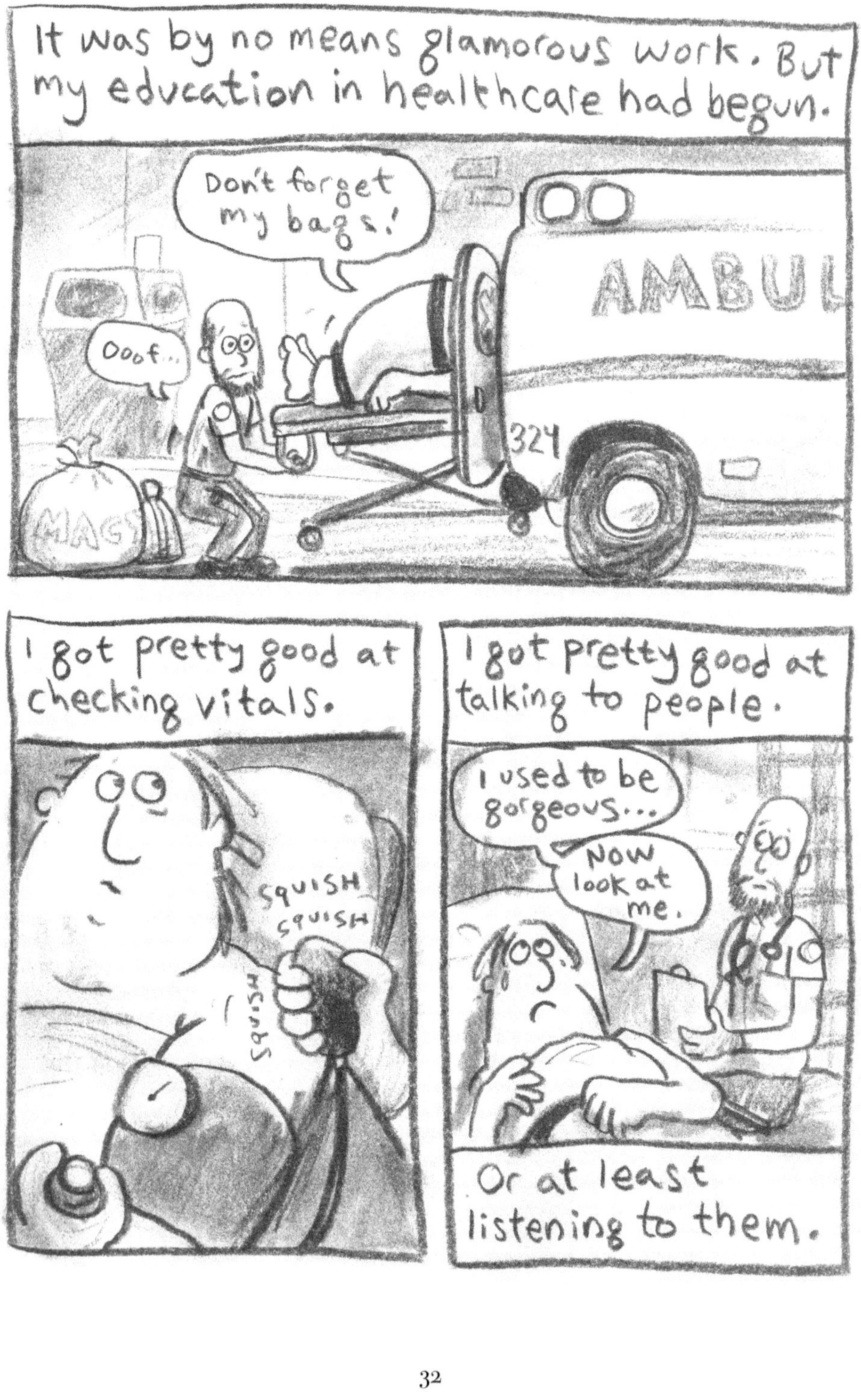

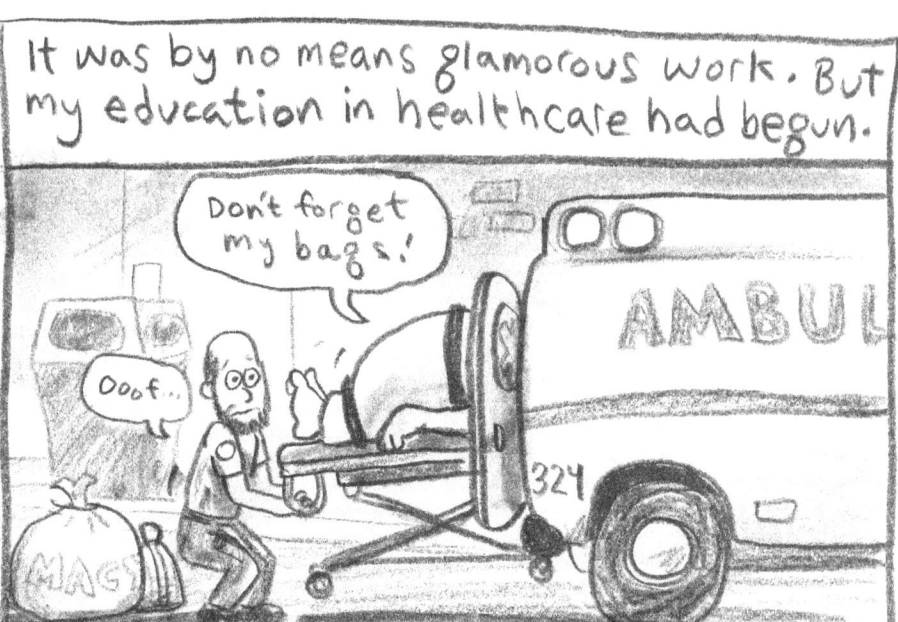

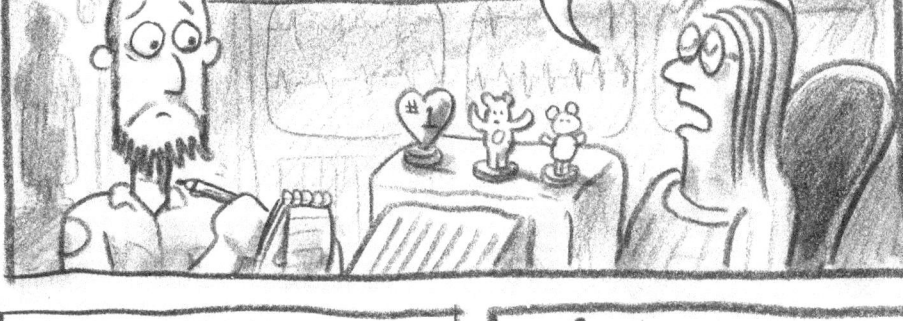

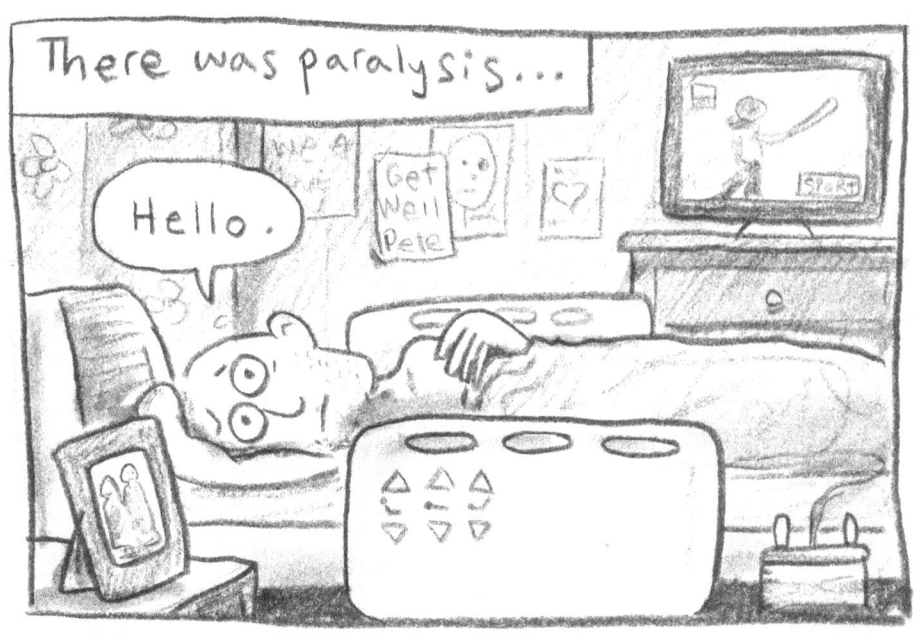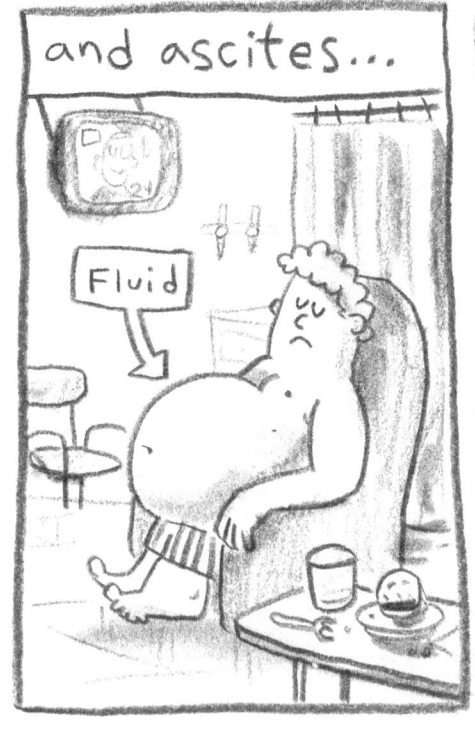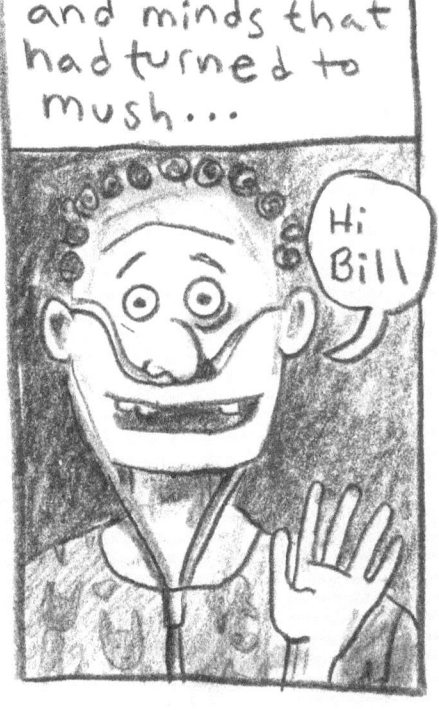

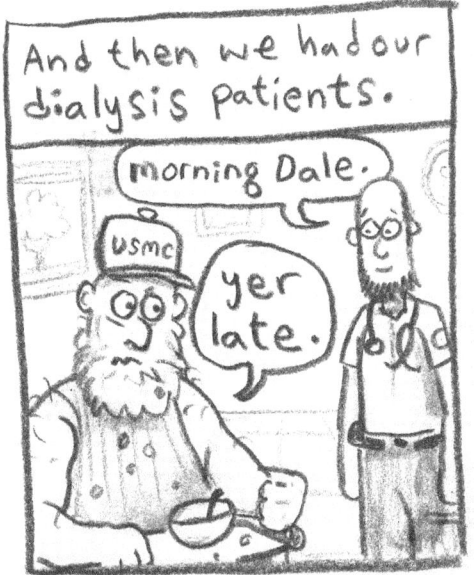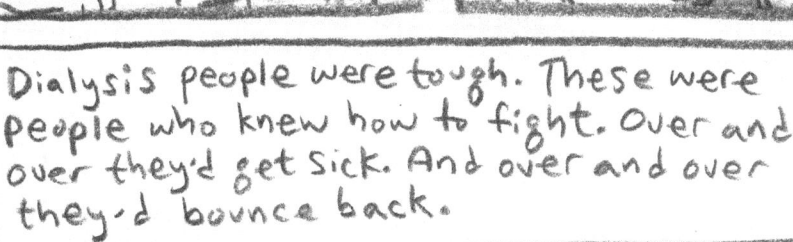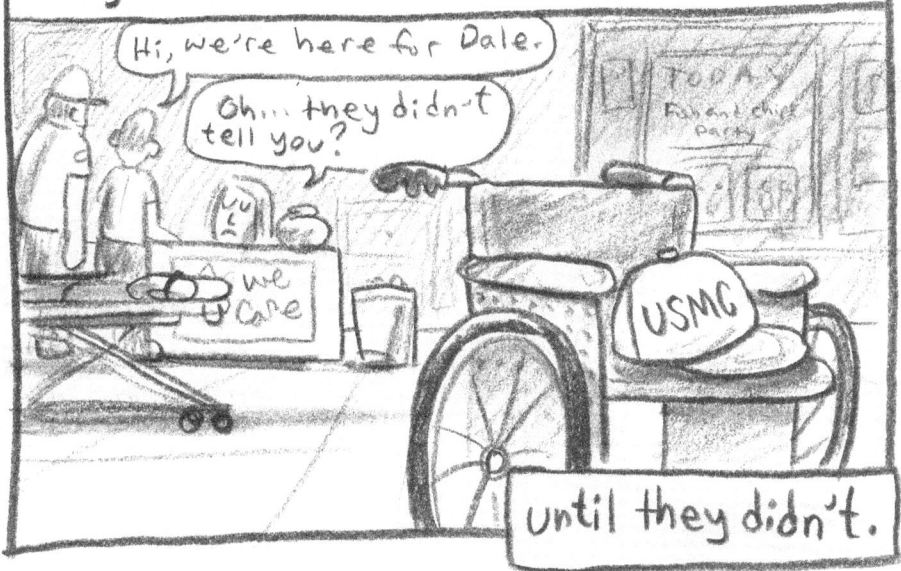

First Time

I had worked at TrashCan for about a year before I finally got a shift on a dedicated 911 truck.

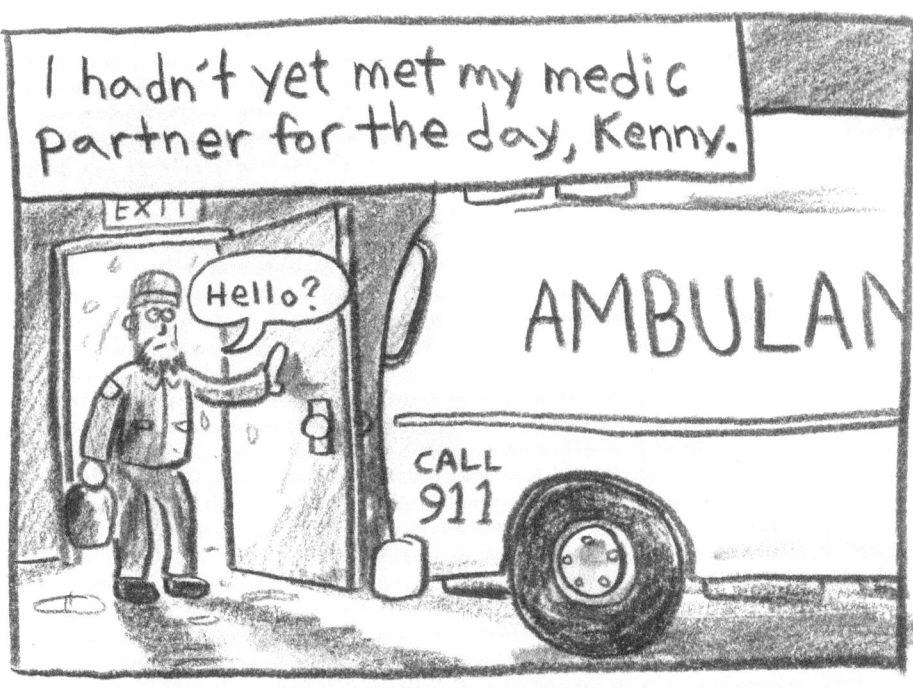

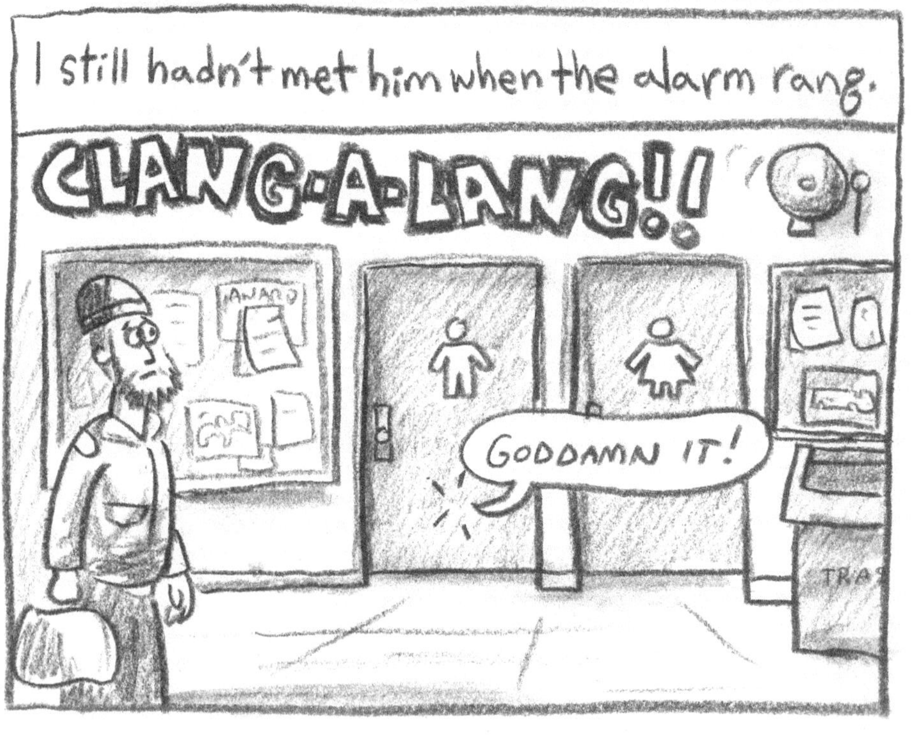

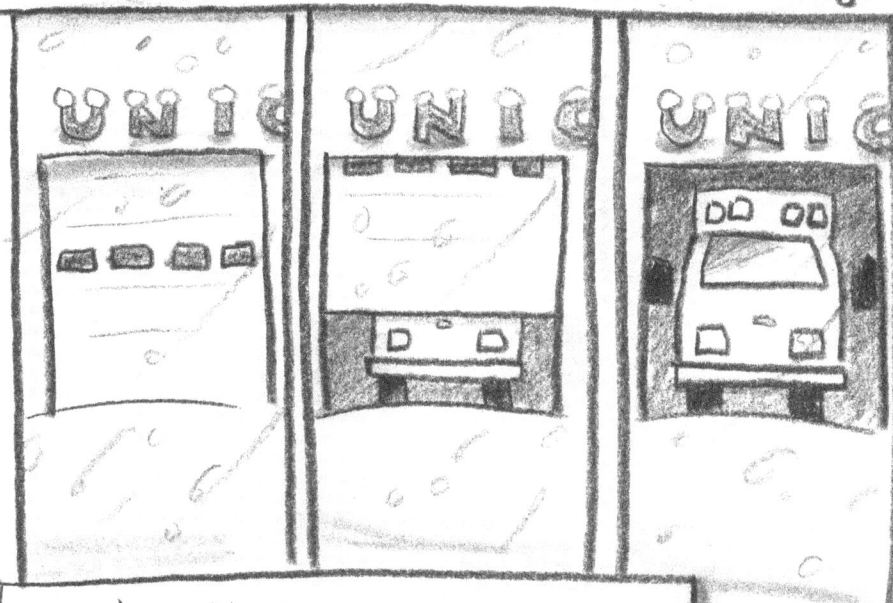

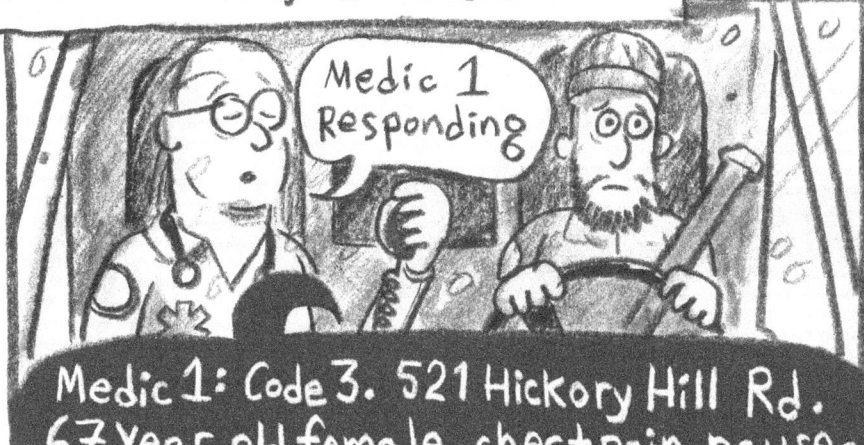

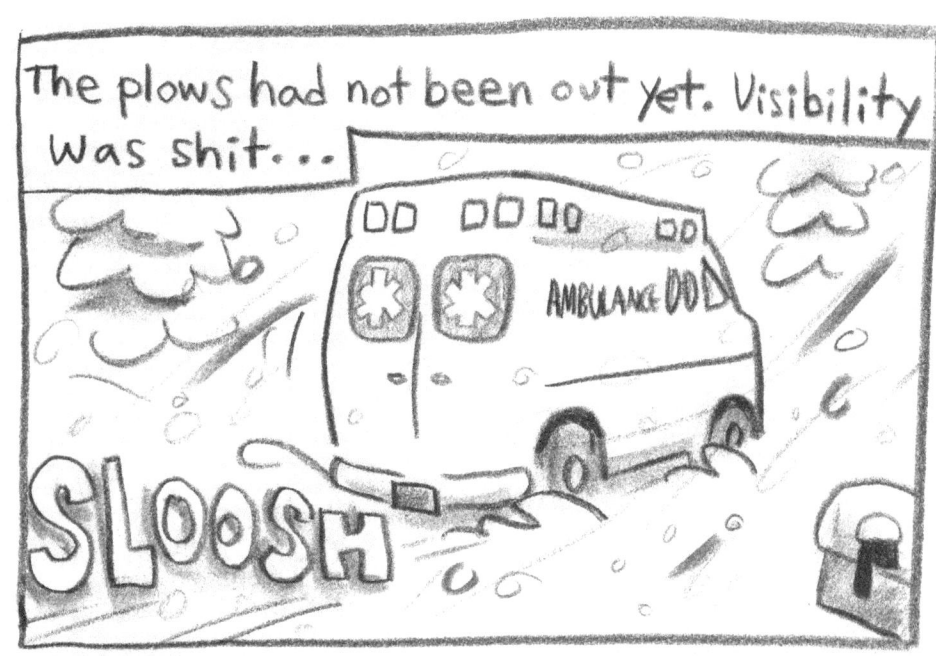
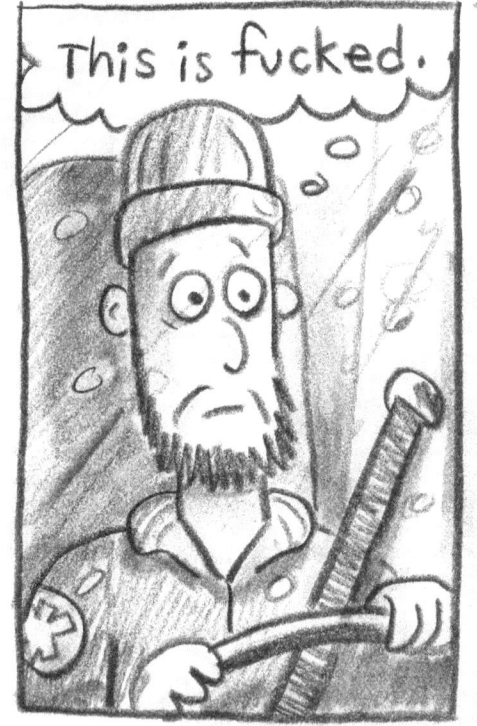
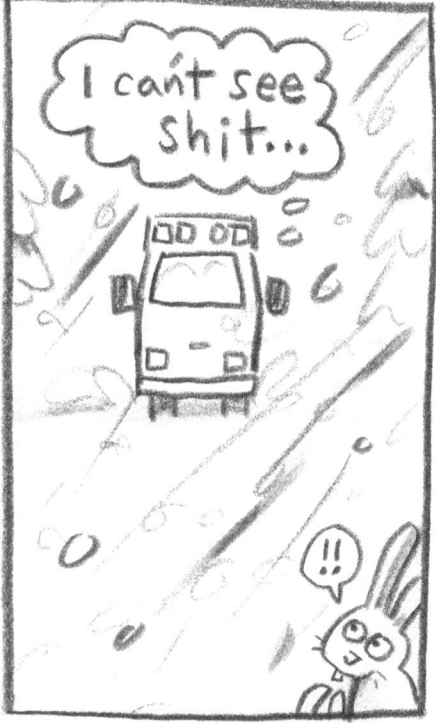

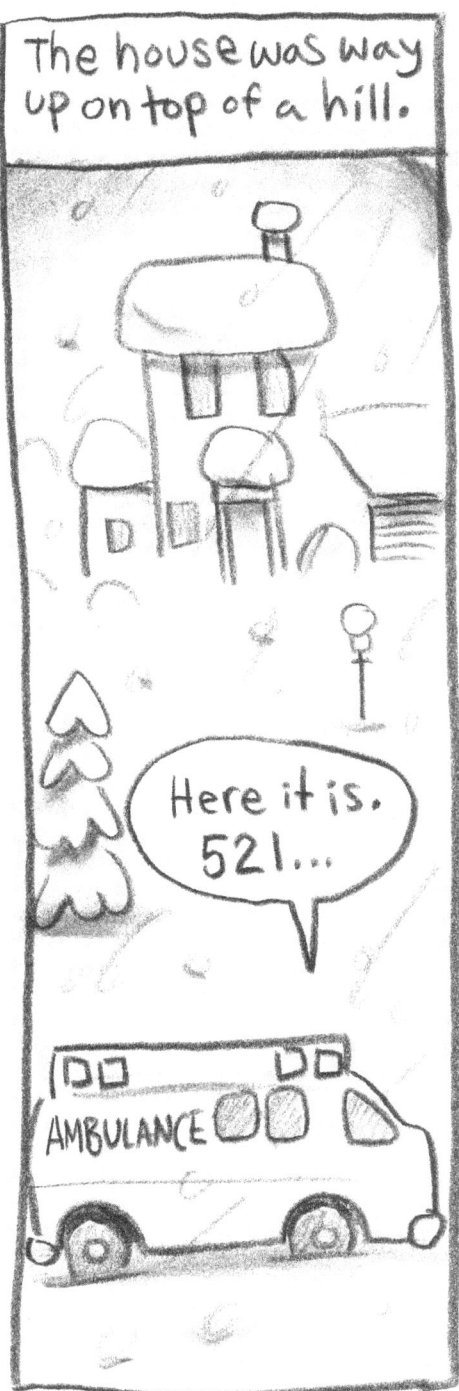
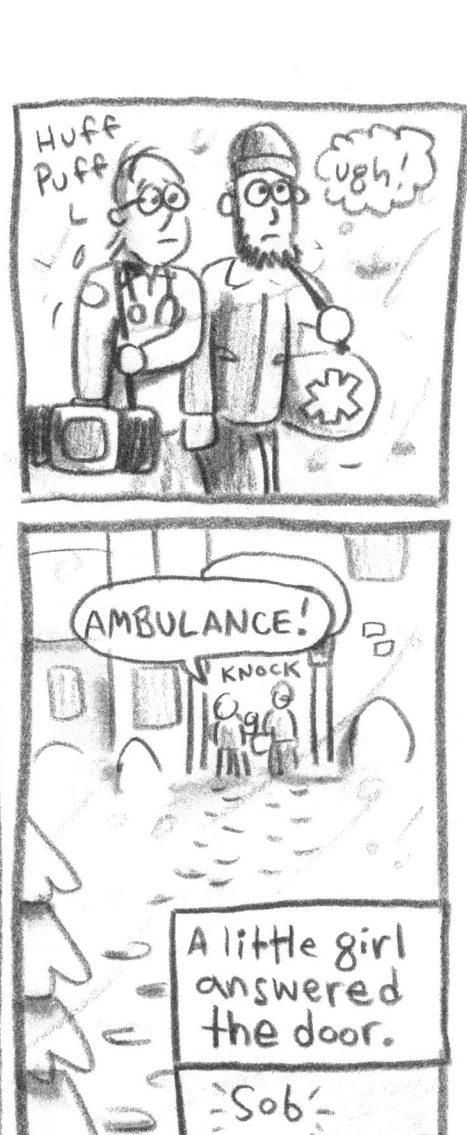

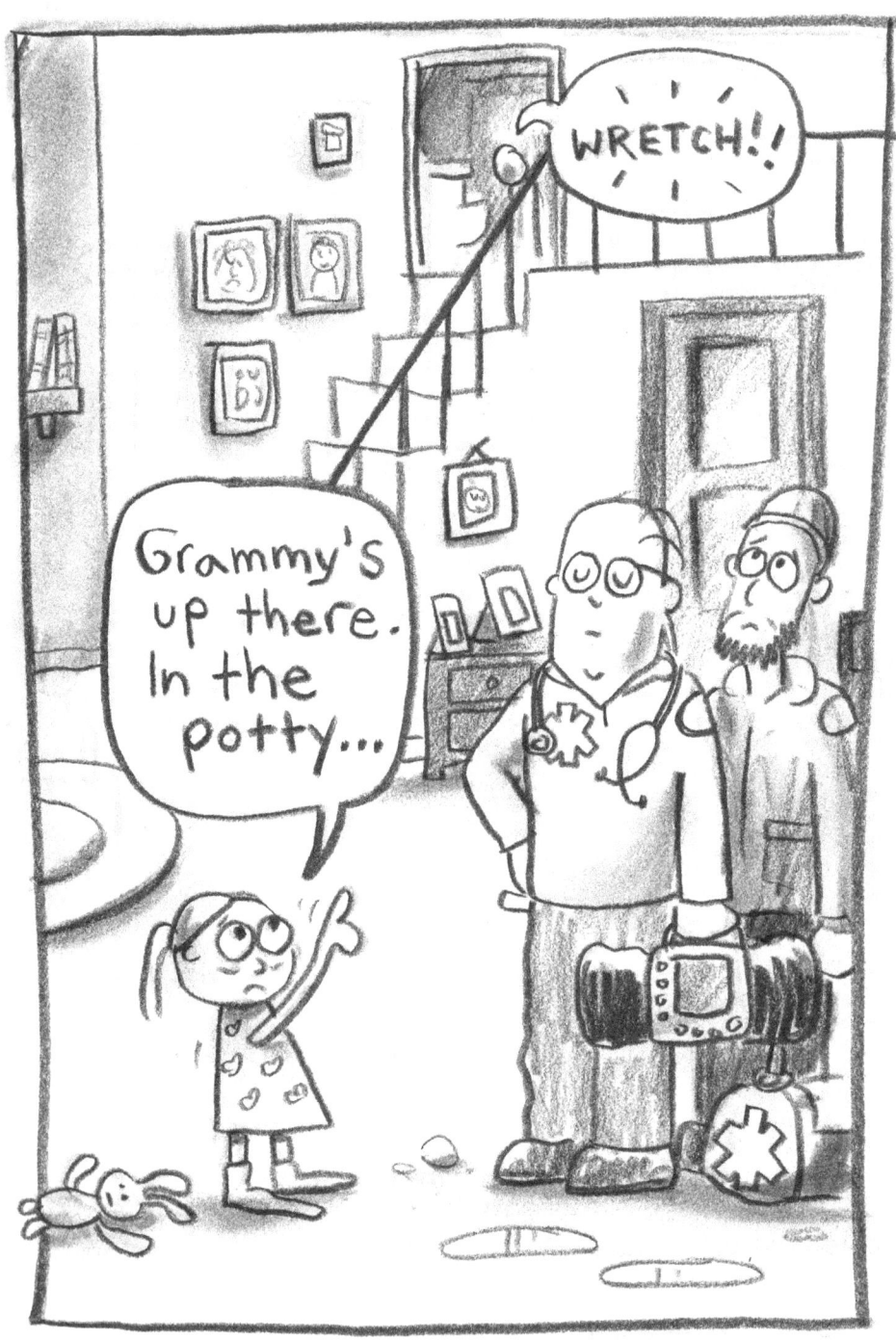

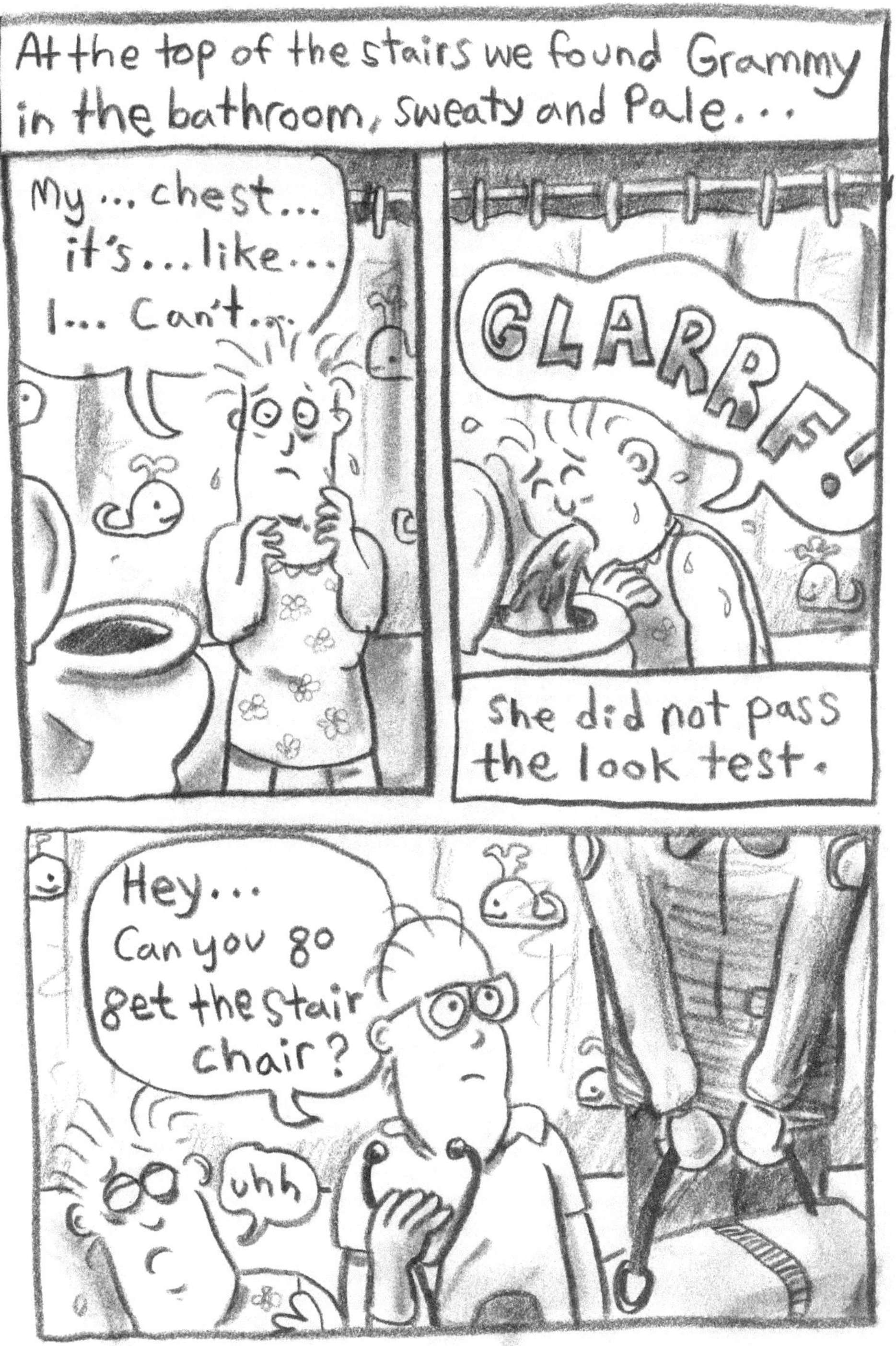

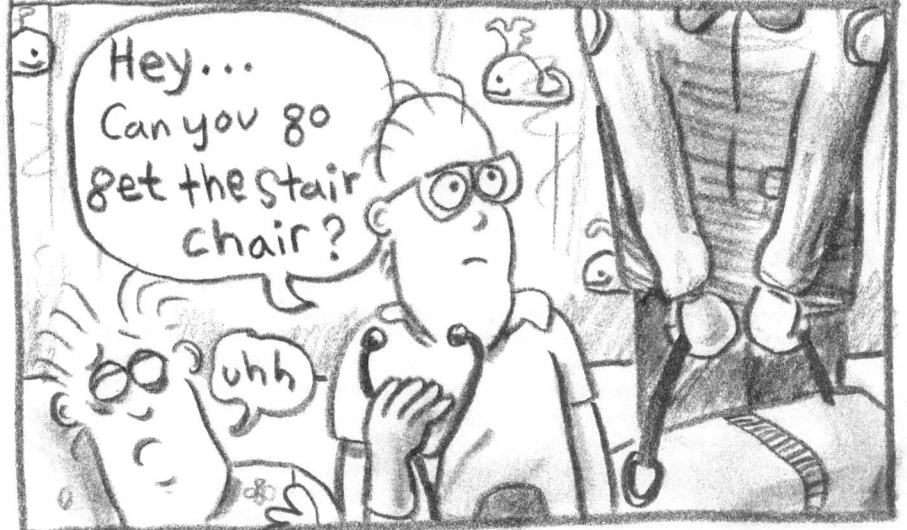

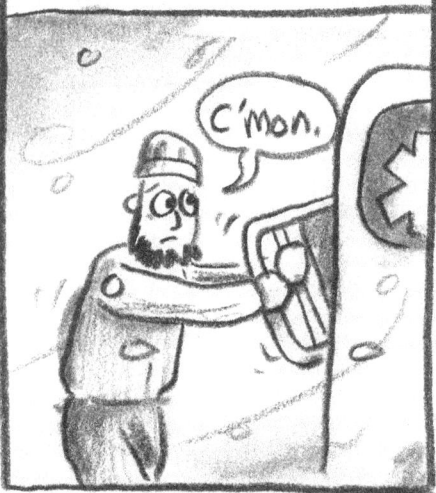
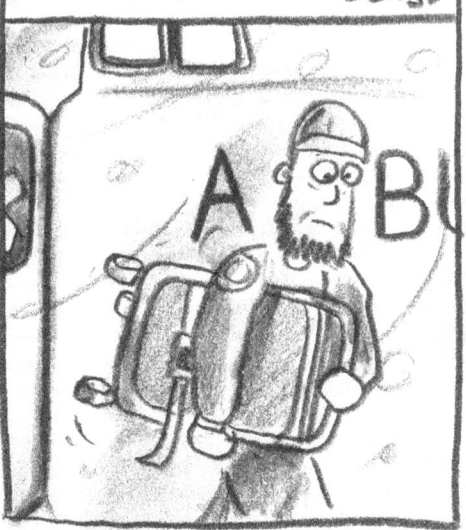
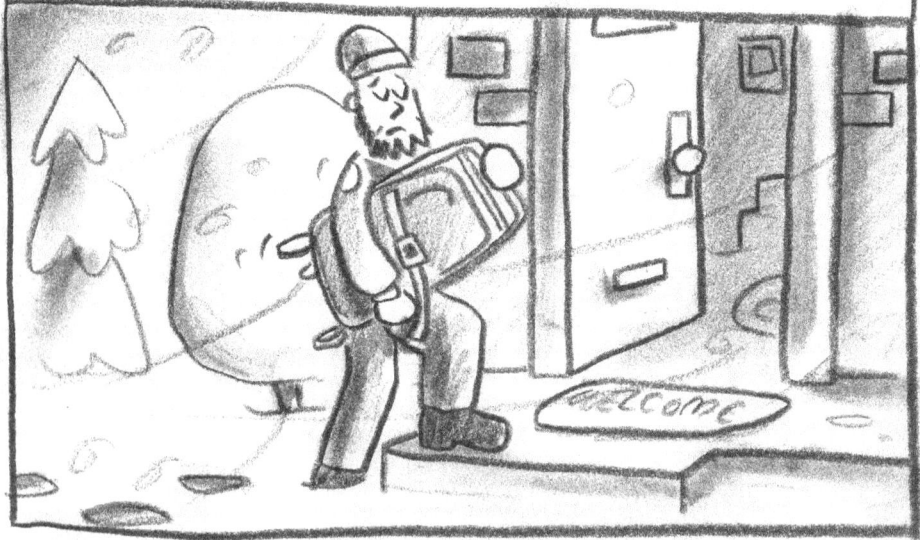

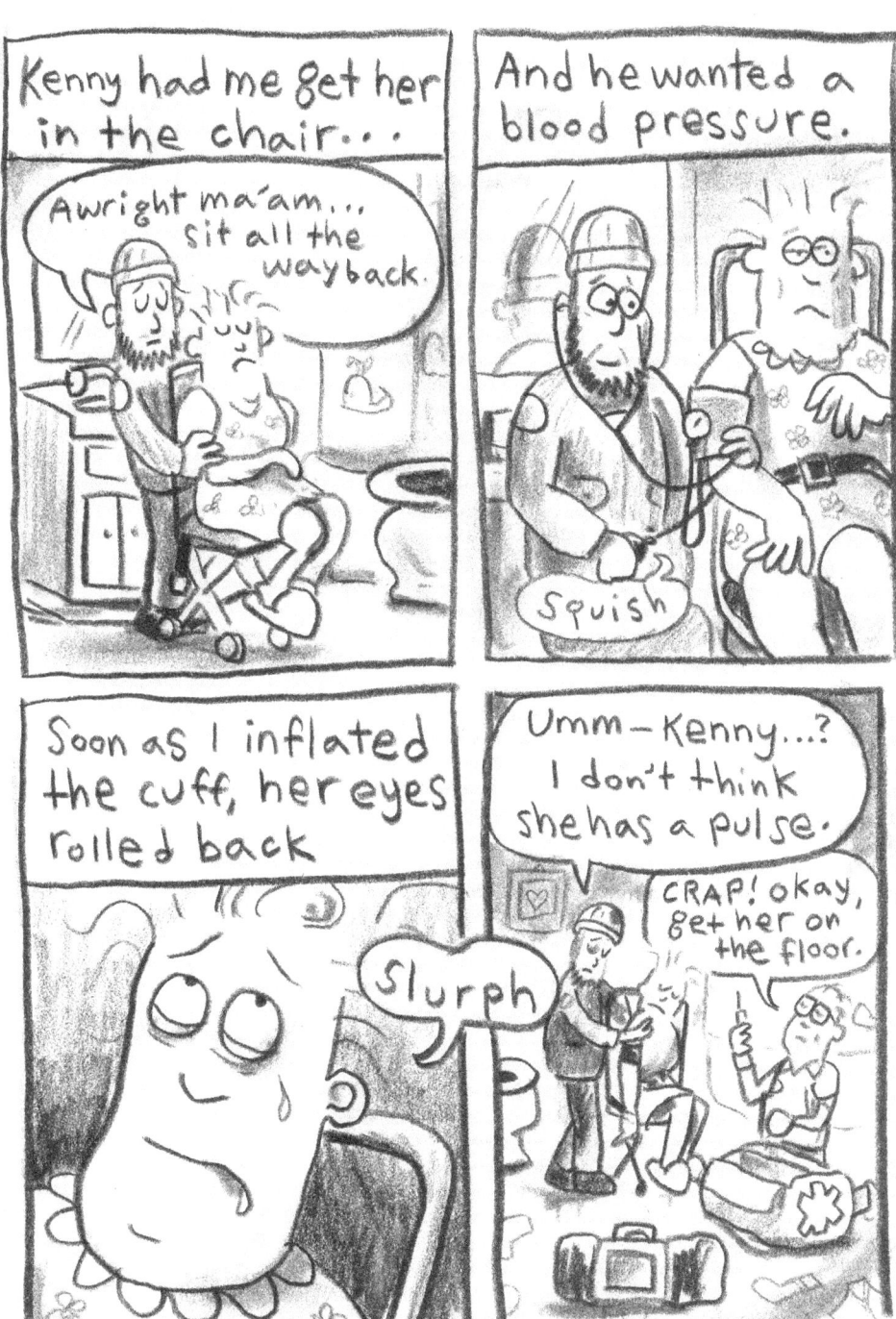

It was not my first time doing CPR. But it was the first time someone died right in front of my face.

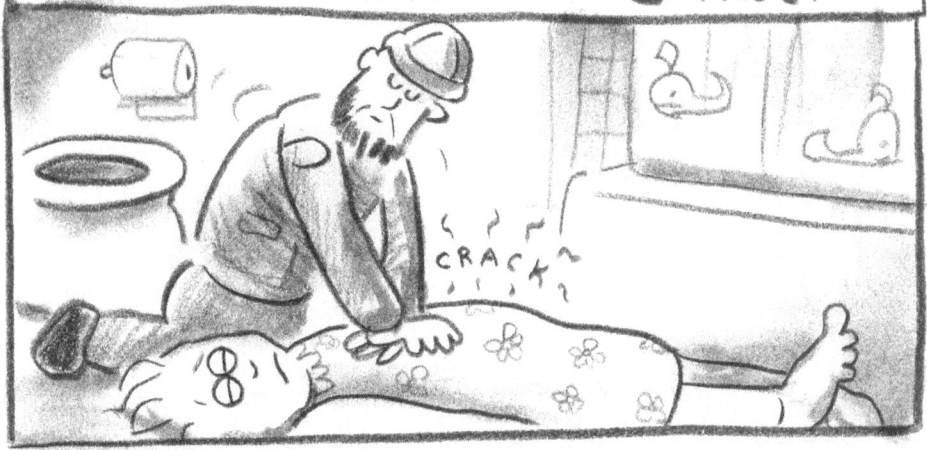

Suddenly a fire-guy was there helping us. I don't know where he came from.

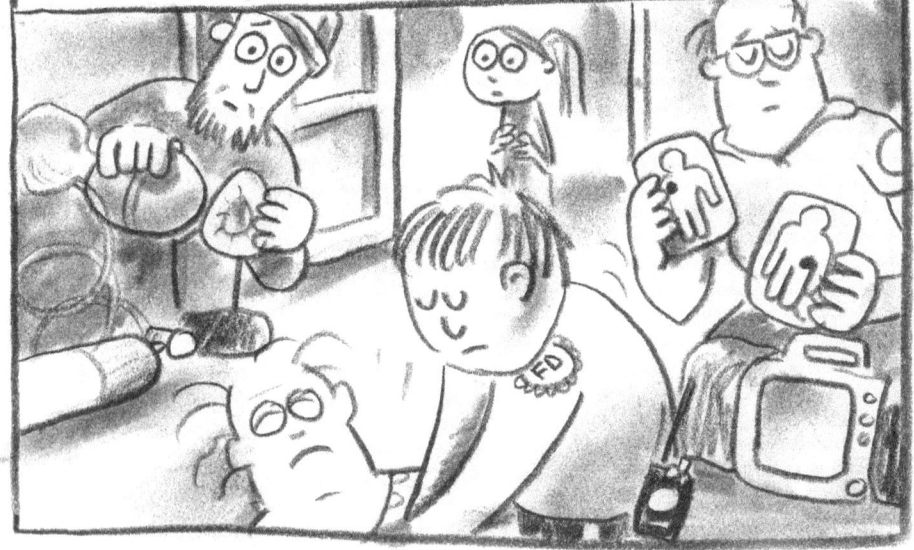

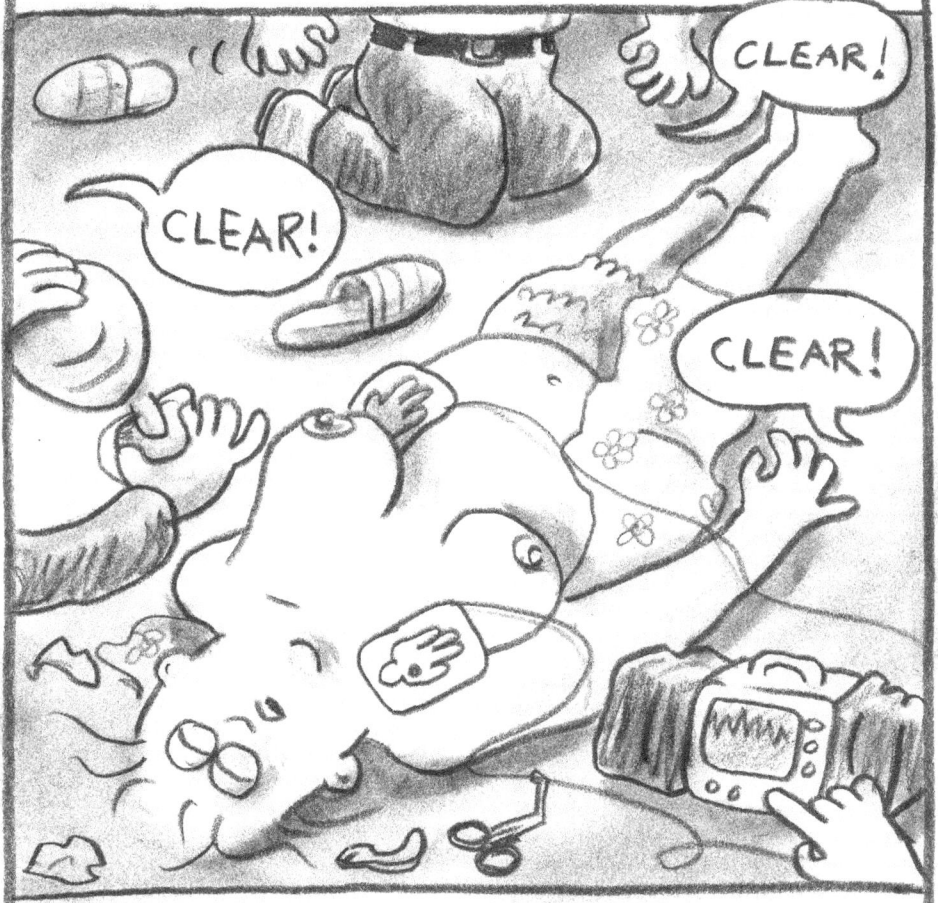

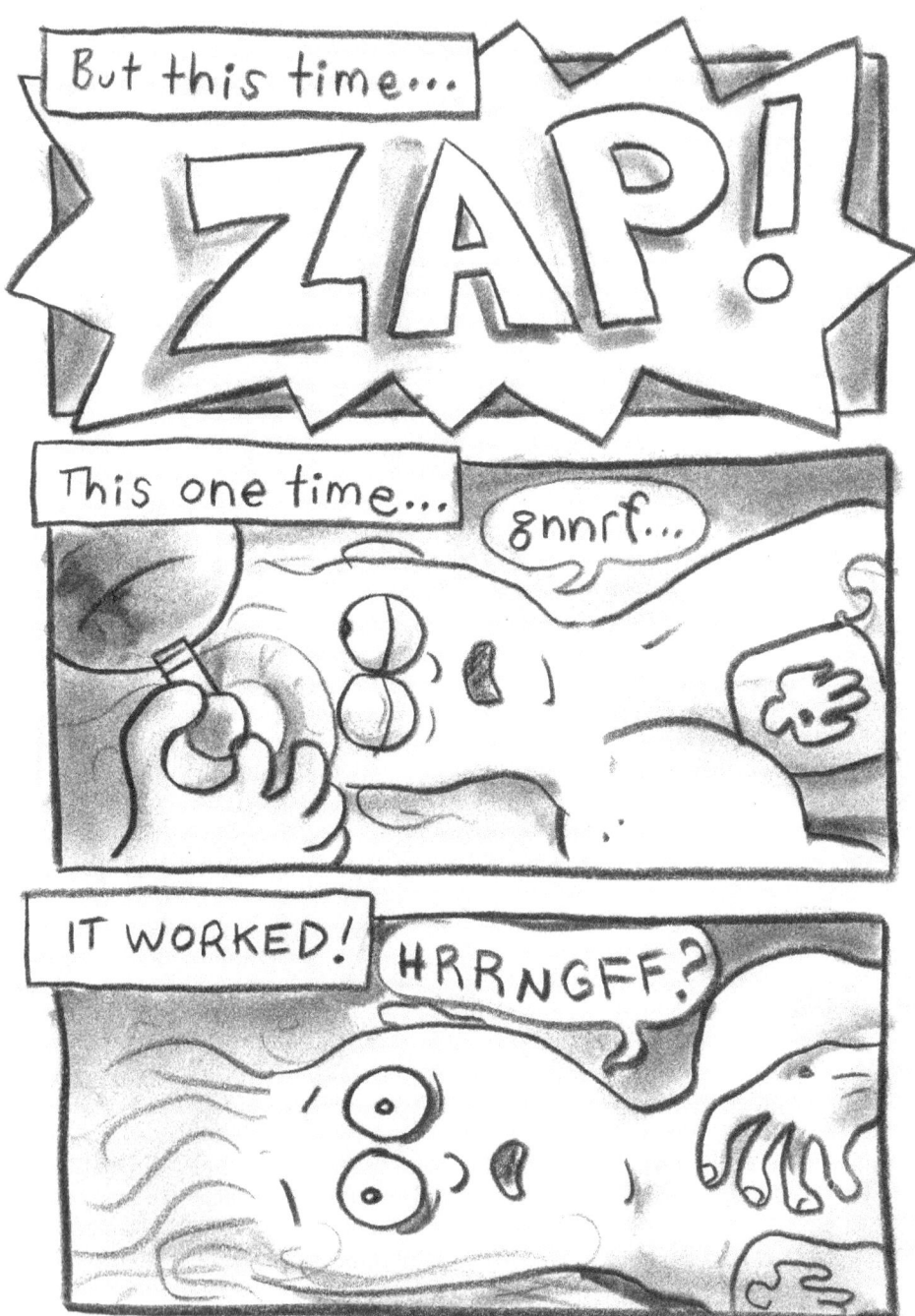

Grammy woke up. But unlike in a movie where the patient is all, like, "Thank you, thank you! You saved my life.", Grammy — whose brain had been without oxygen for a minute or two — wanted to kill us.

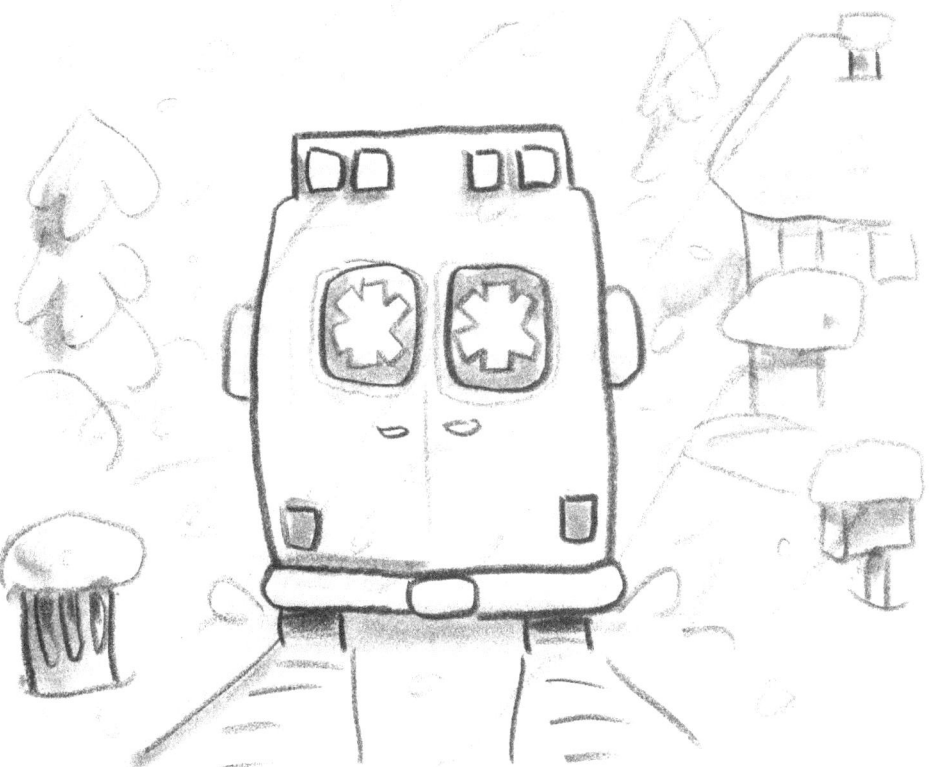

Still, we managed to get her down the stairs, into the truck, and off to the hospital. All before the plows ever even got out.

wednesdays with Bob

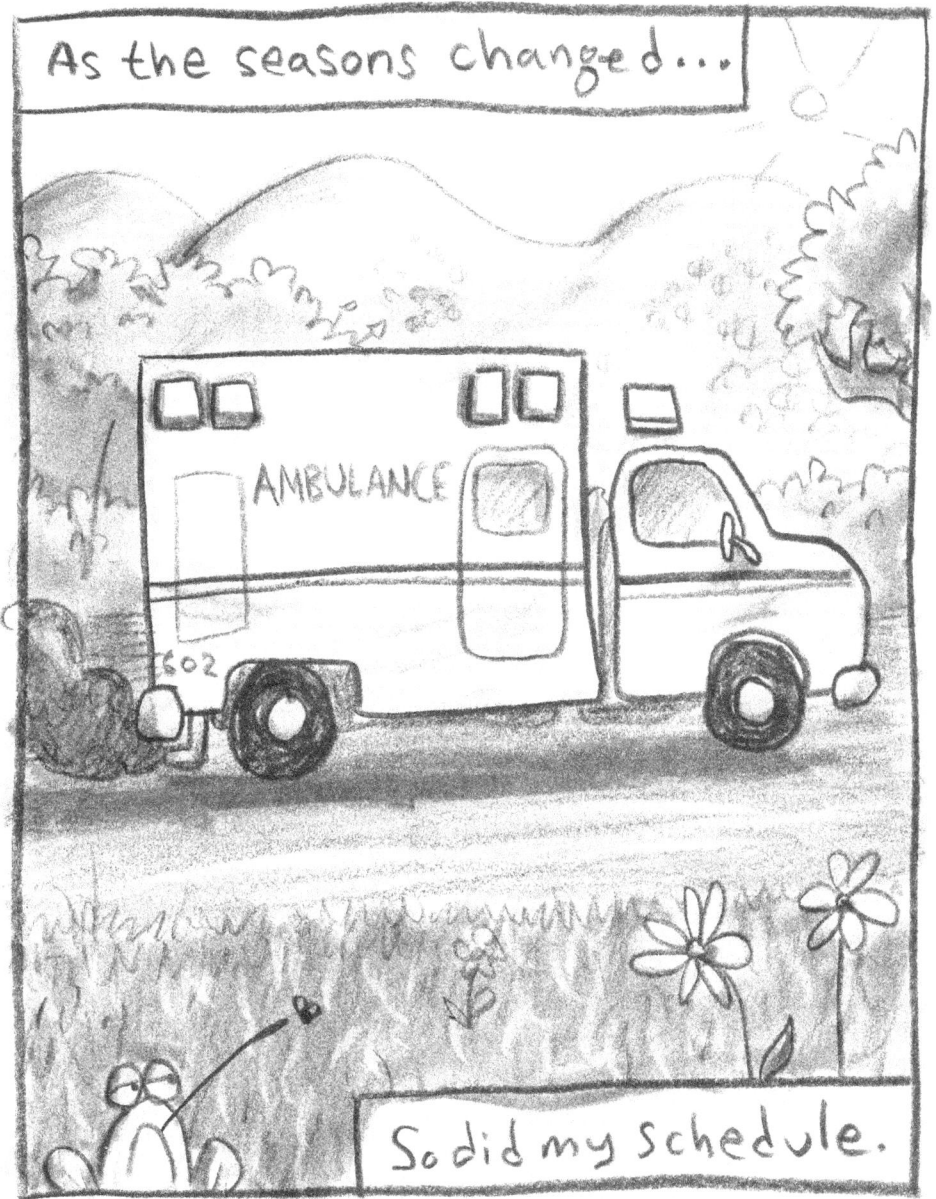

As the seasons changed...

So did my schedule.

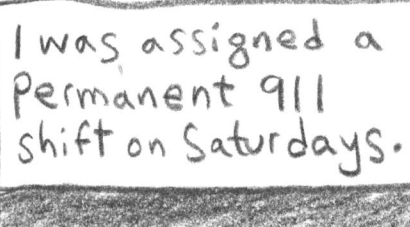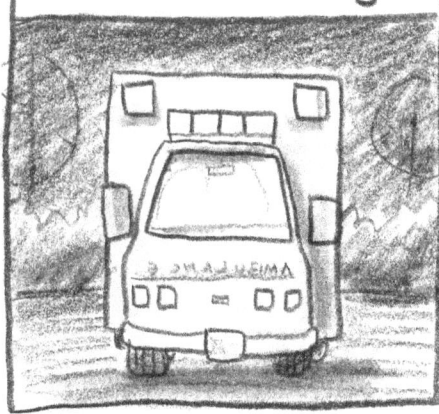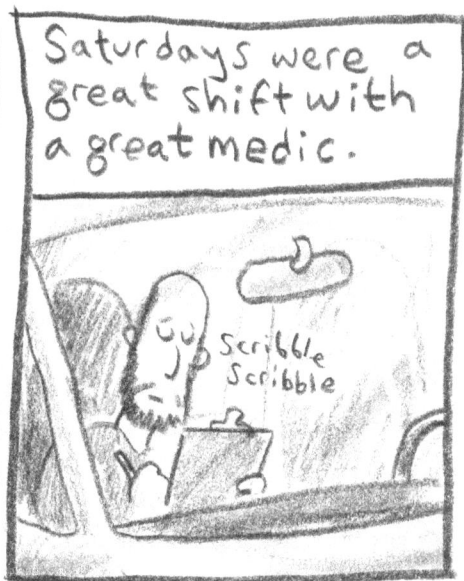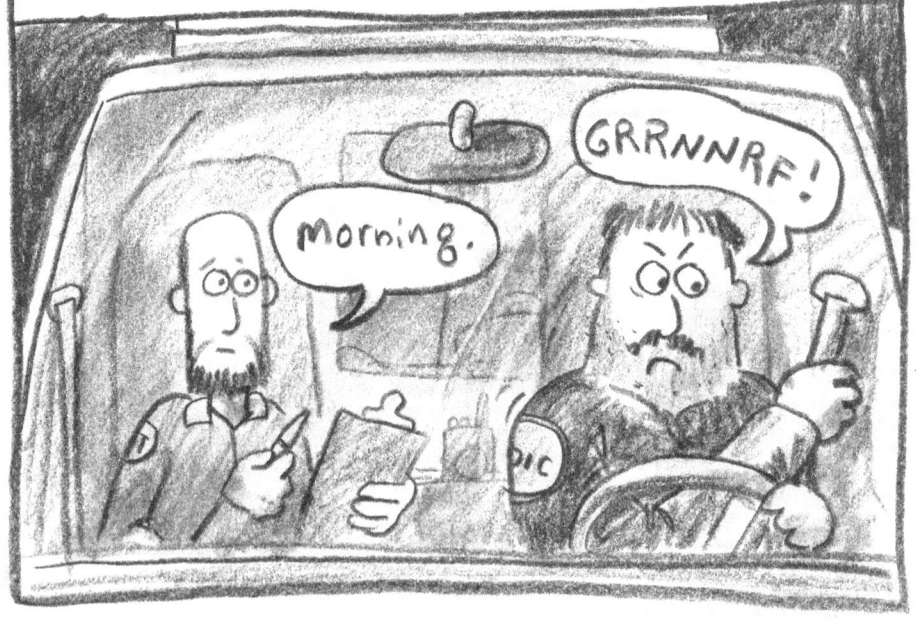

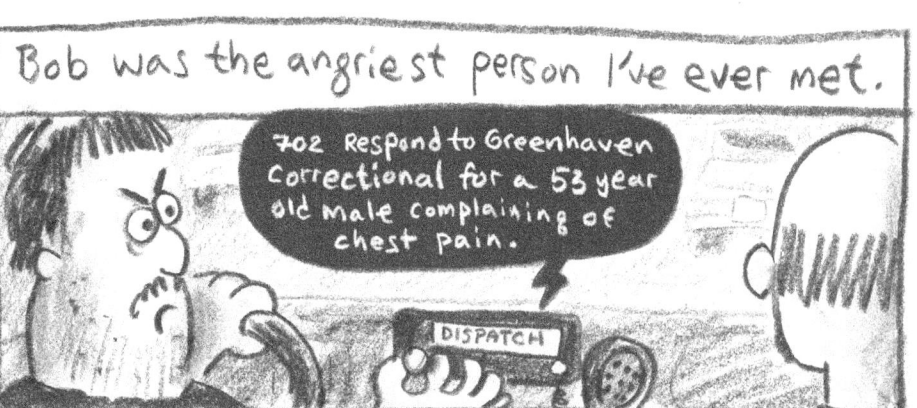
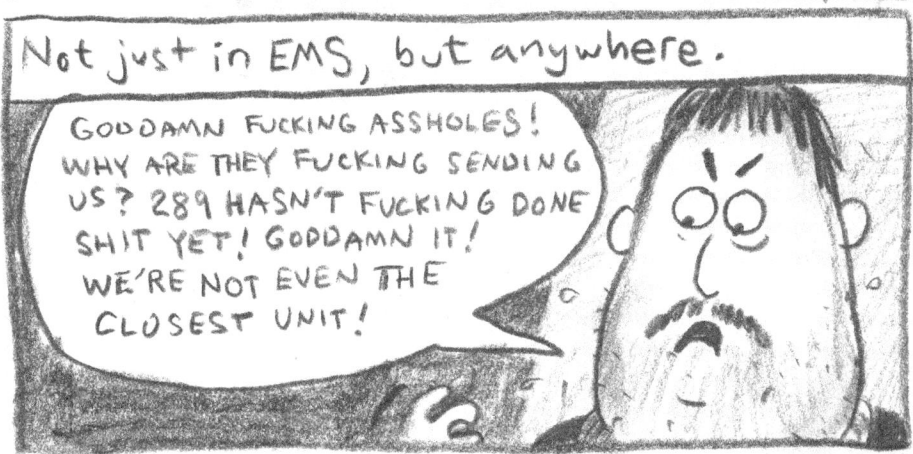
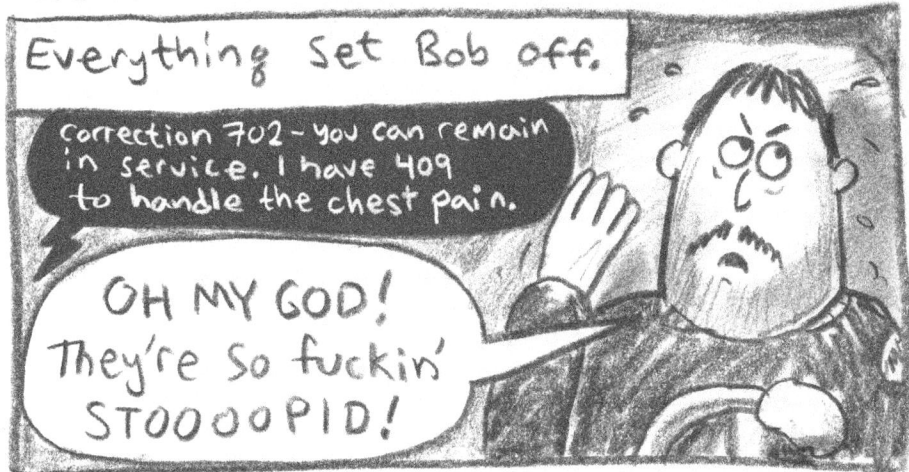

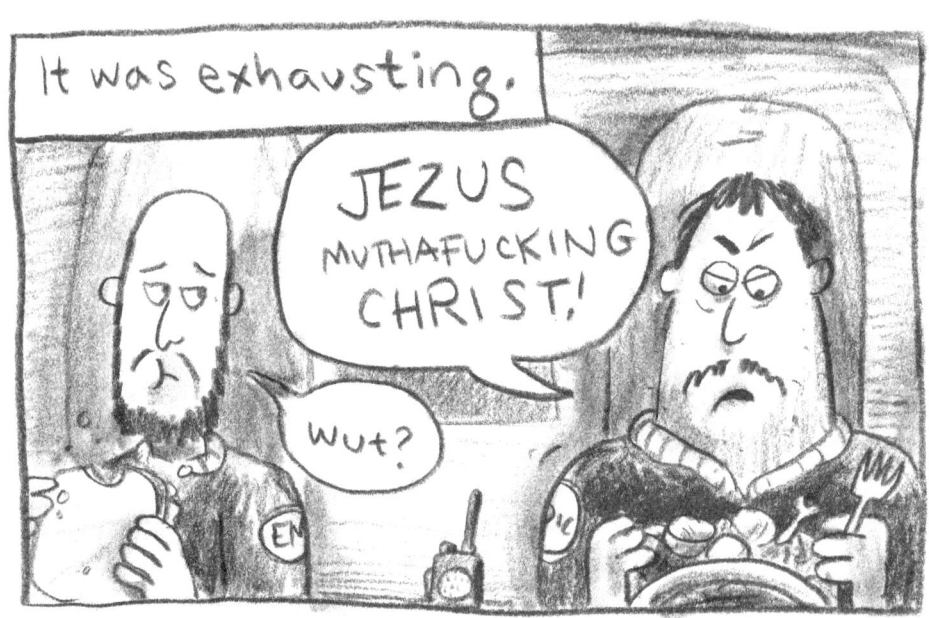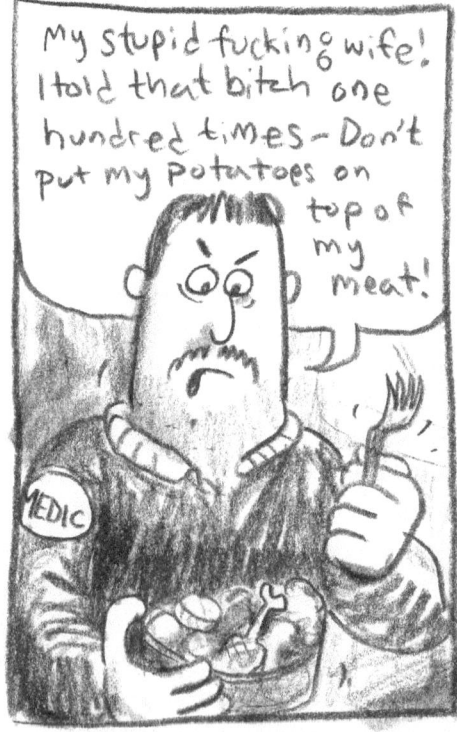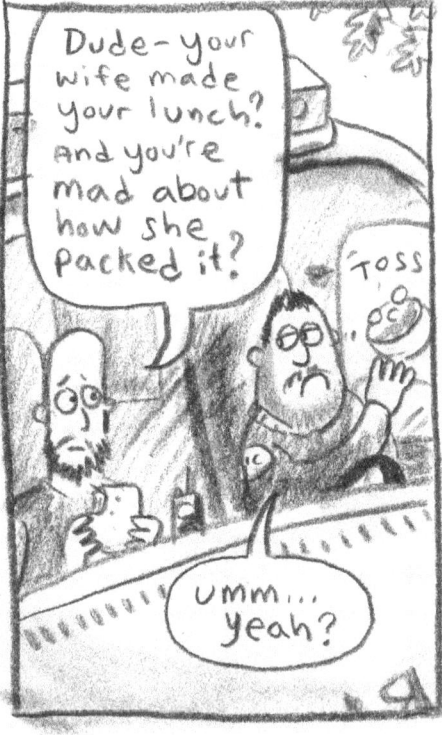

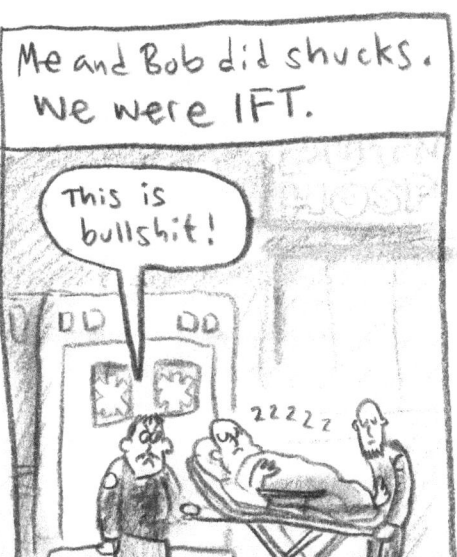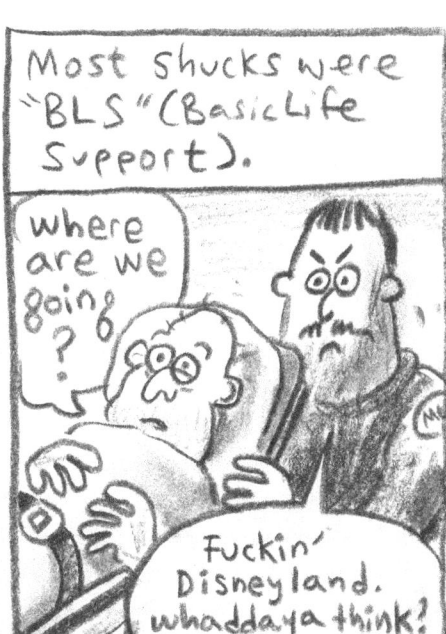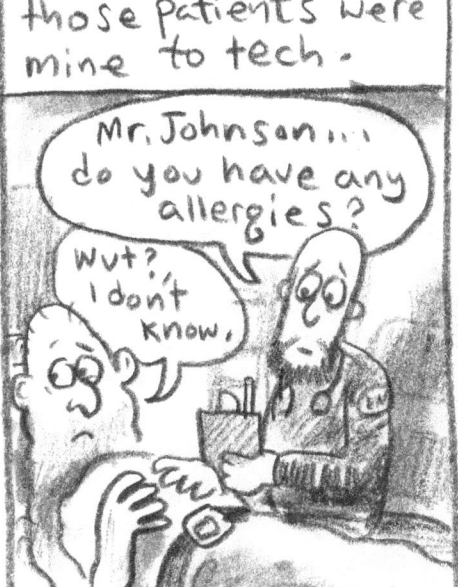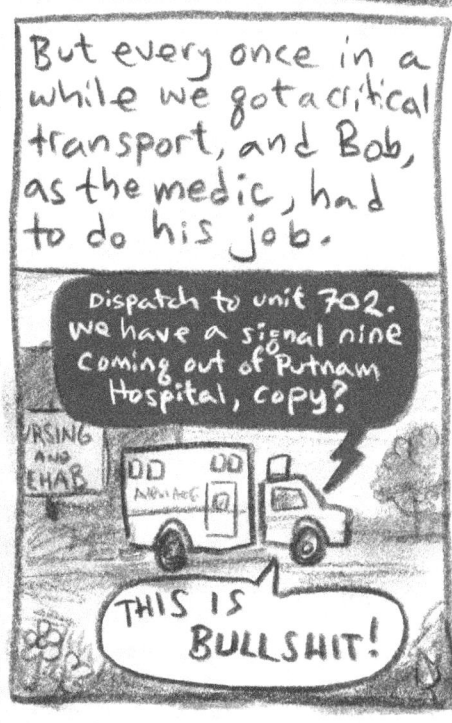

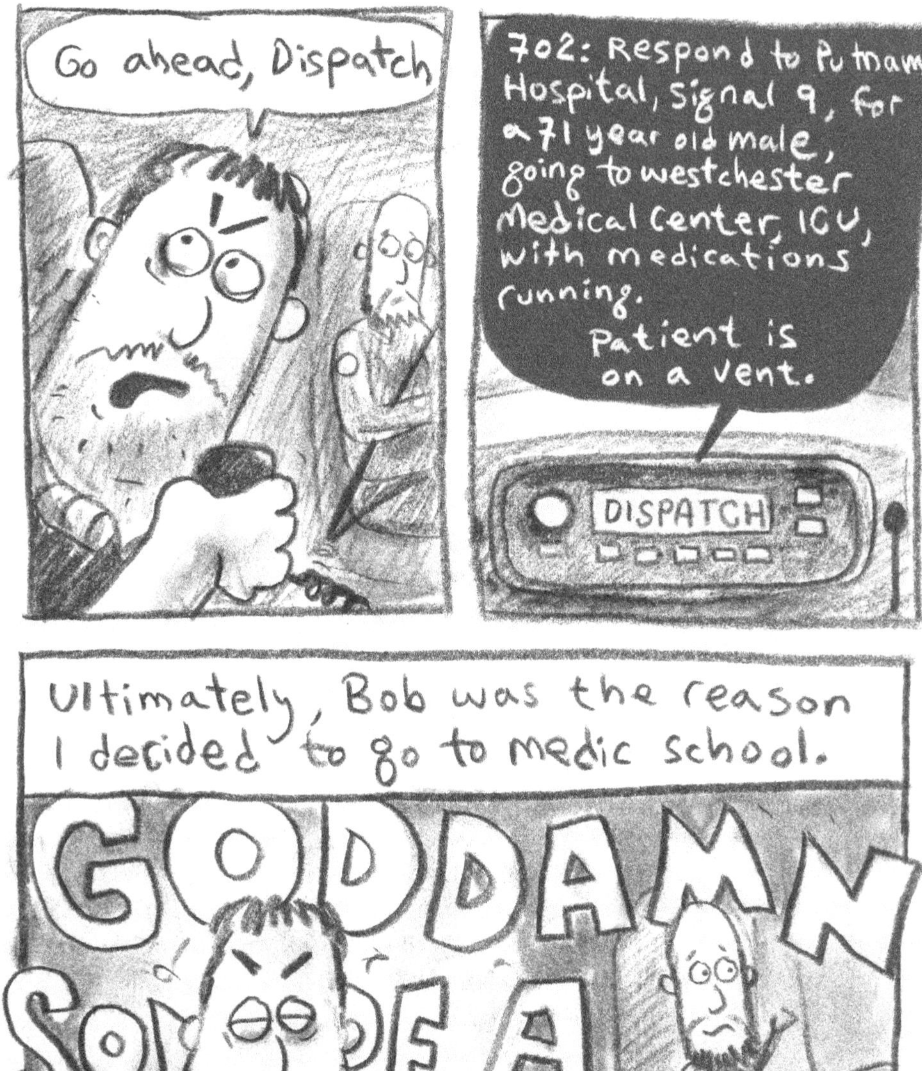

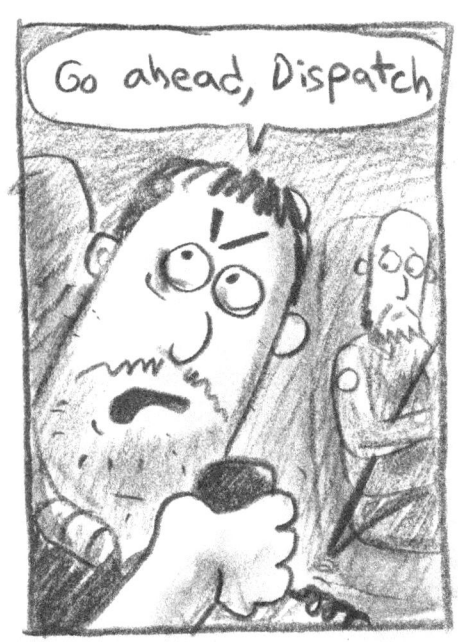
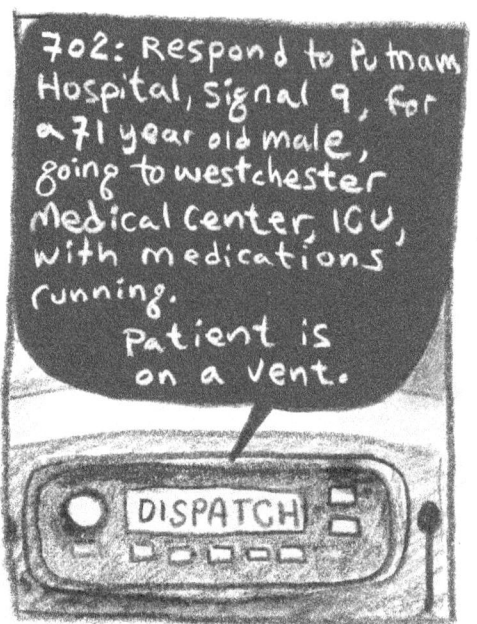

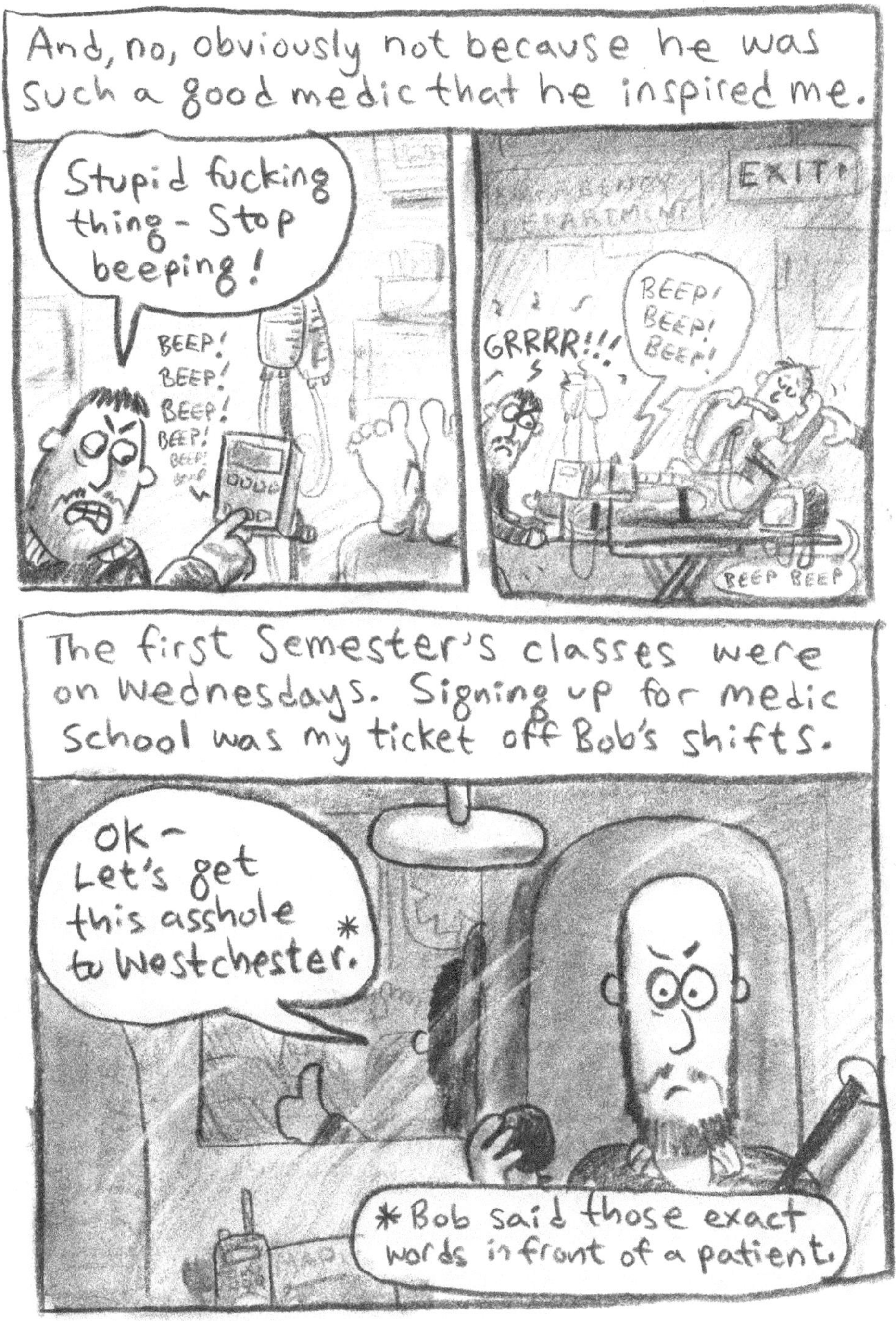

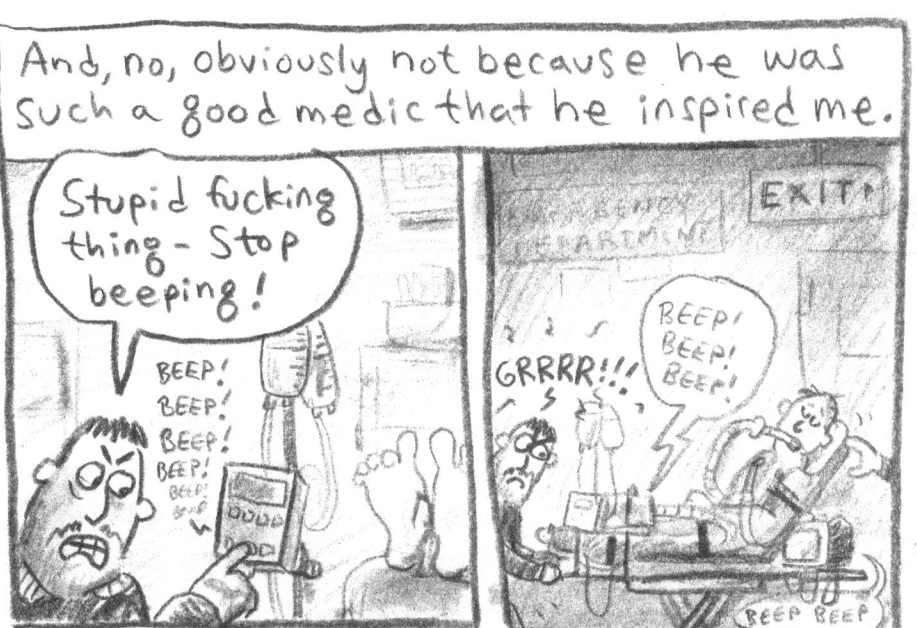

Getting Schooled

I hadn't been in school in over 20 years. The medic program was a cold bucket of water. I mean sure, I had taken an EMT class—but this was for real.

HTN

ING'S RIAD

$$\frac{Volume (mL)}{Minutes} \times Drop\ factor\ (gtt/mL) = Flow\ Rate\ (gtt/min)$$

$CO = HR \times SV$
CO = Cardiac Output
HR = Heart Rate
SV = Stroke Volume

$GFR = 39.1 \times \left(\frac{hei}{se}\right)$
Glomerular Filt

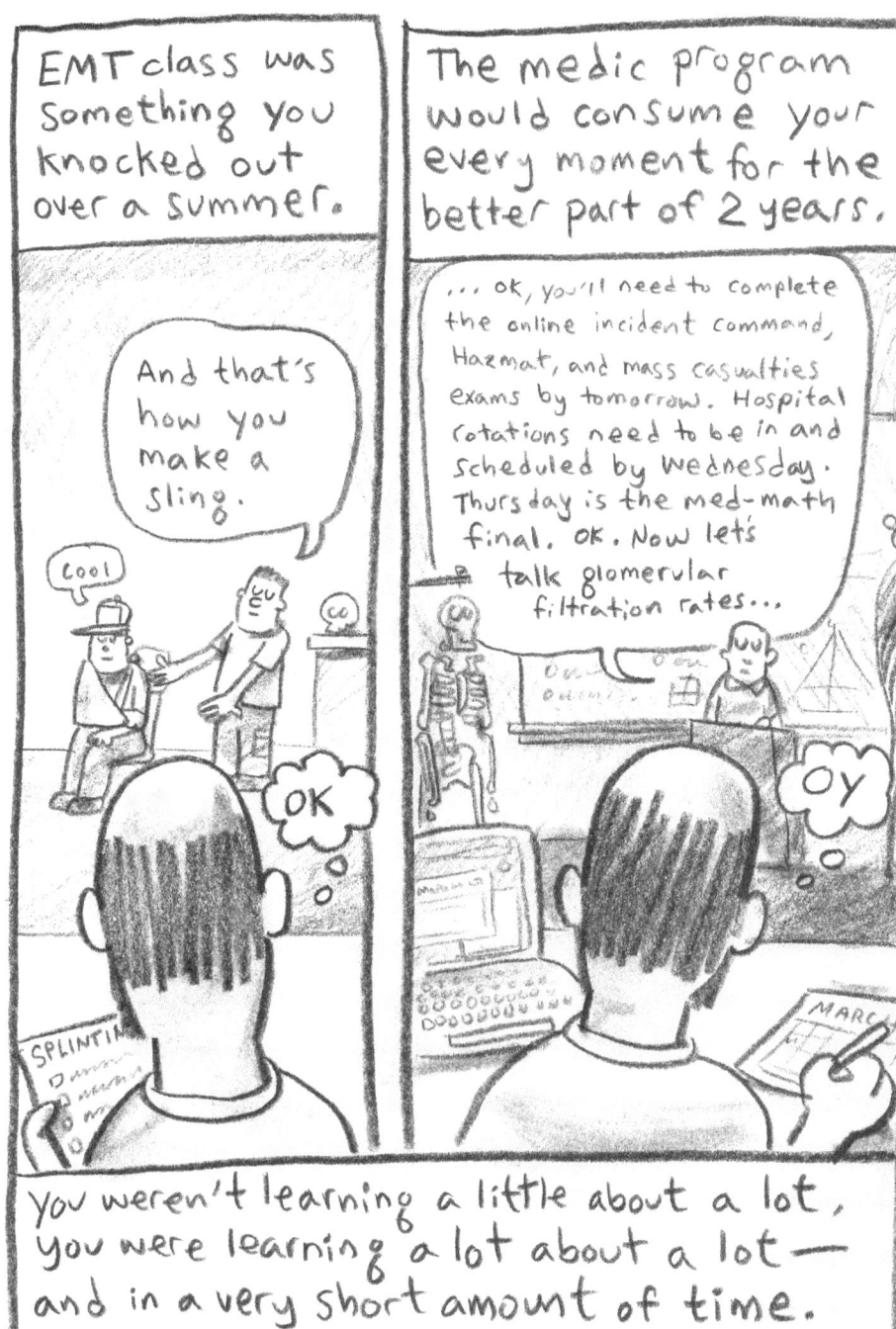

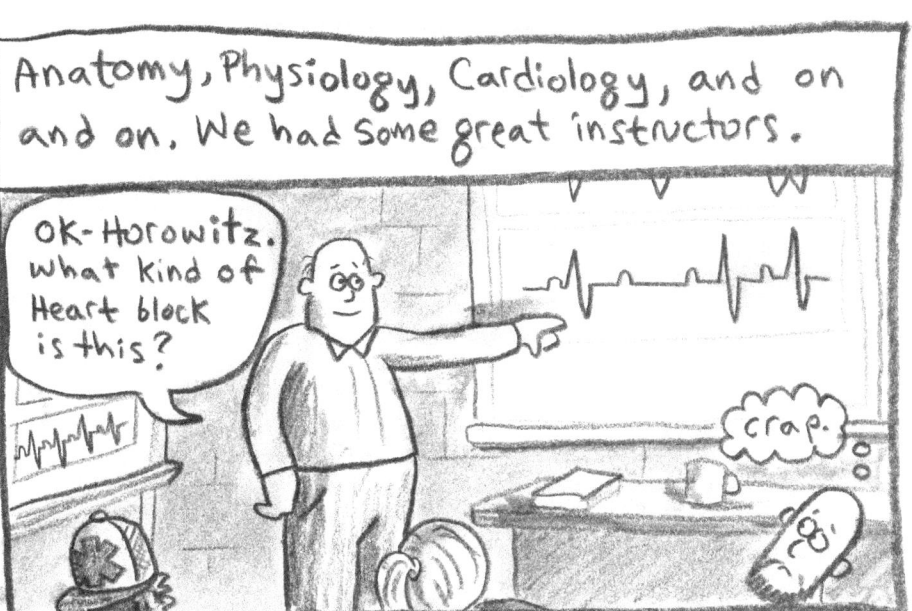

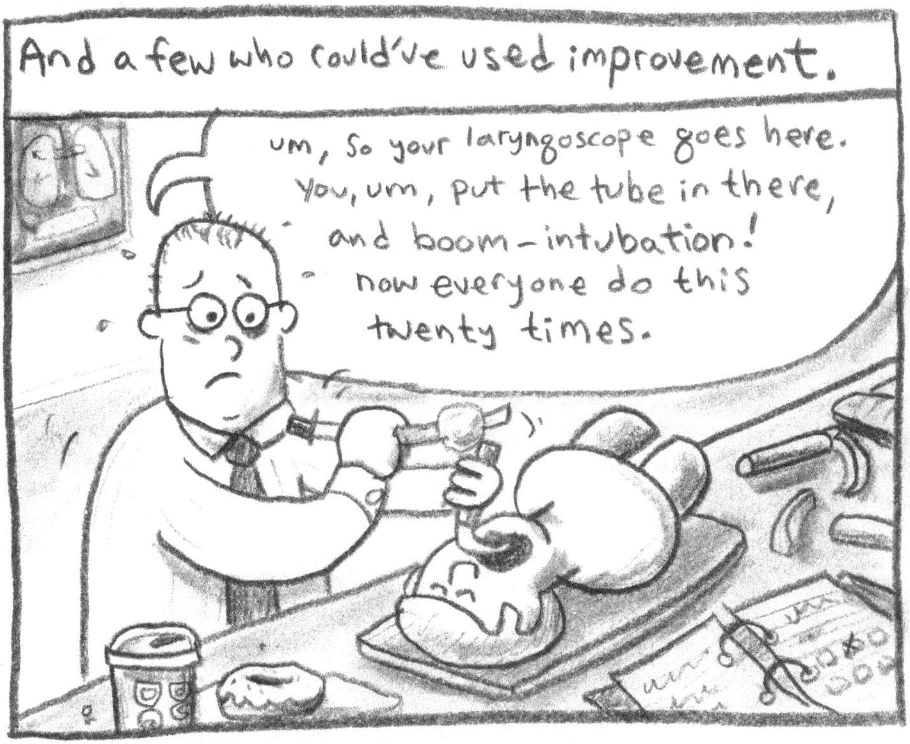

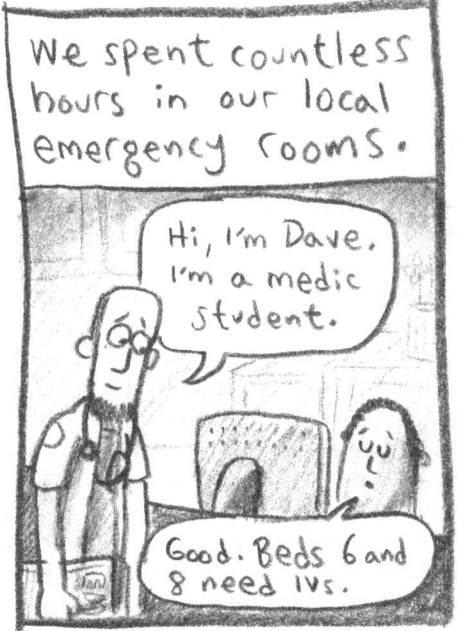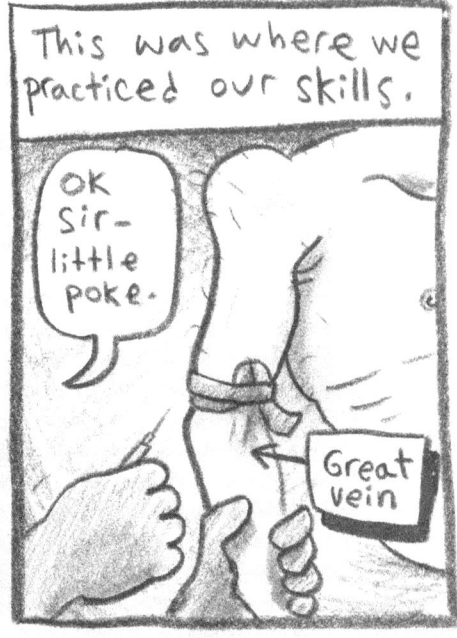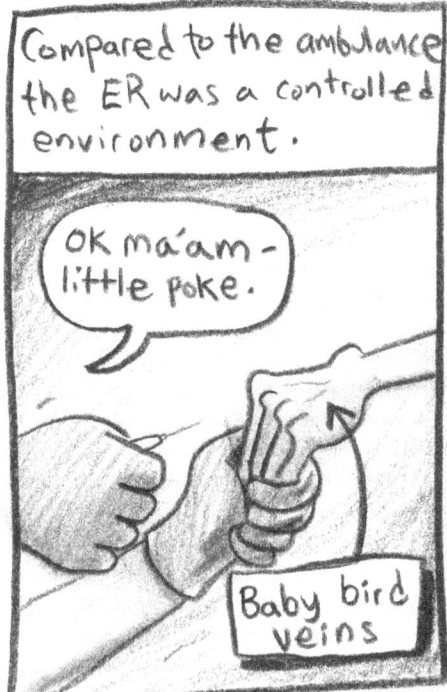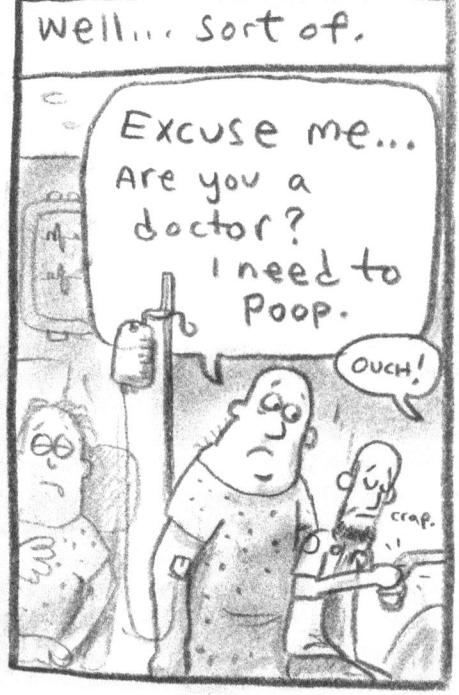

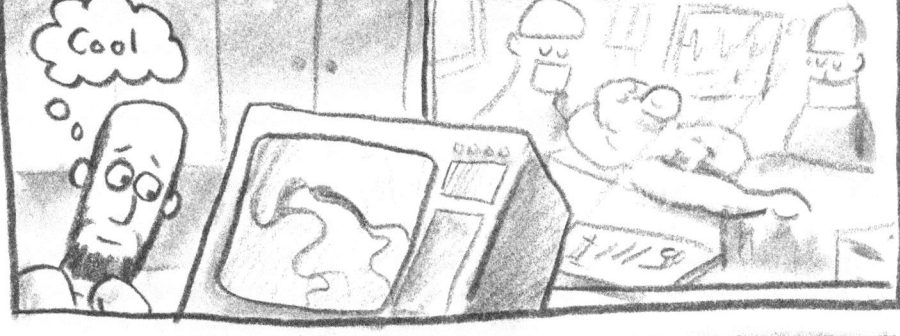

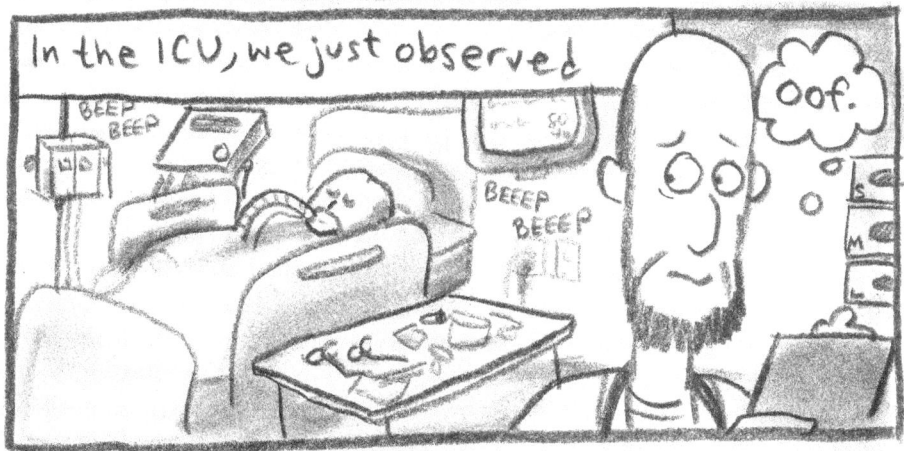

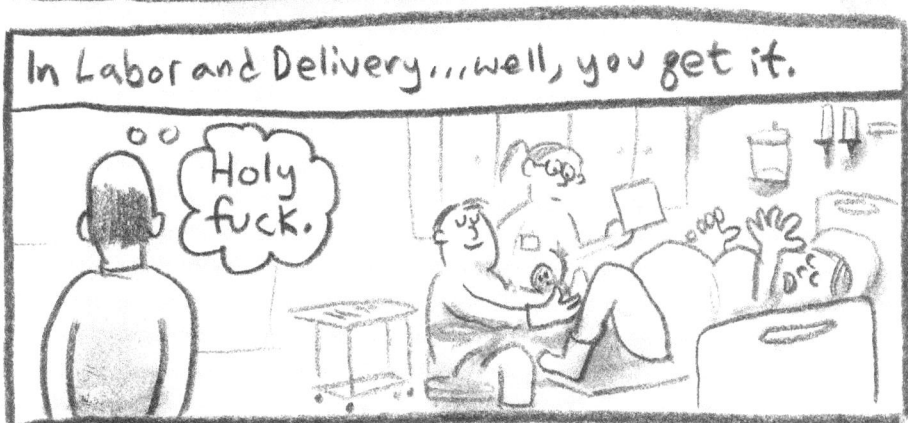

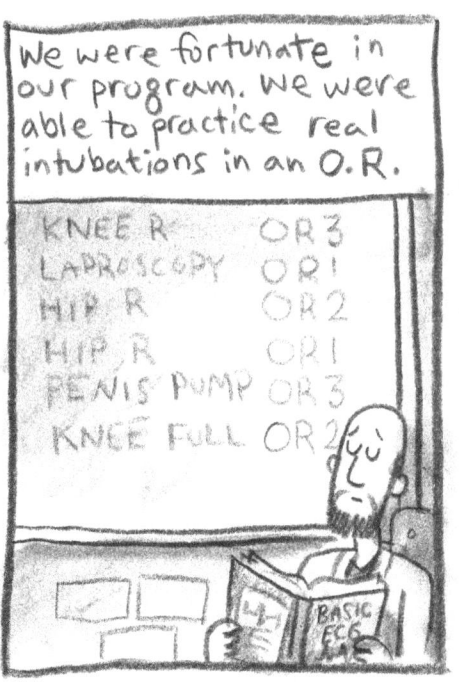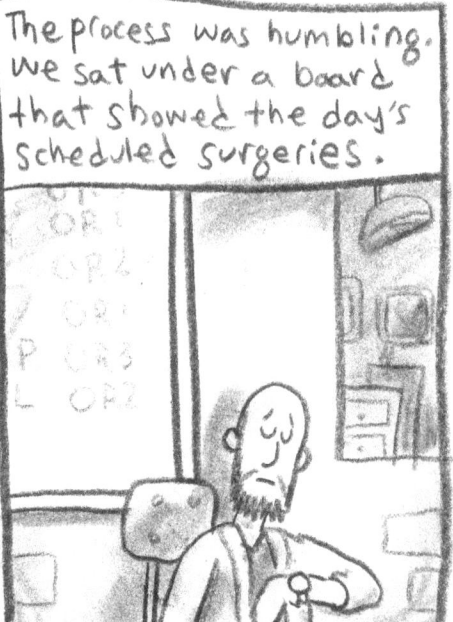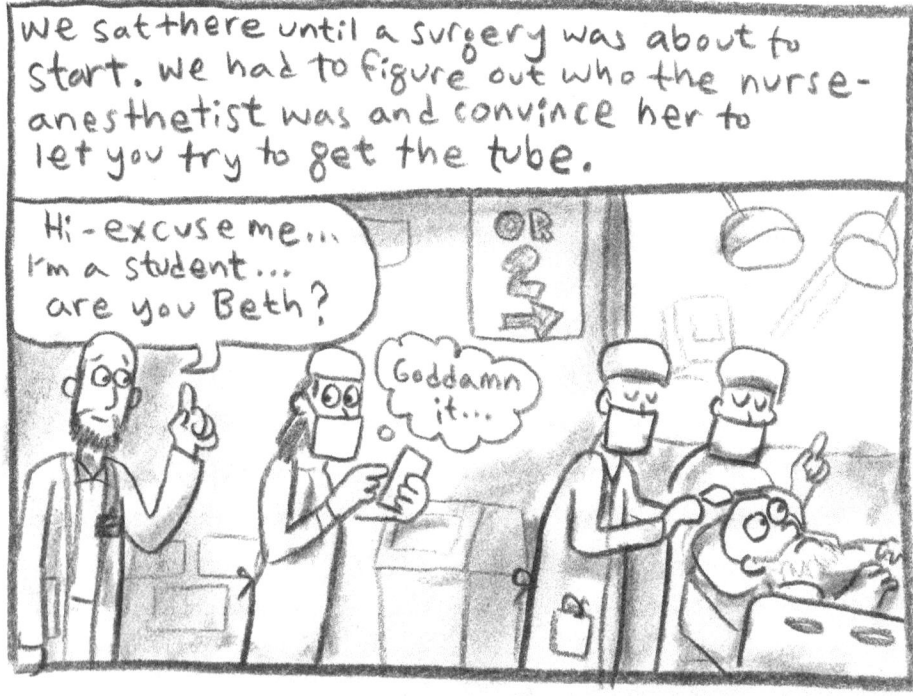

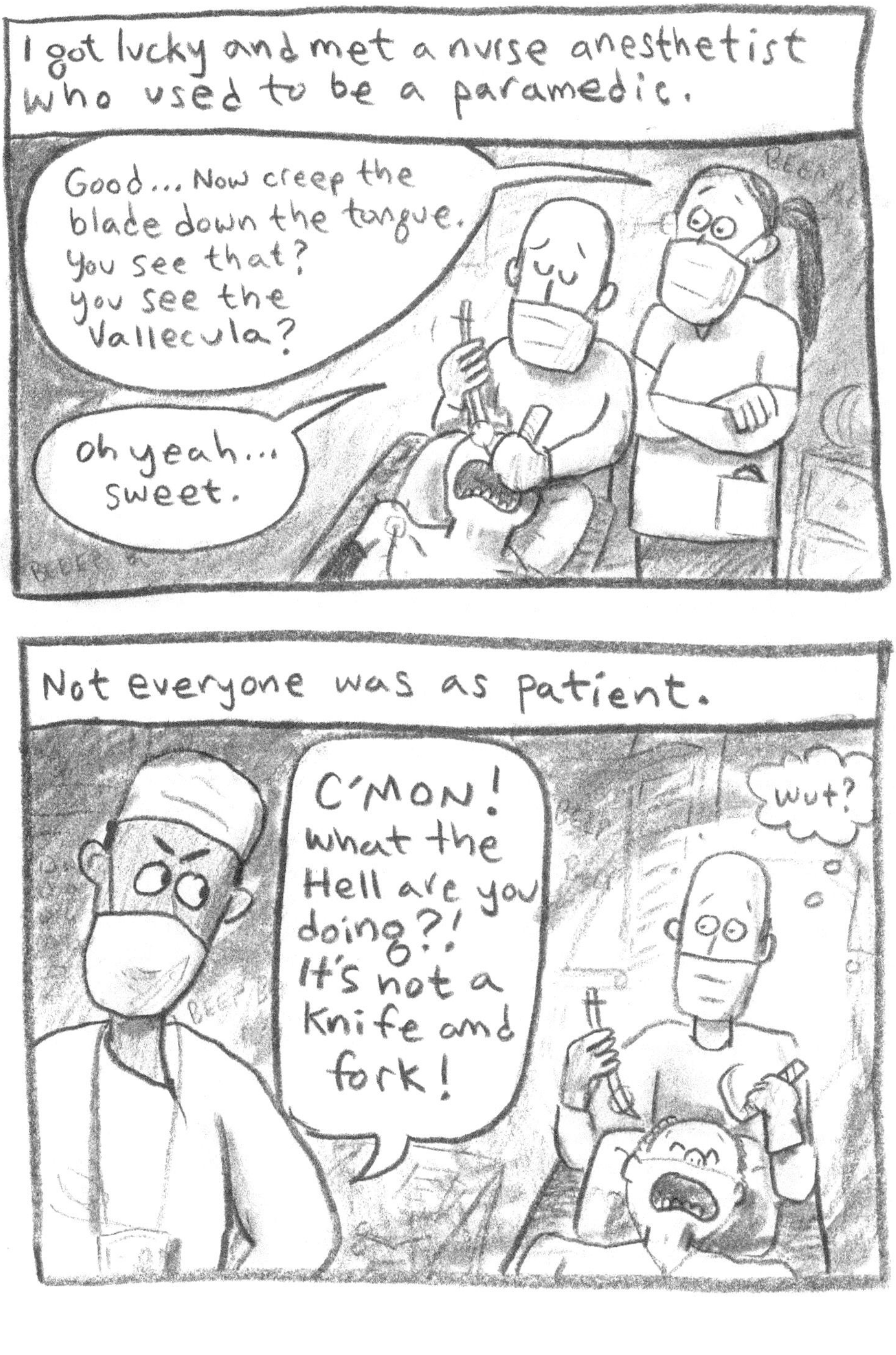

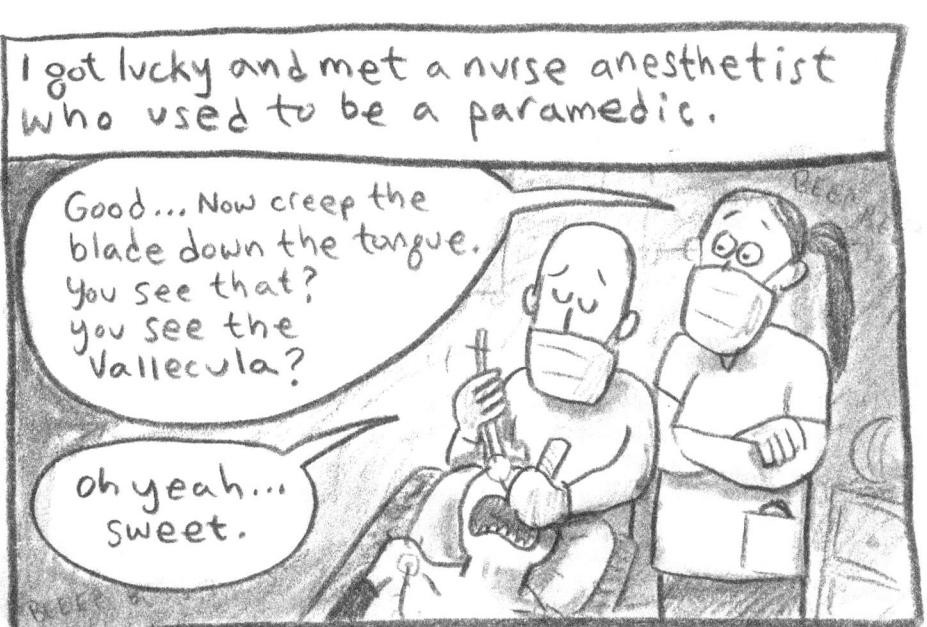

Ride On

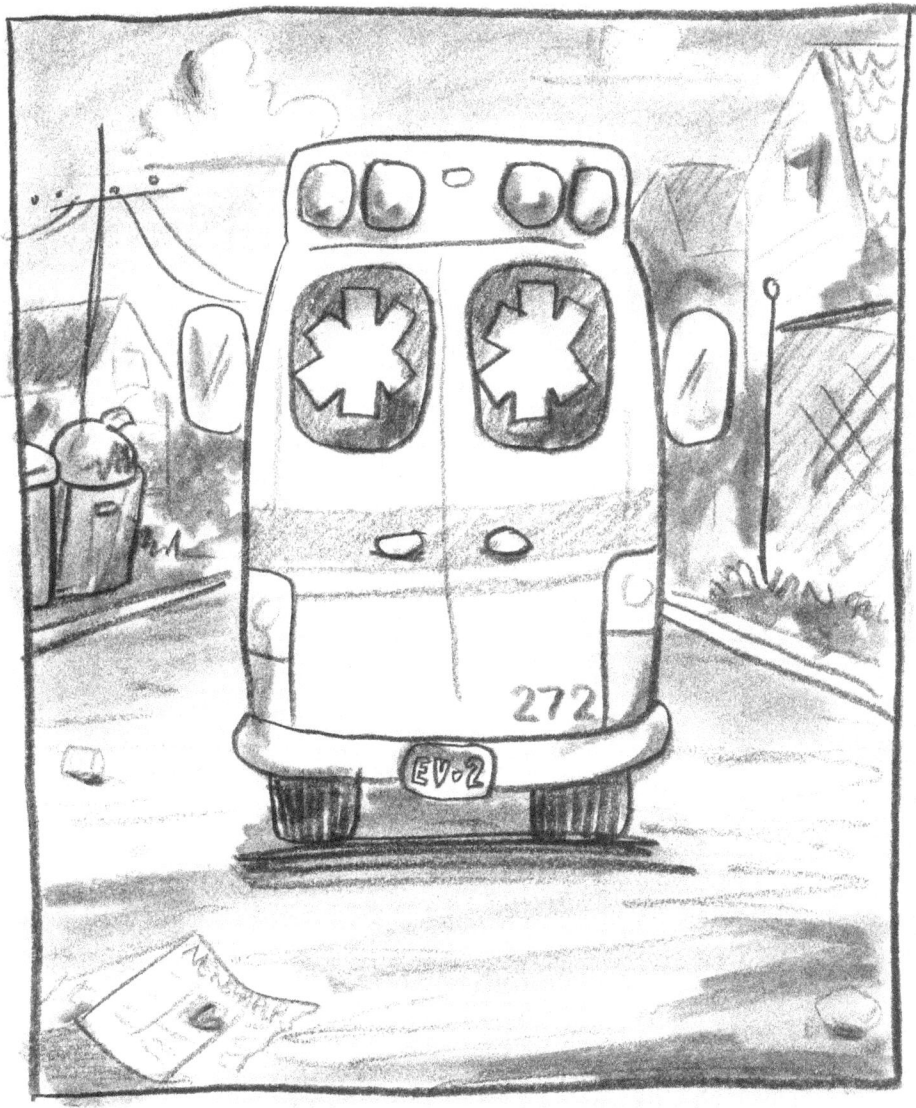

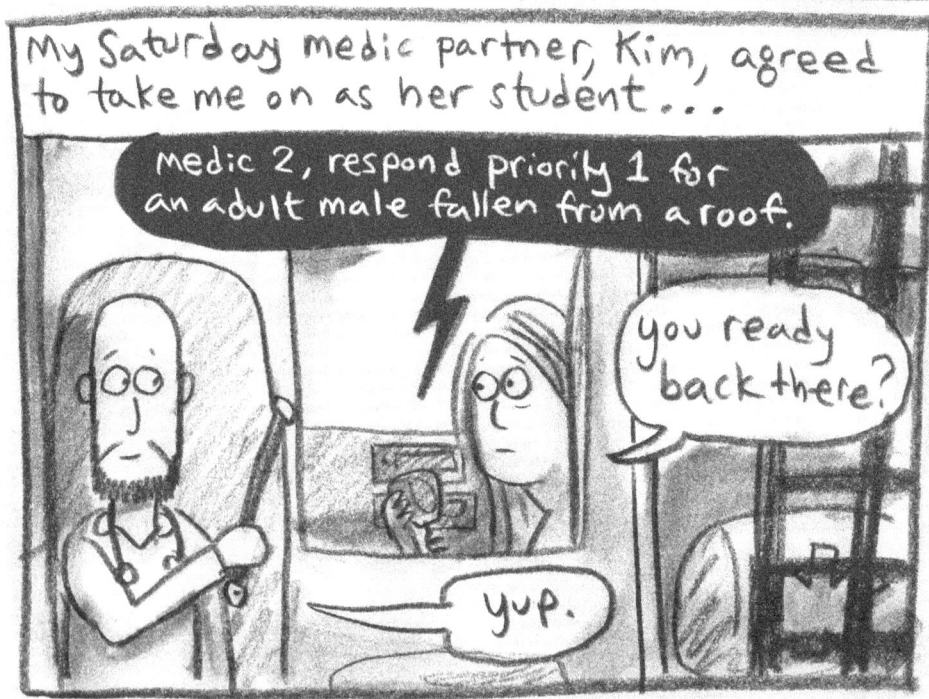

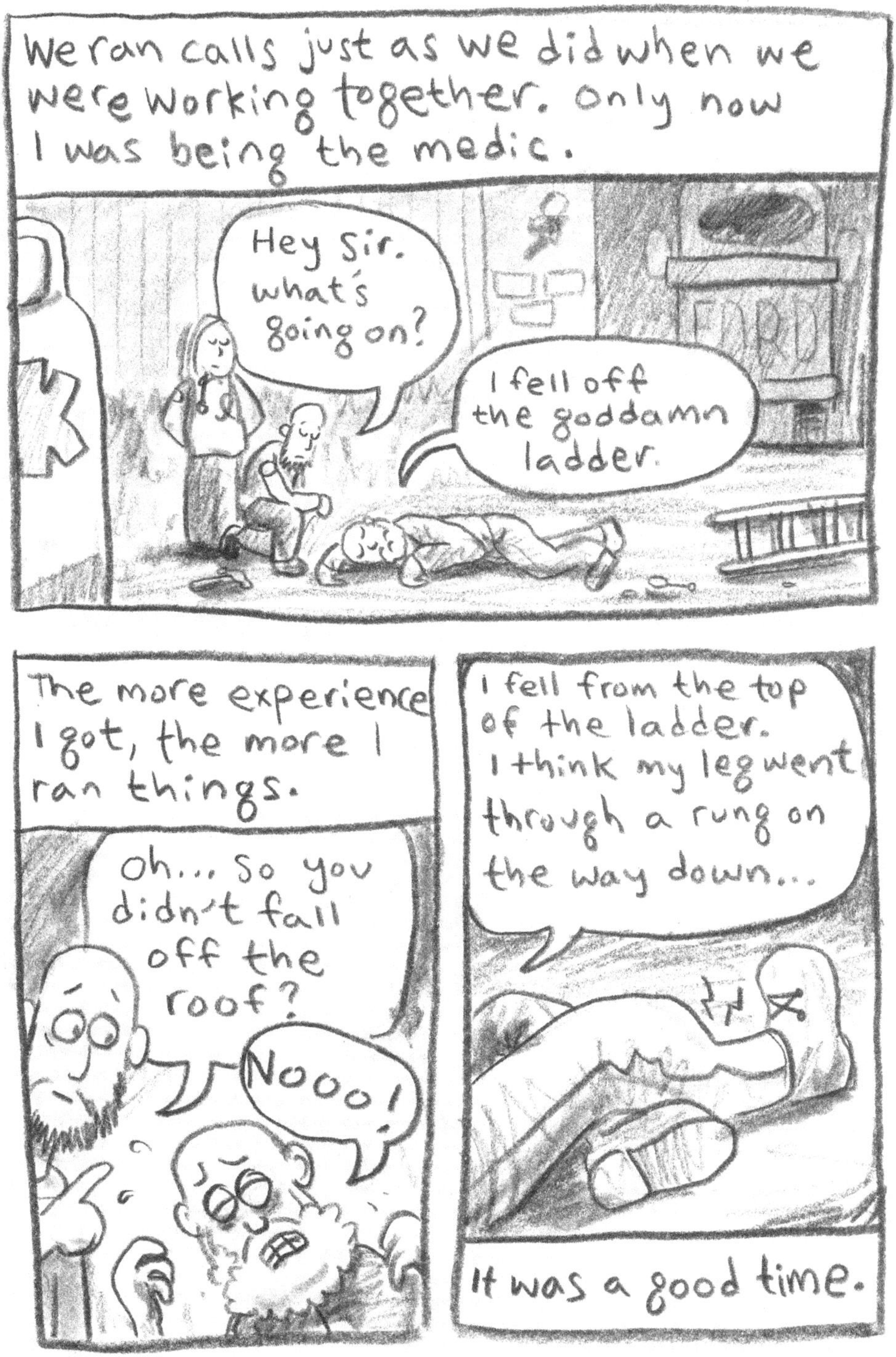

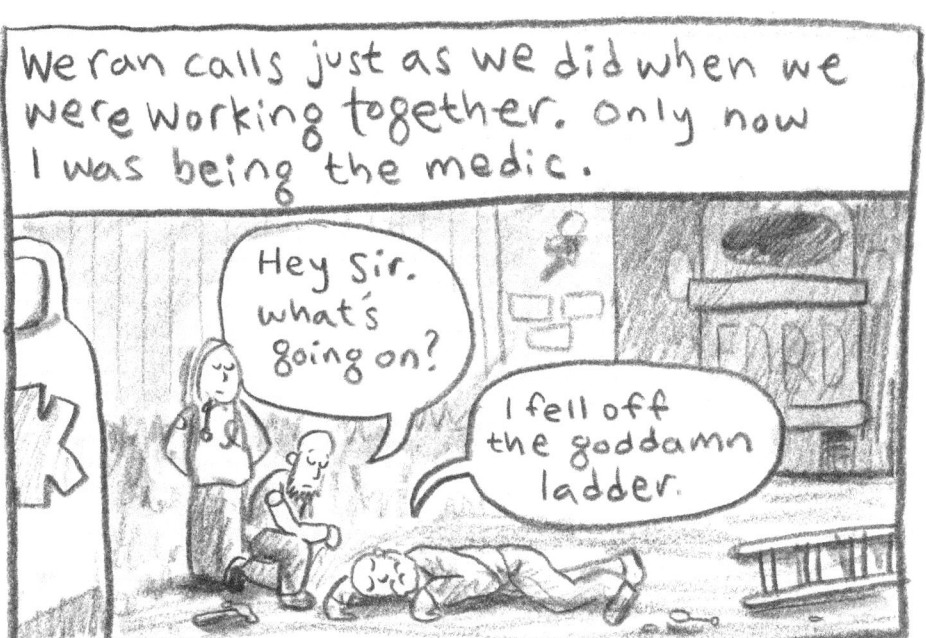

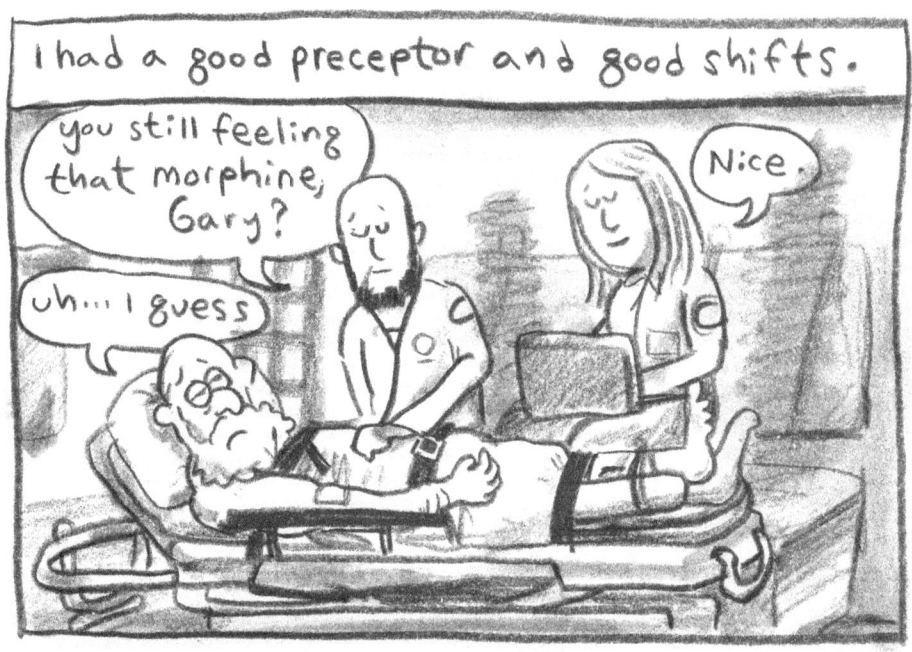

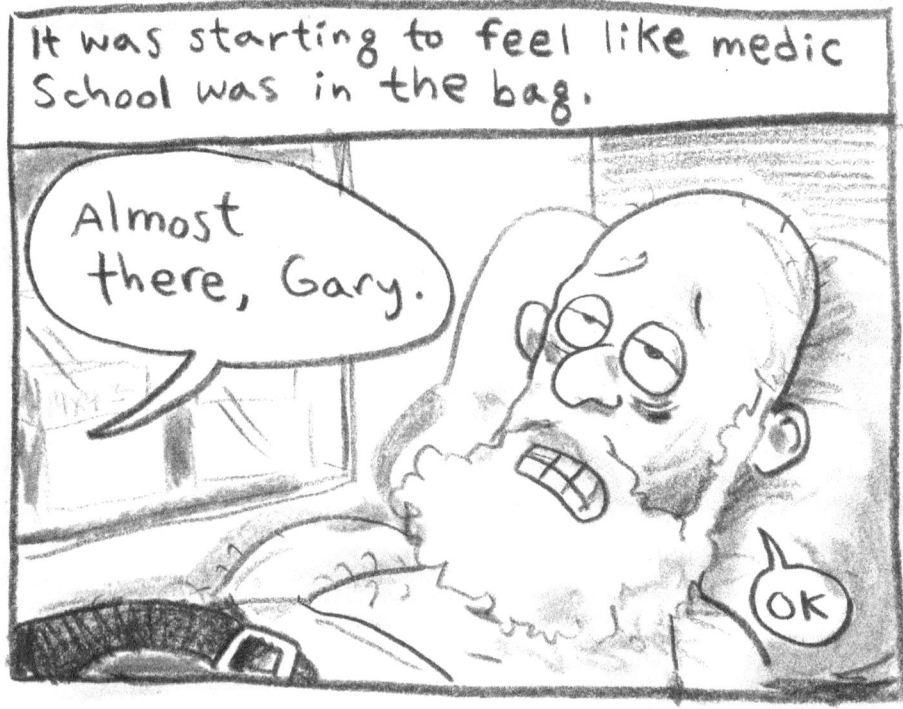

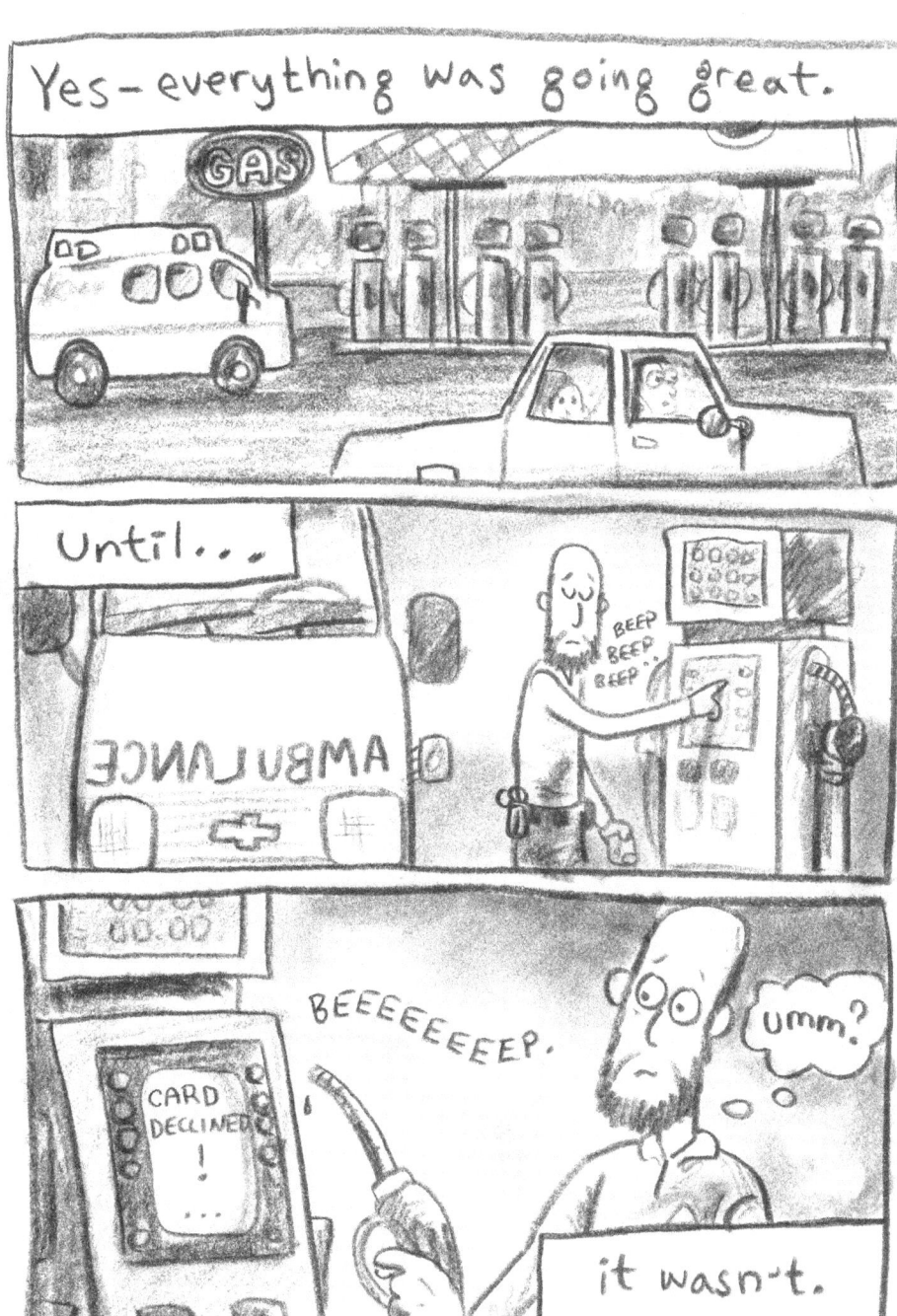

TransCare - the worst ambulance service in the region - the place I worked: The place I had scheduled the whole year's ride times, was about to shit the bed...

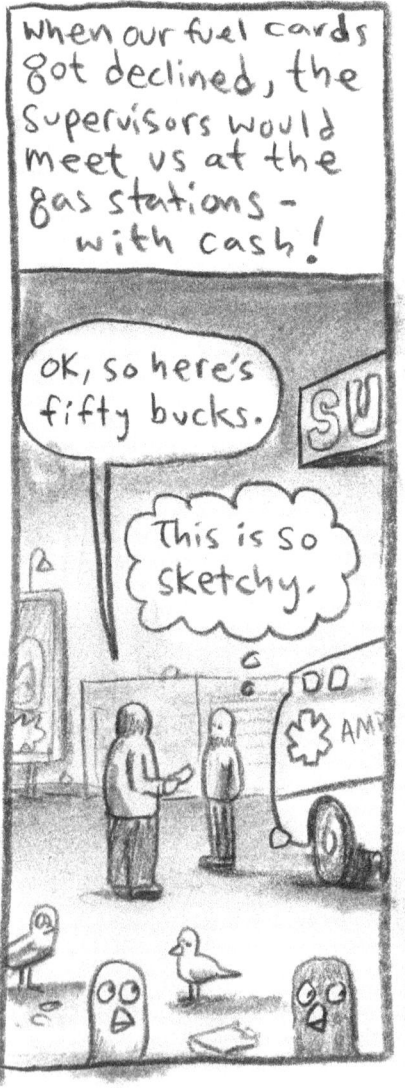

When our fuel cards got declined, the supervisors would meet us at the gas stations - with cash!

"OK, so here's fifty bucks."

This is so sketchy.

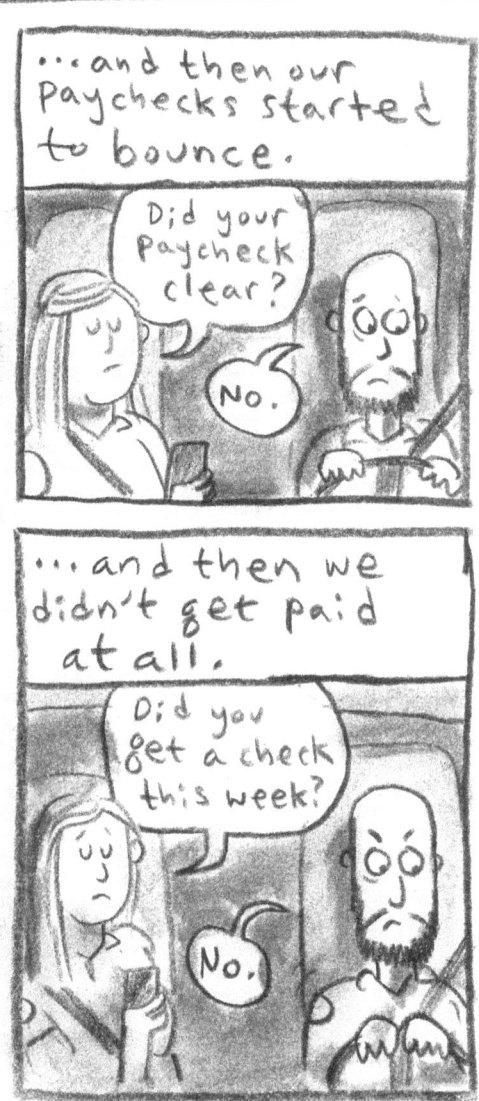

...and then our paychecks started to bounce.

"Did your paycheck clear?"

"No."

...and then we didn't get paid at all.

"Did you get a check this week?"

"No."

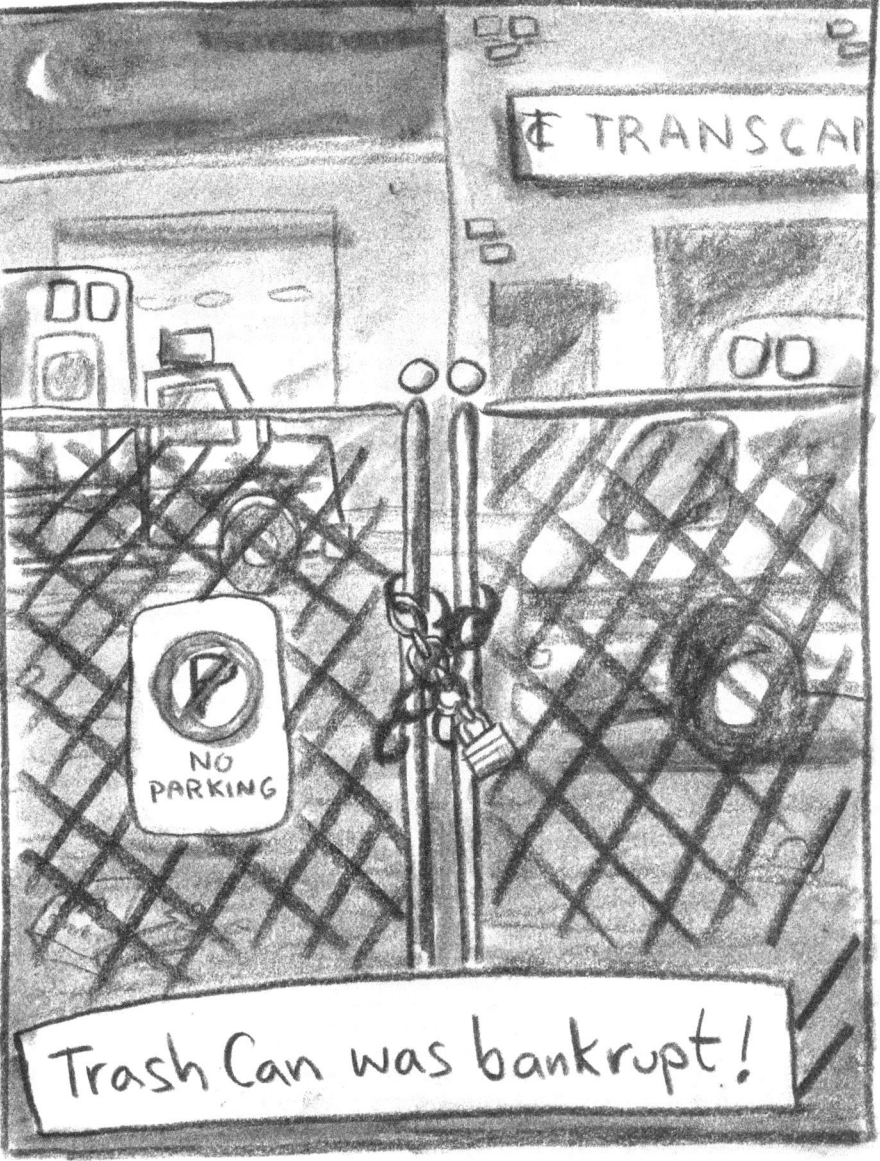

Part II

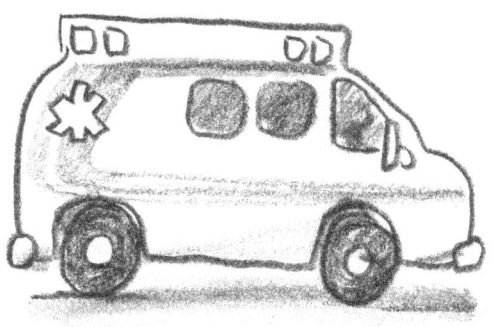

Clean Slate

No one shed a tear when TransCare went under. I sure didn't. It was actually the best thing that could have happened to me.

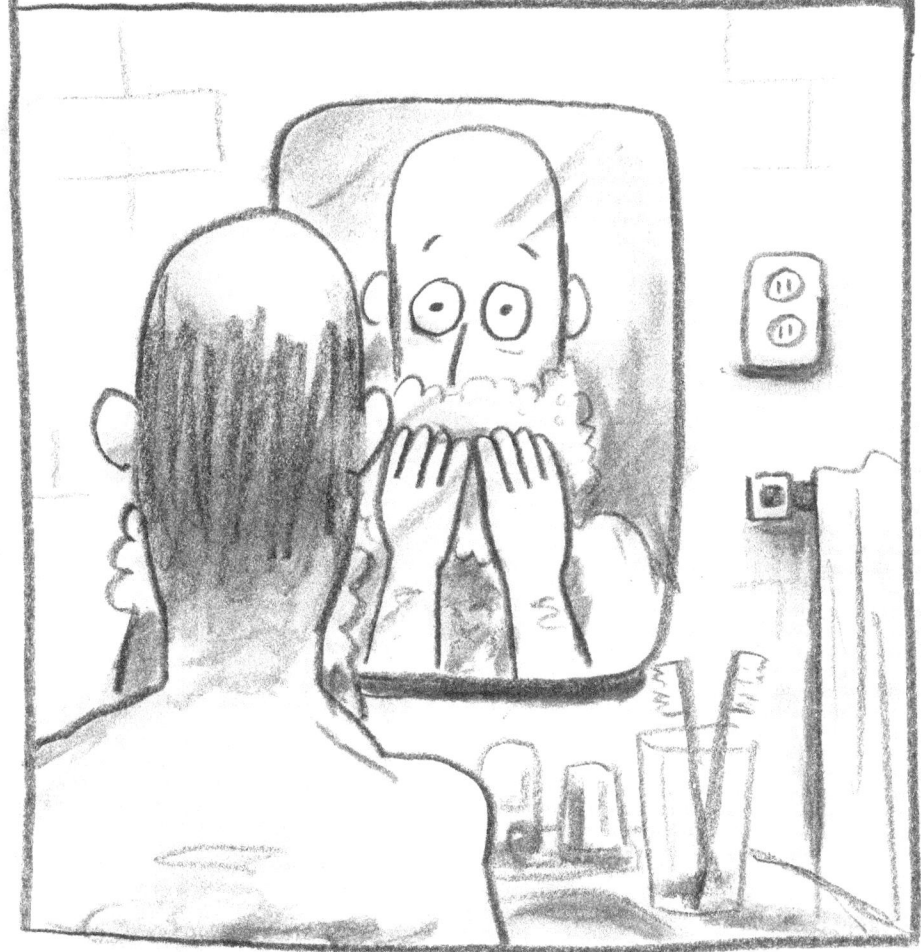

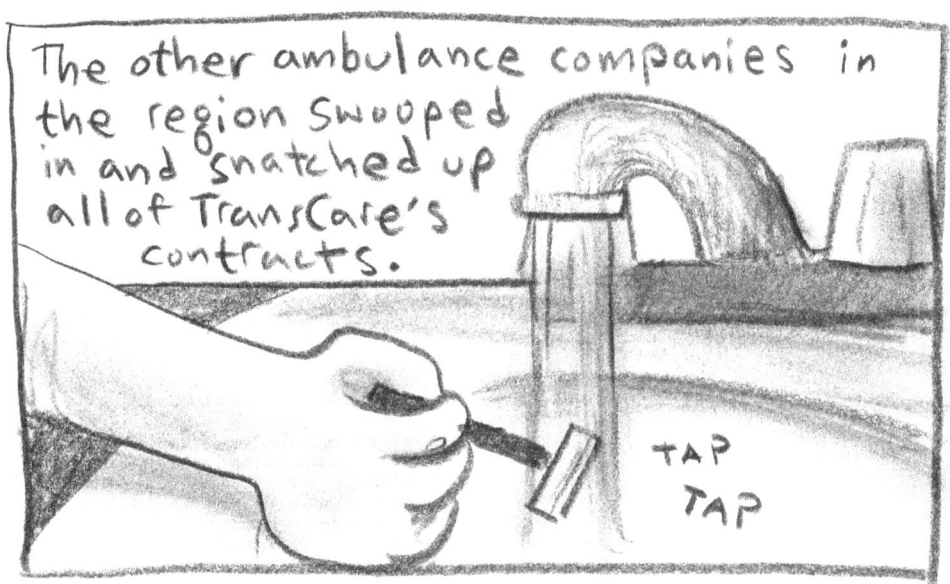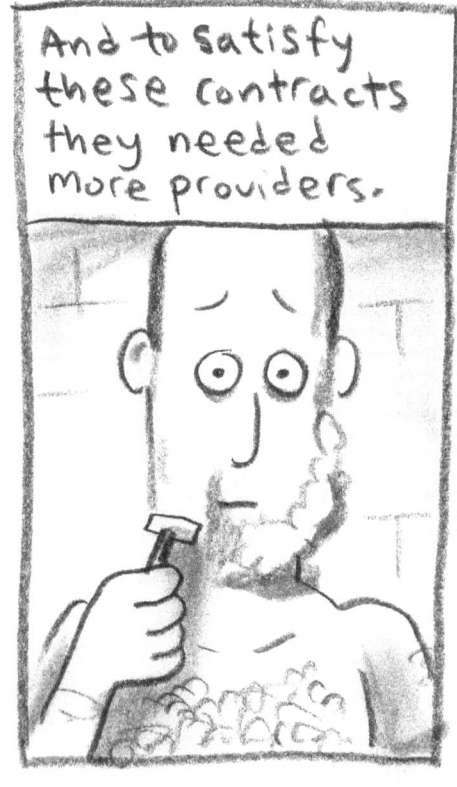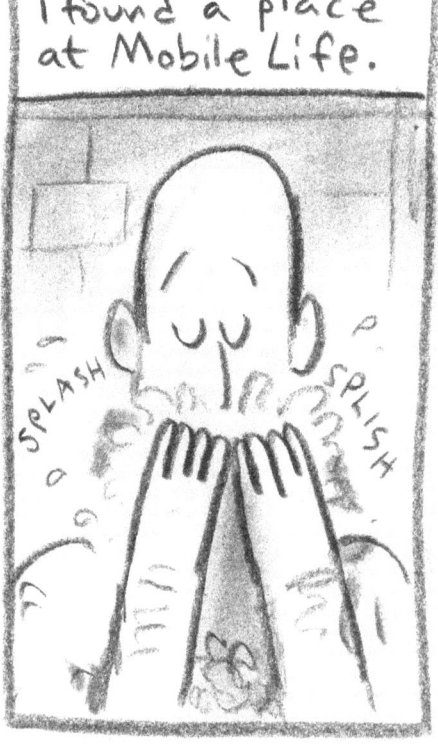

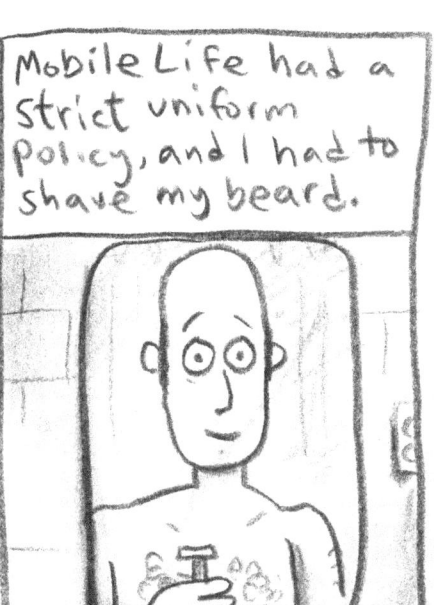
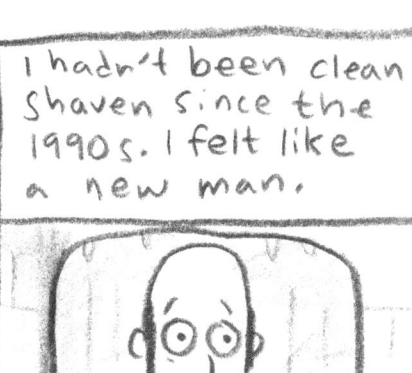
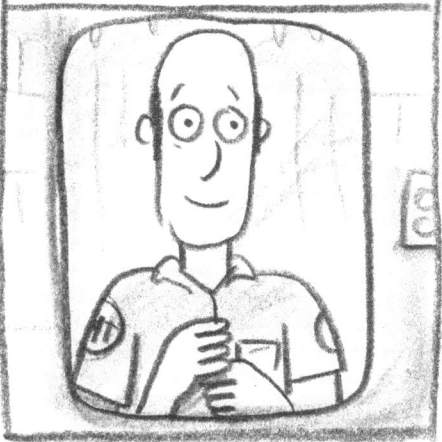
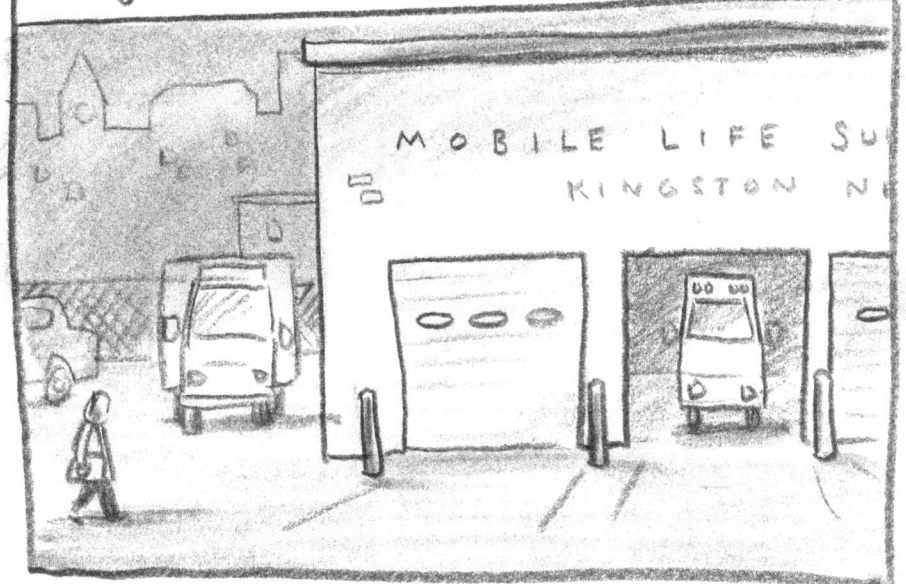

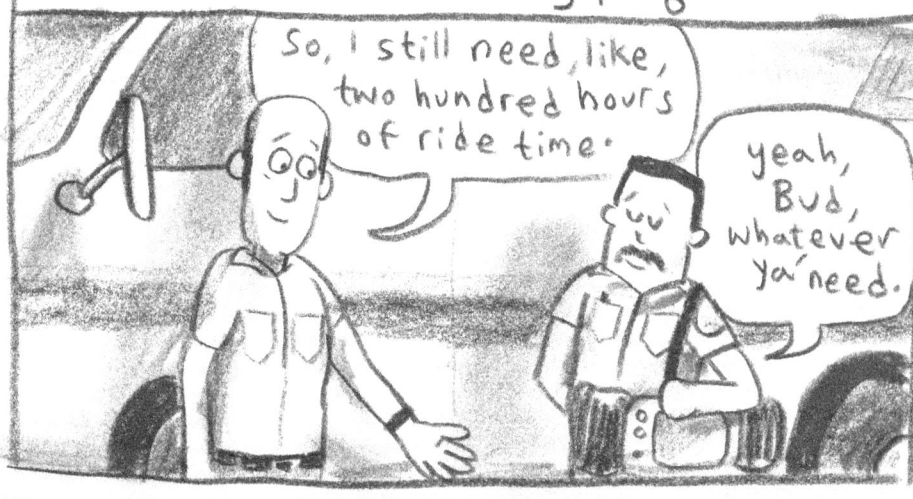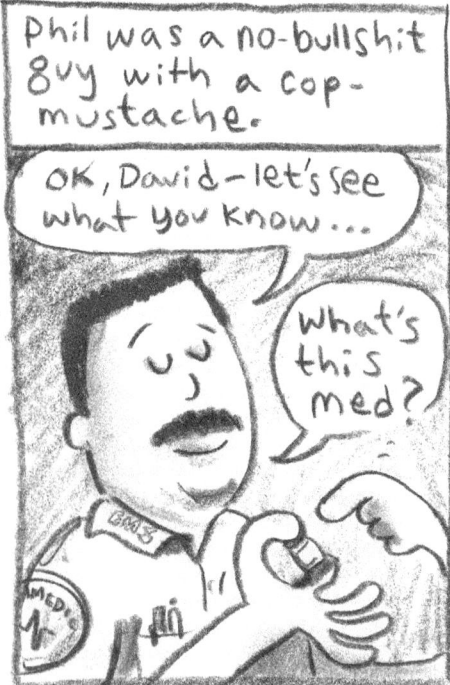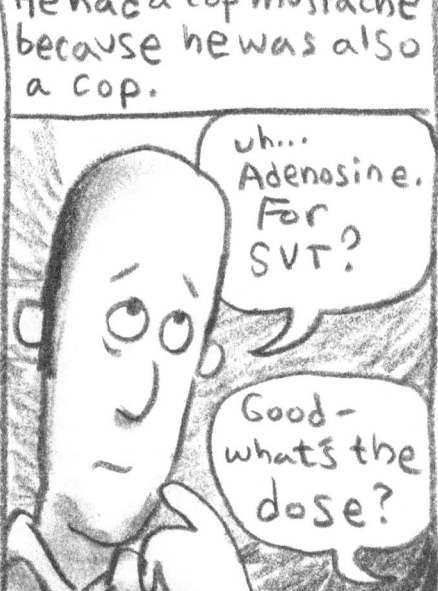

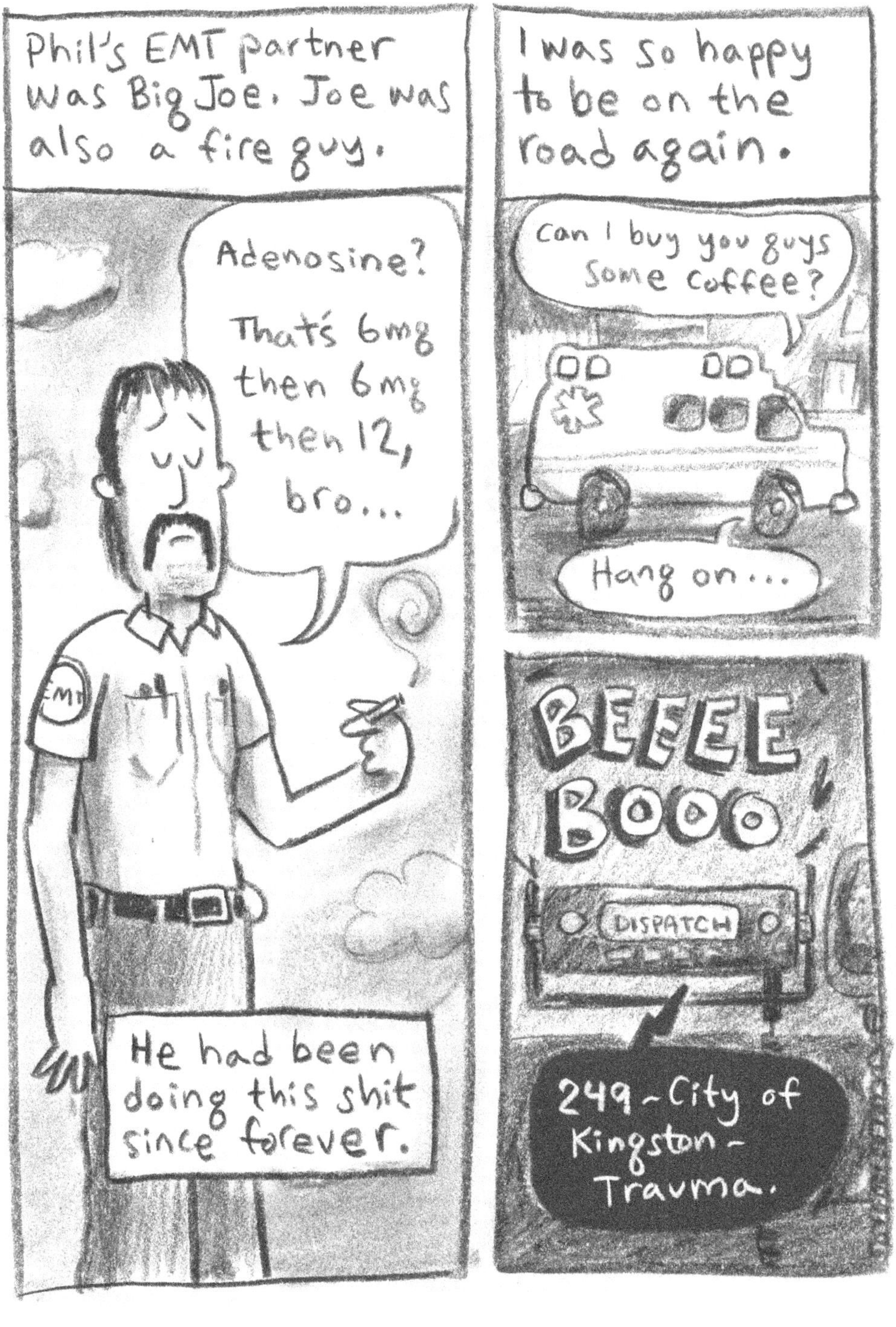

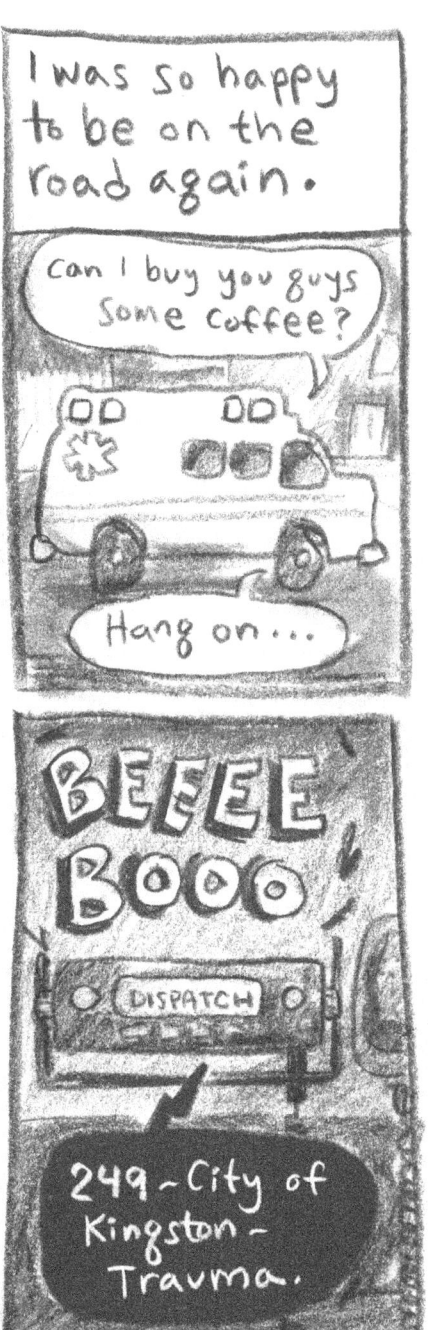

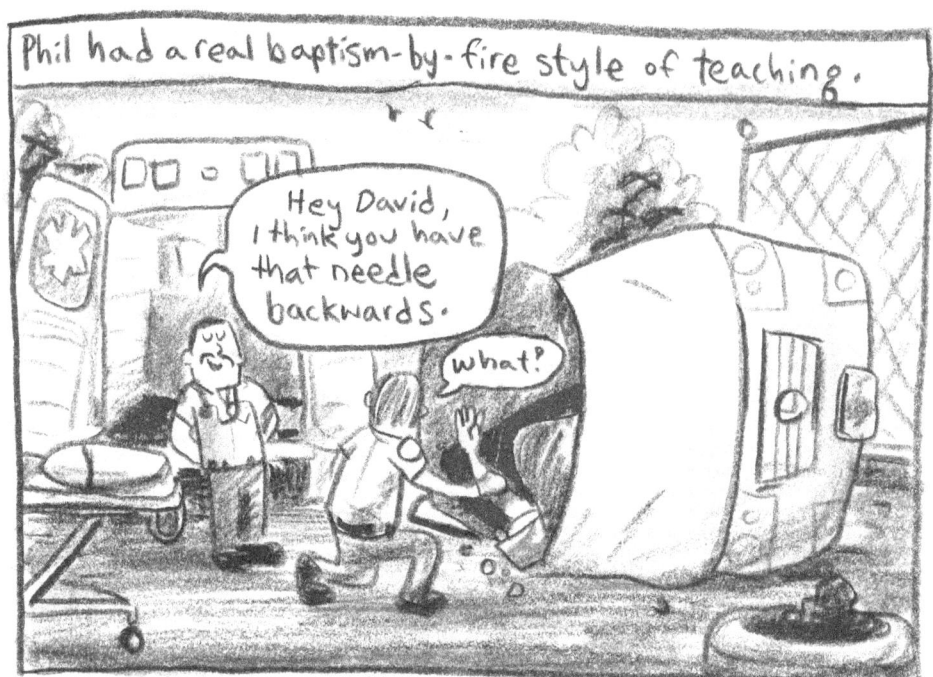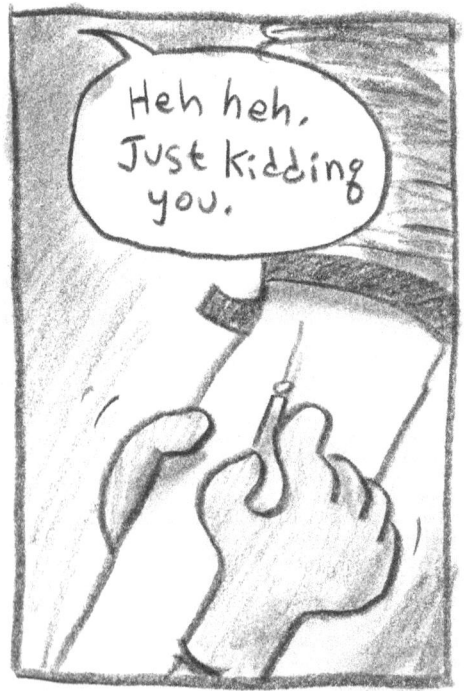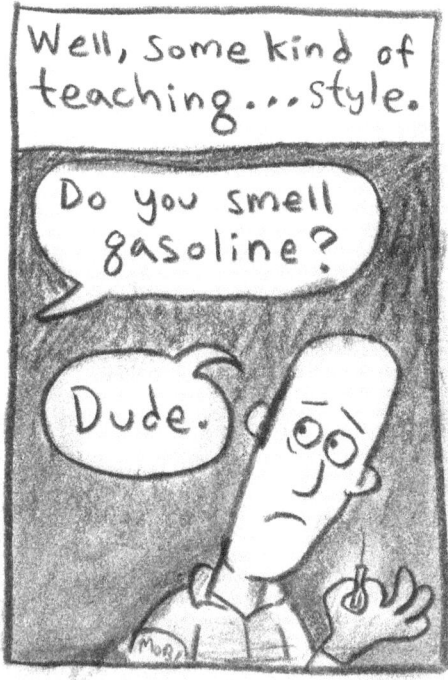

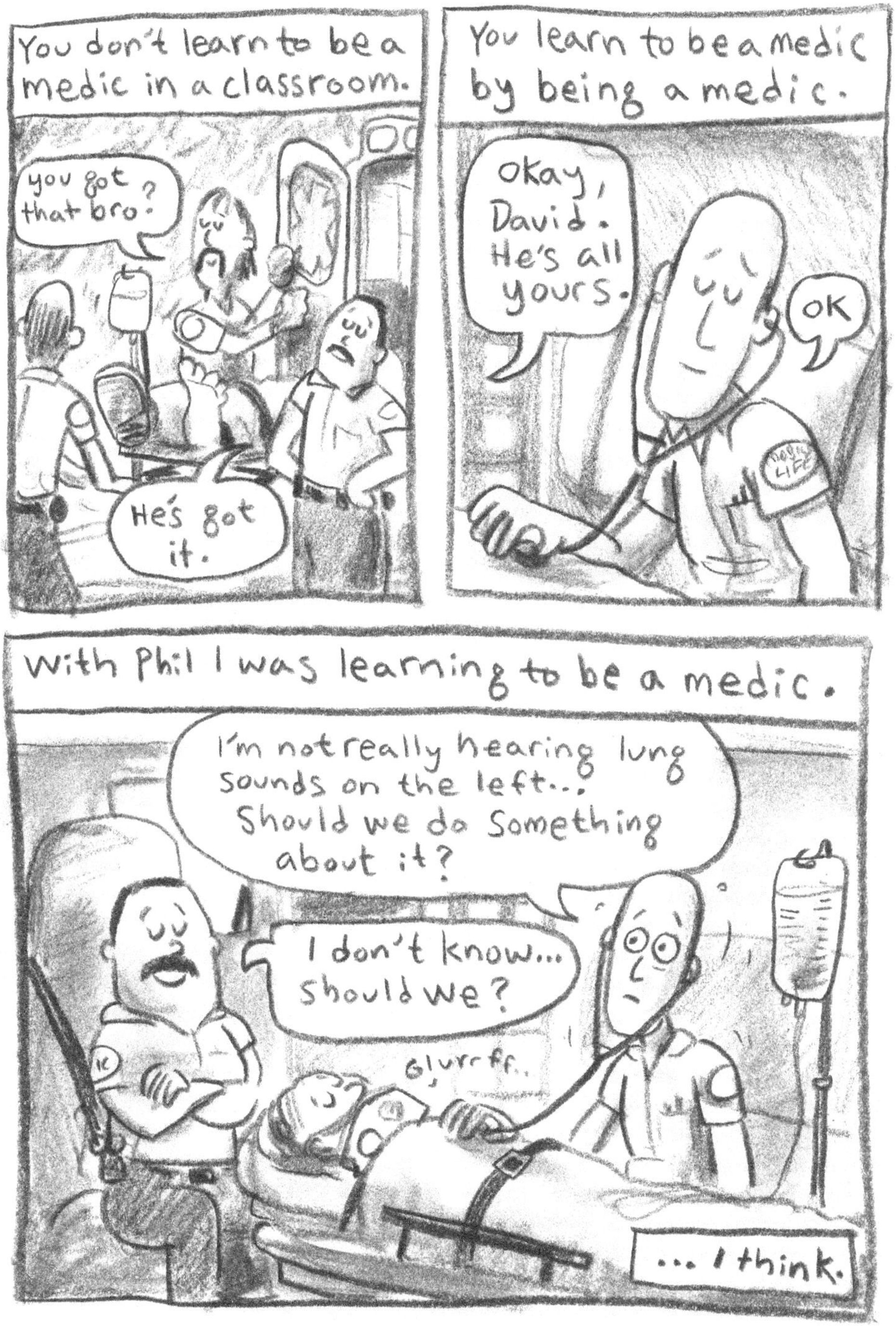

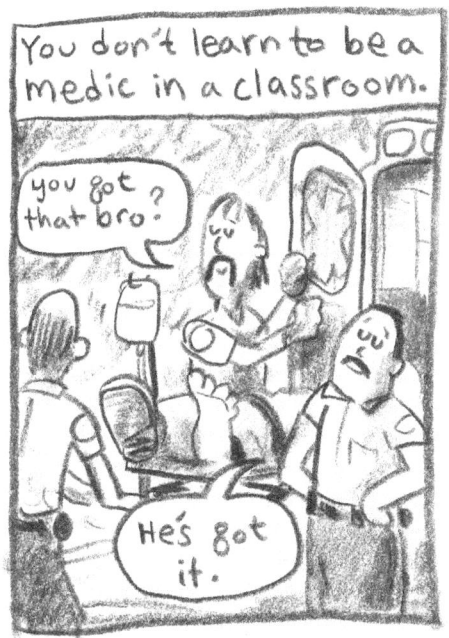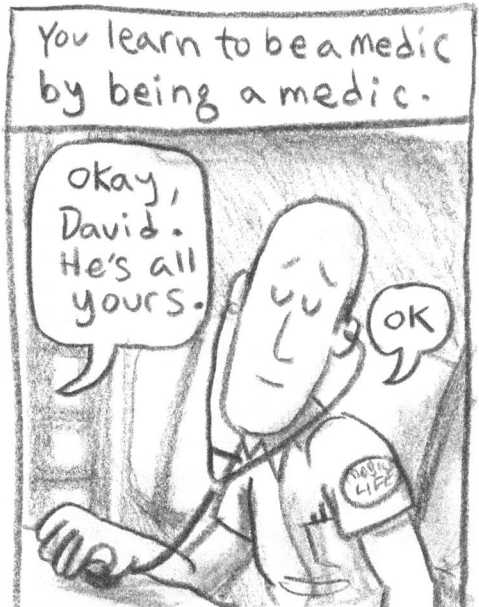

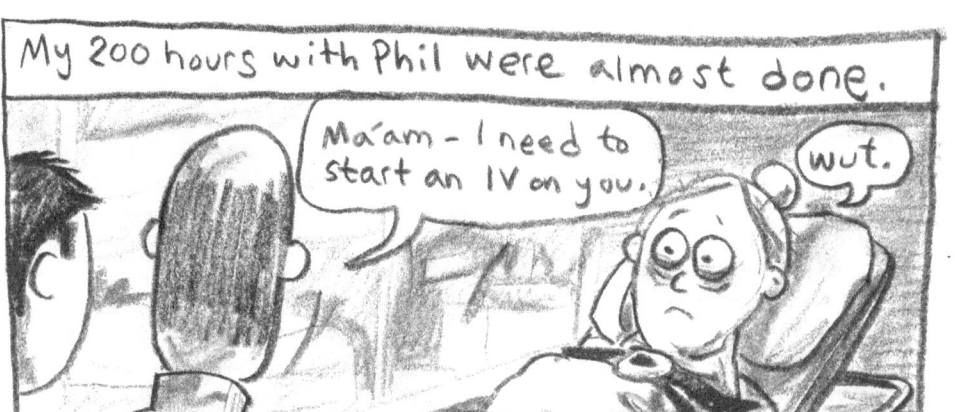
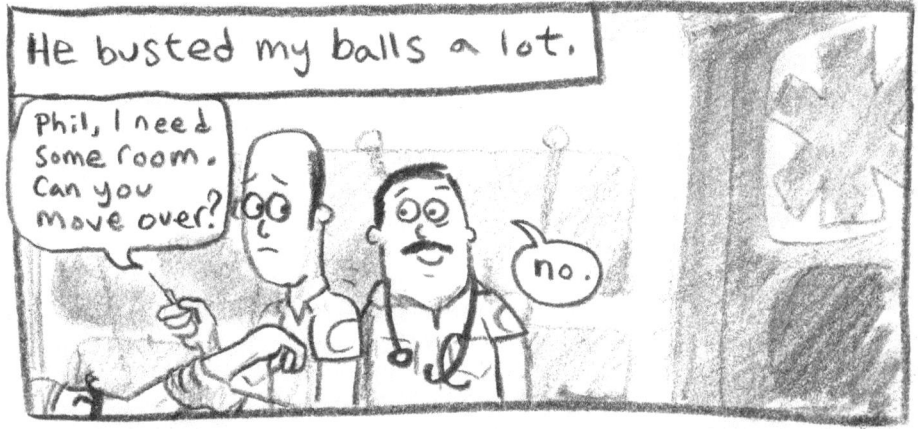
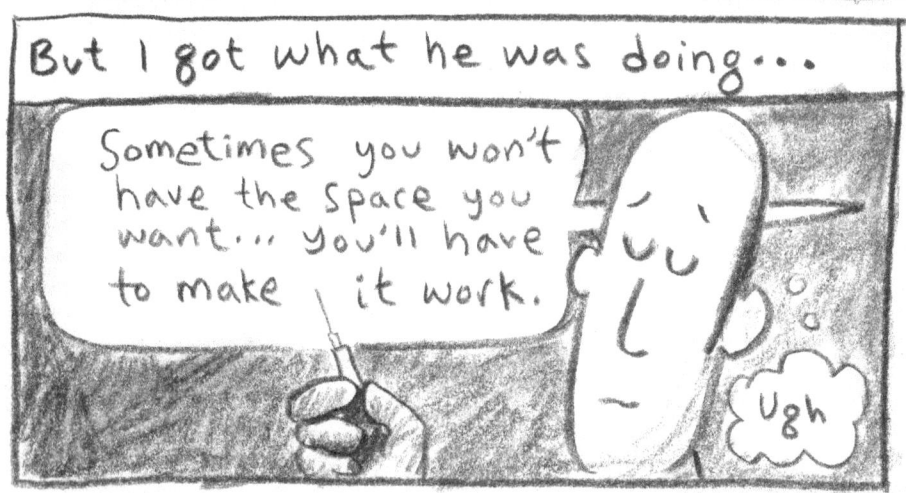

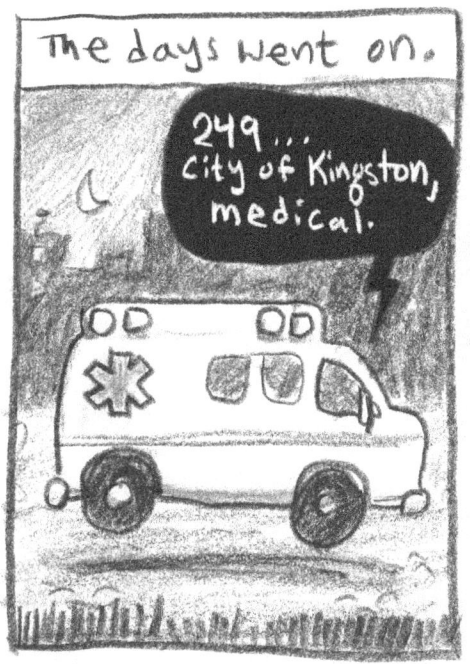
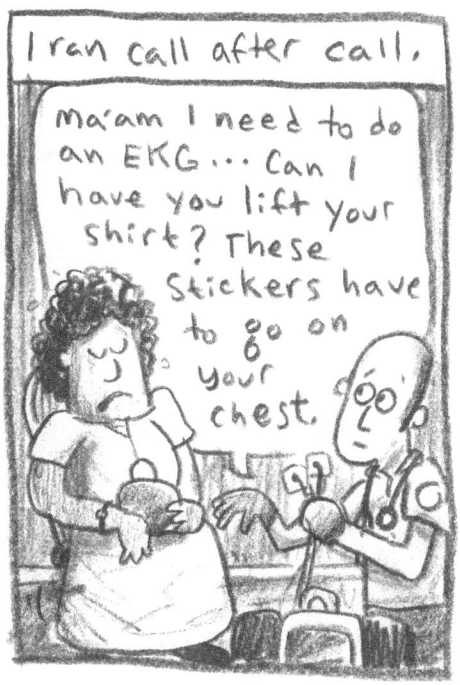
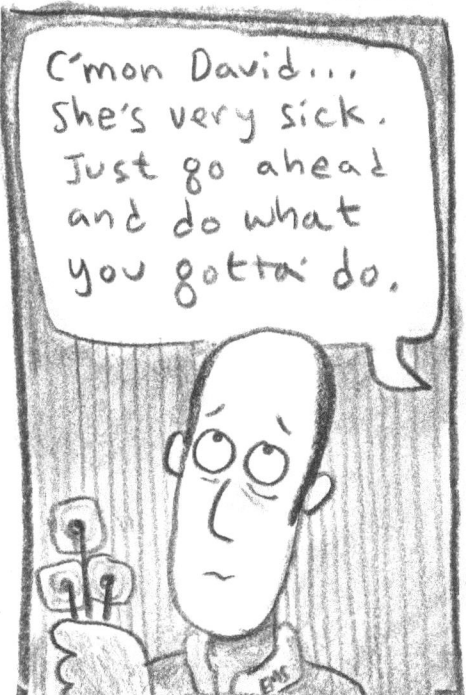
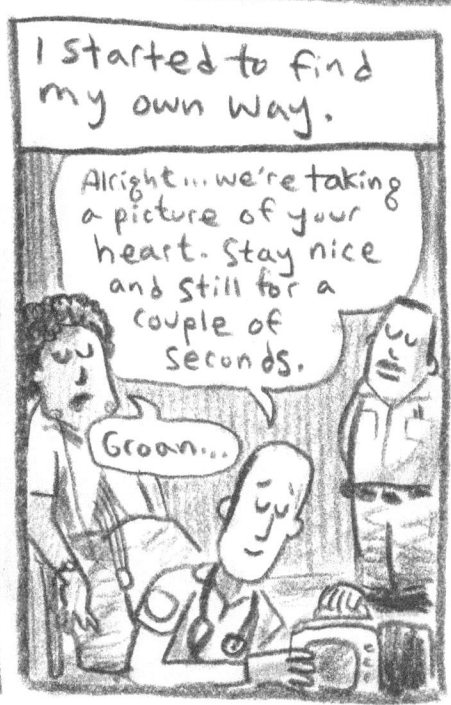

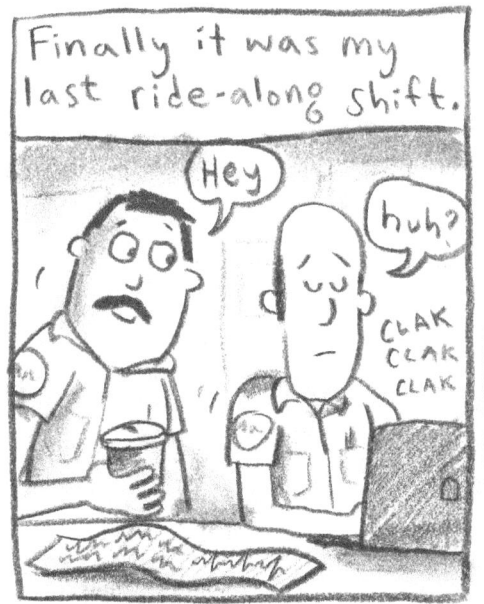

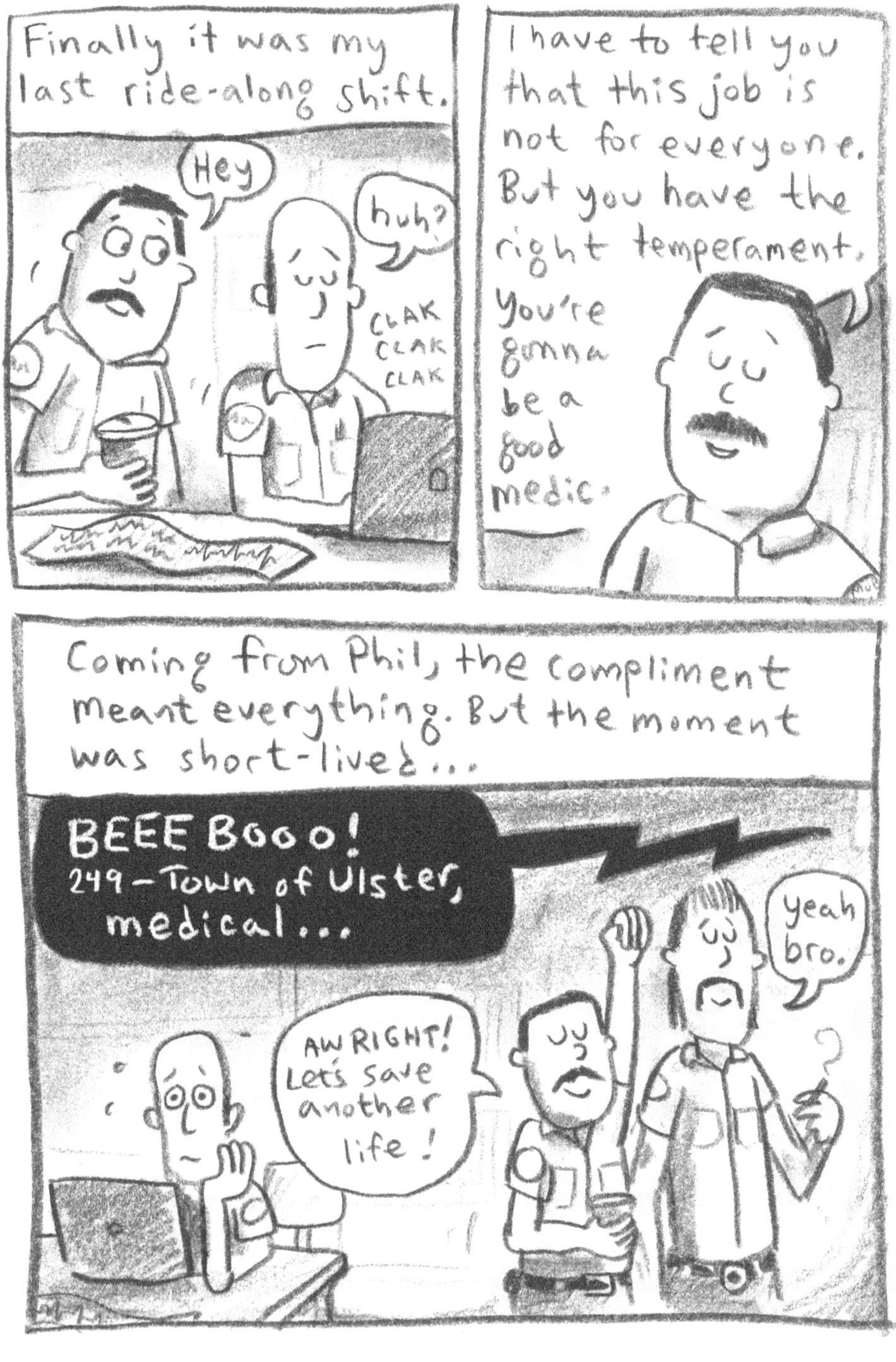

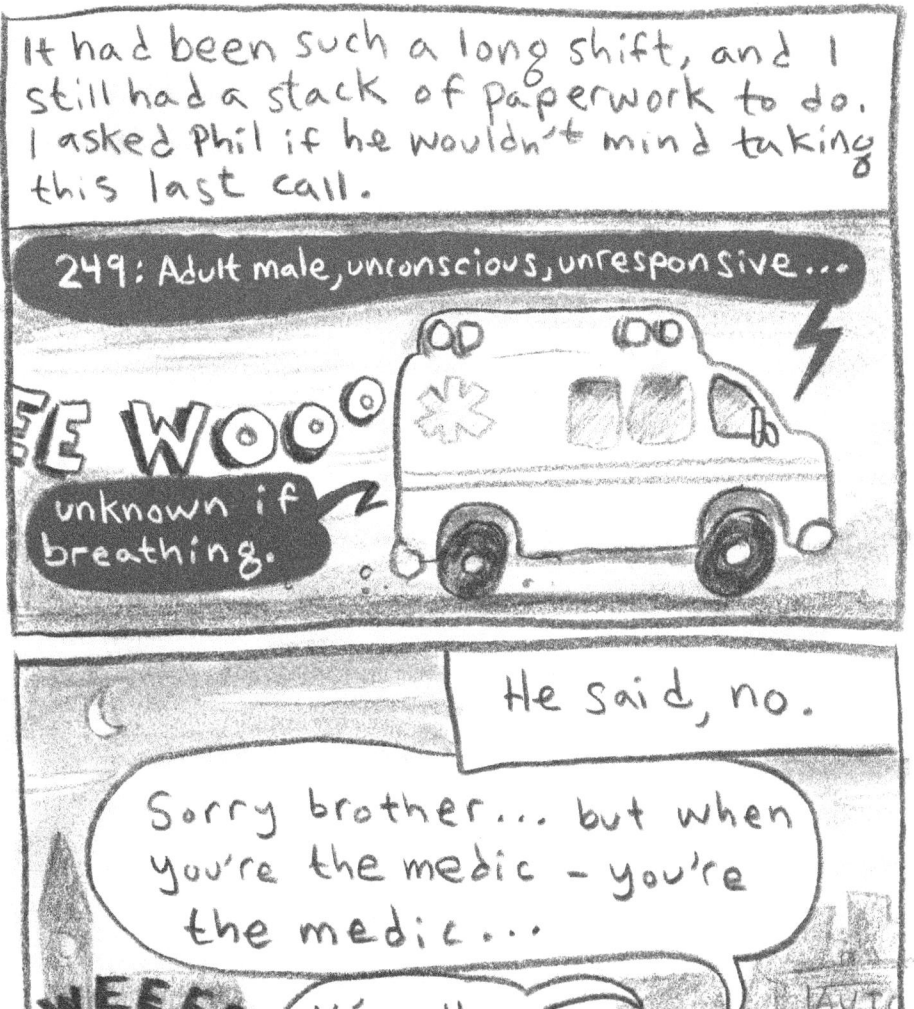

Bad Tacos

Just after the holidays I took and passed the state exam.

oh boy...

I had become a paramedic.

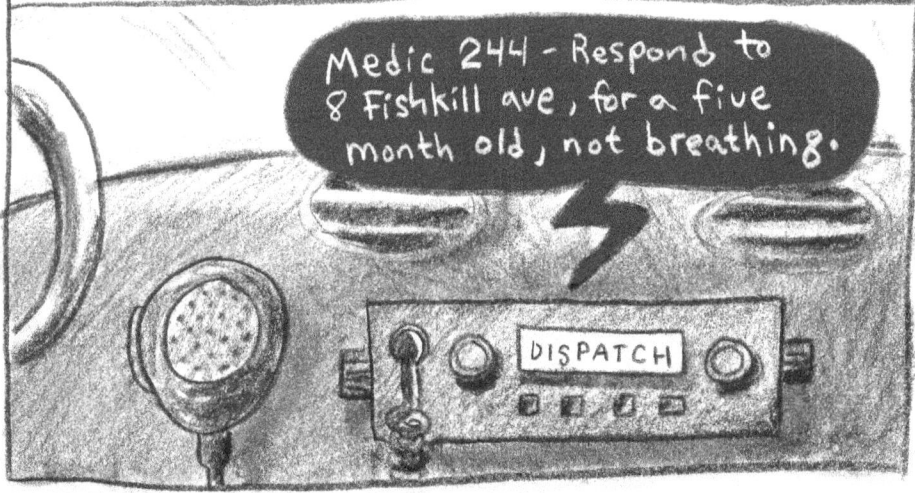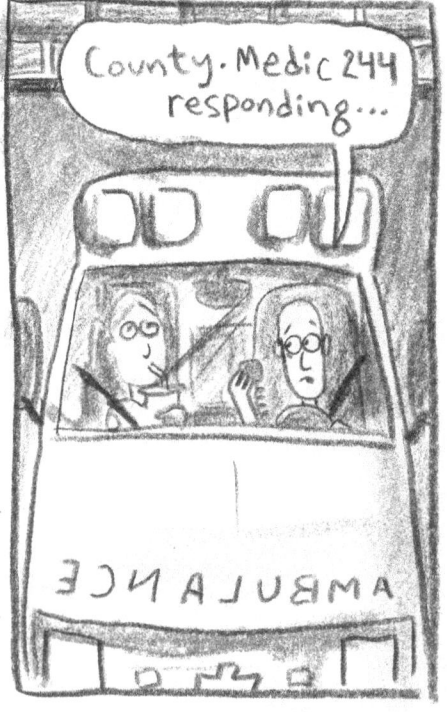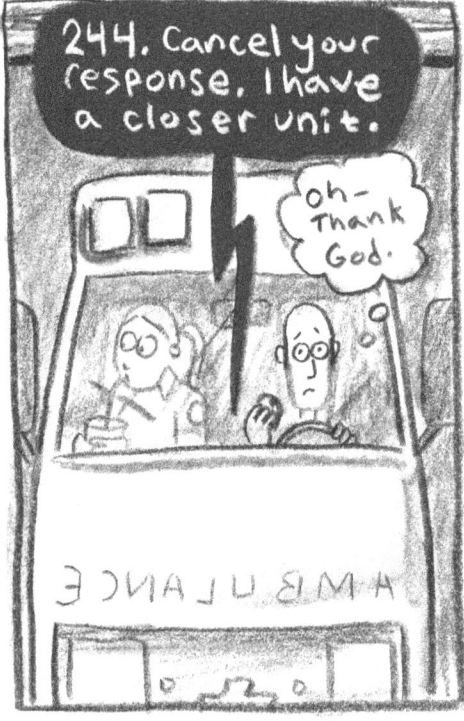

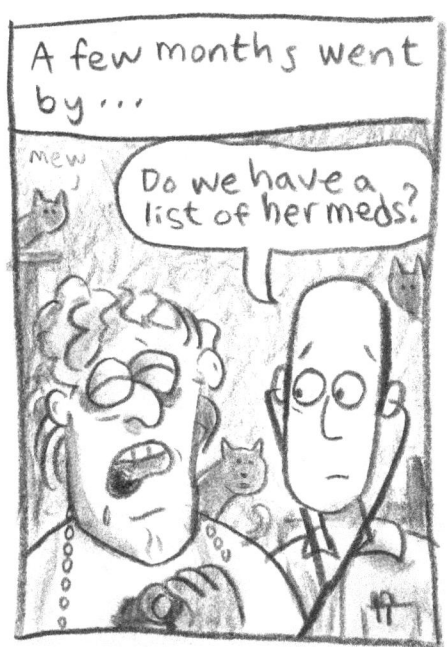
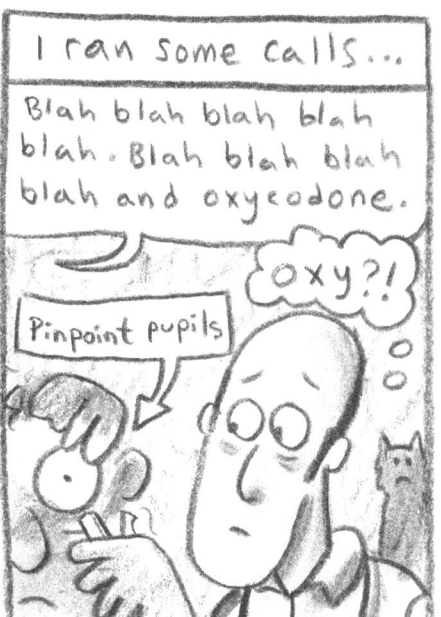
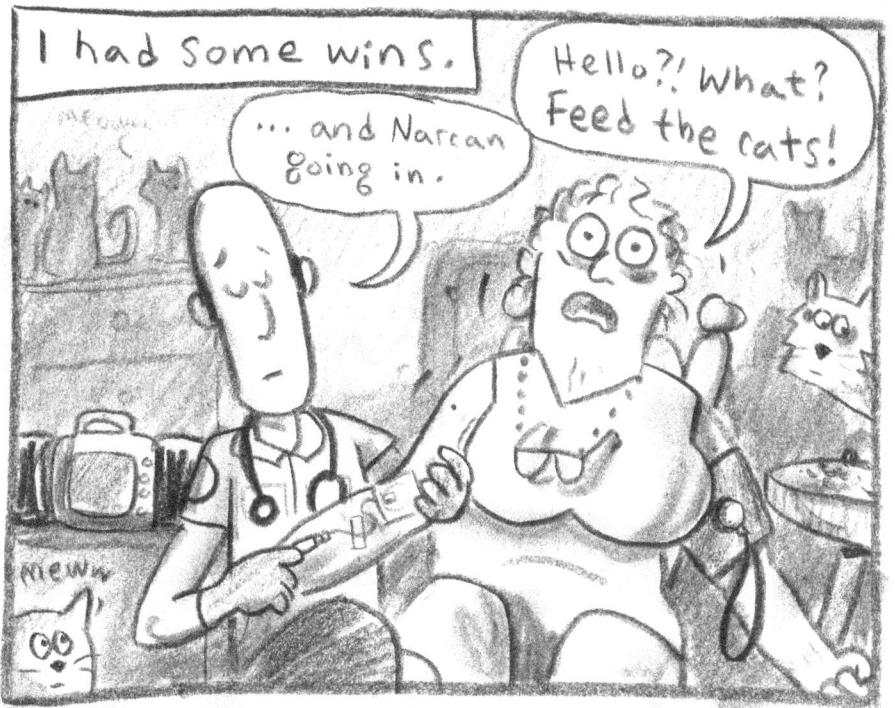

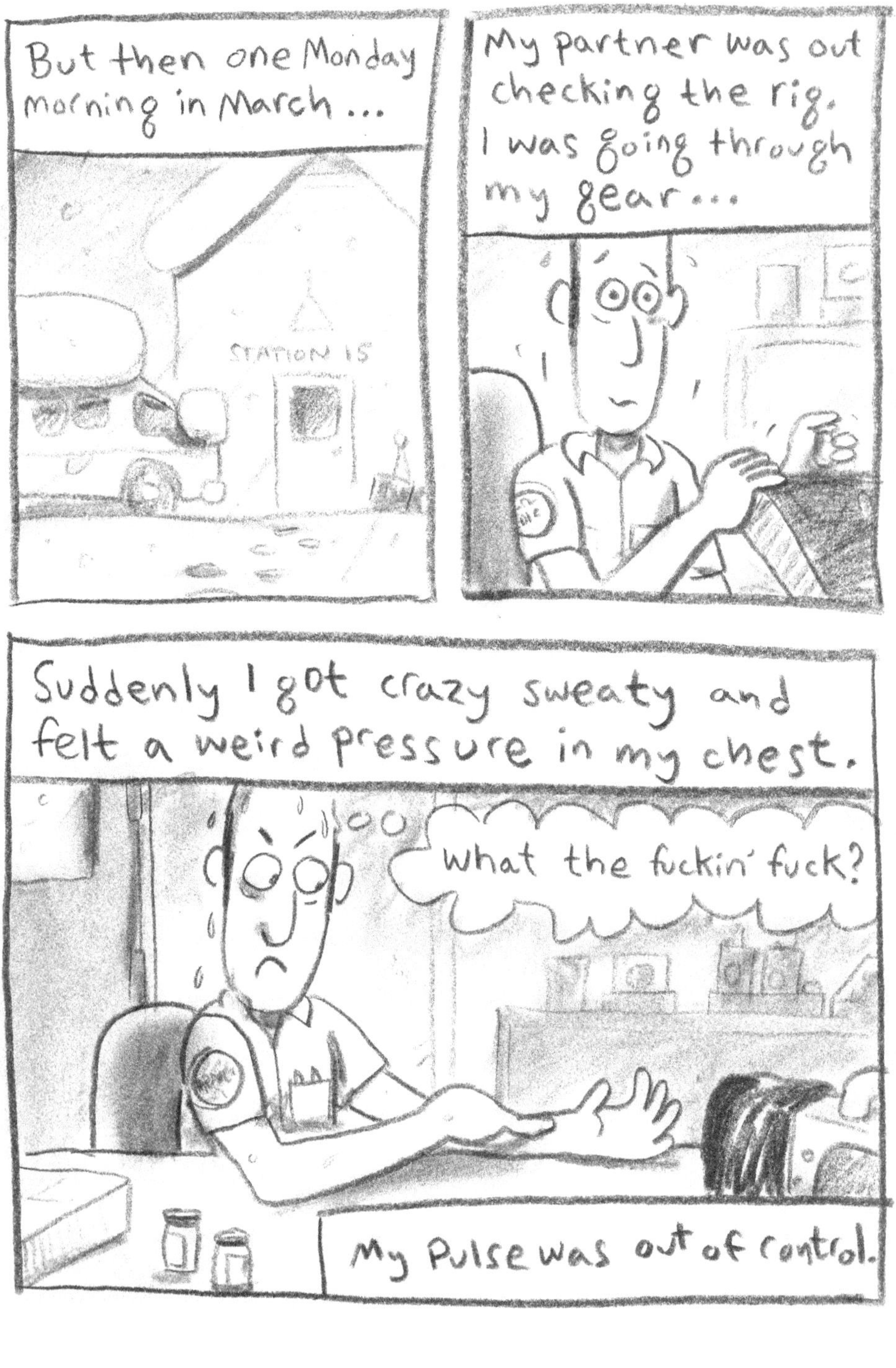

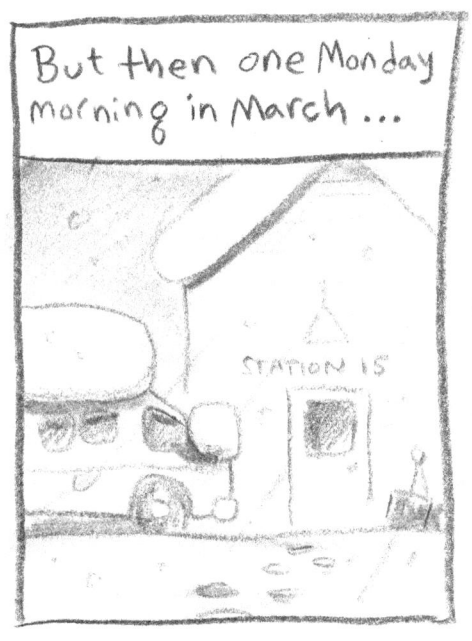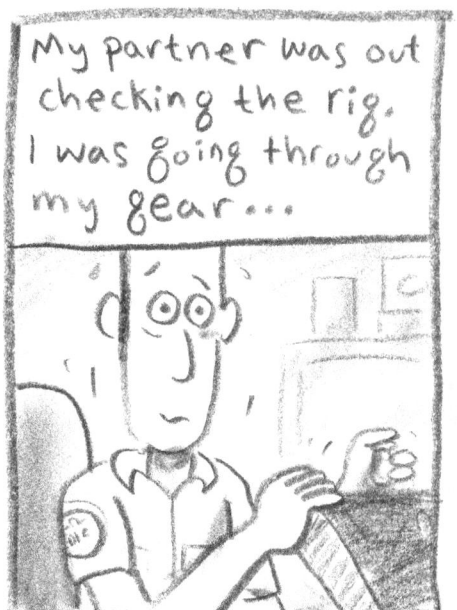

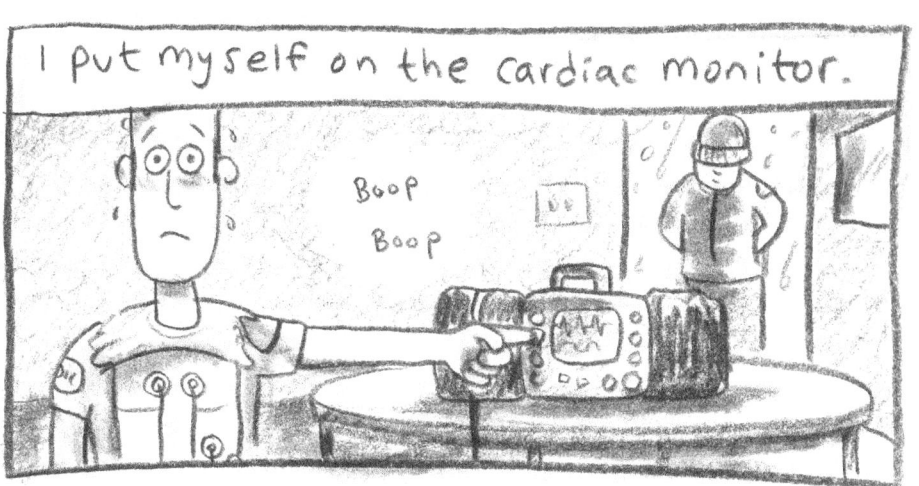

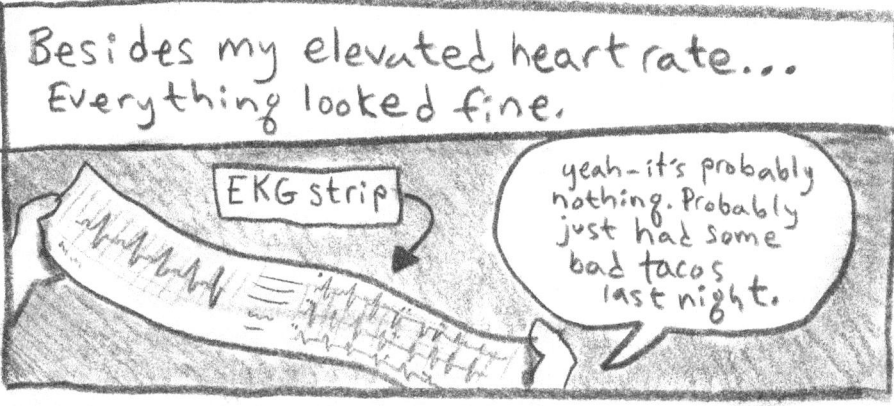

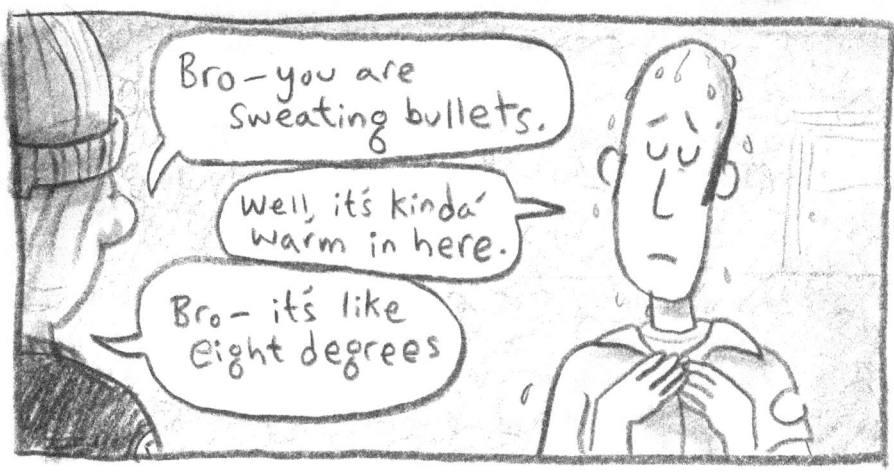

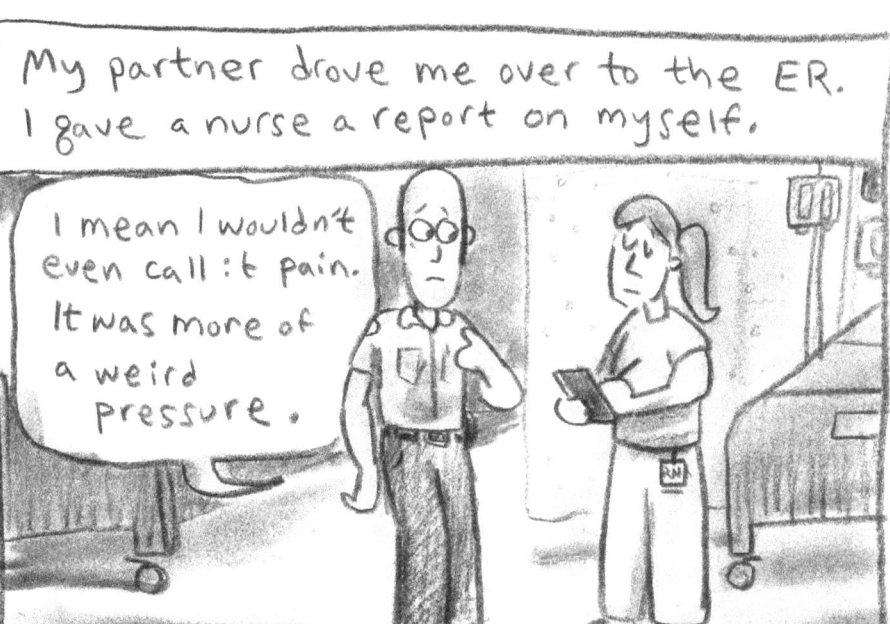

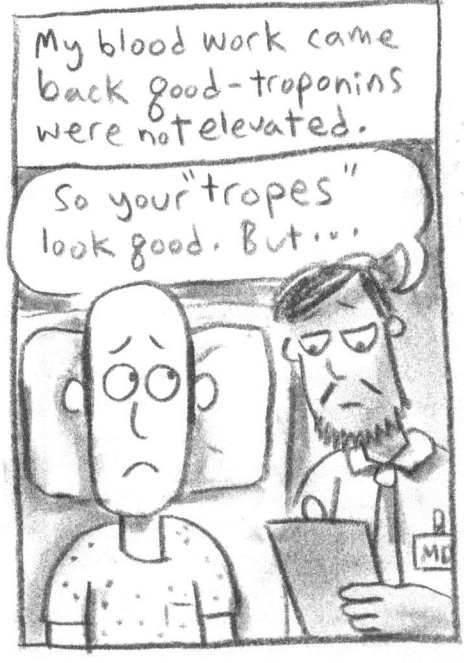
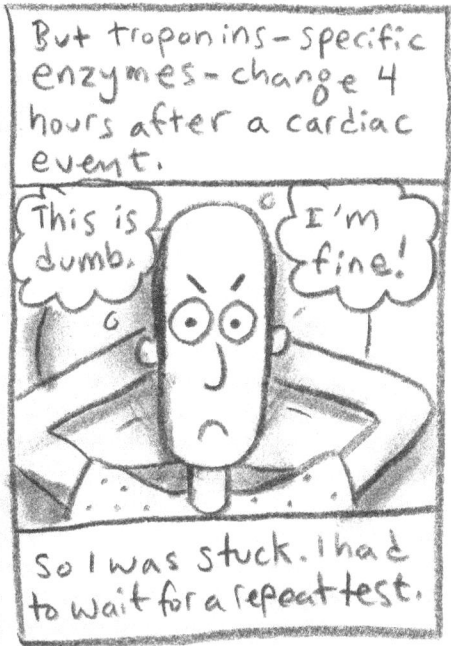
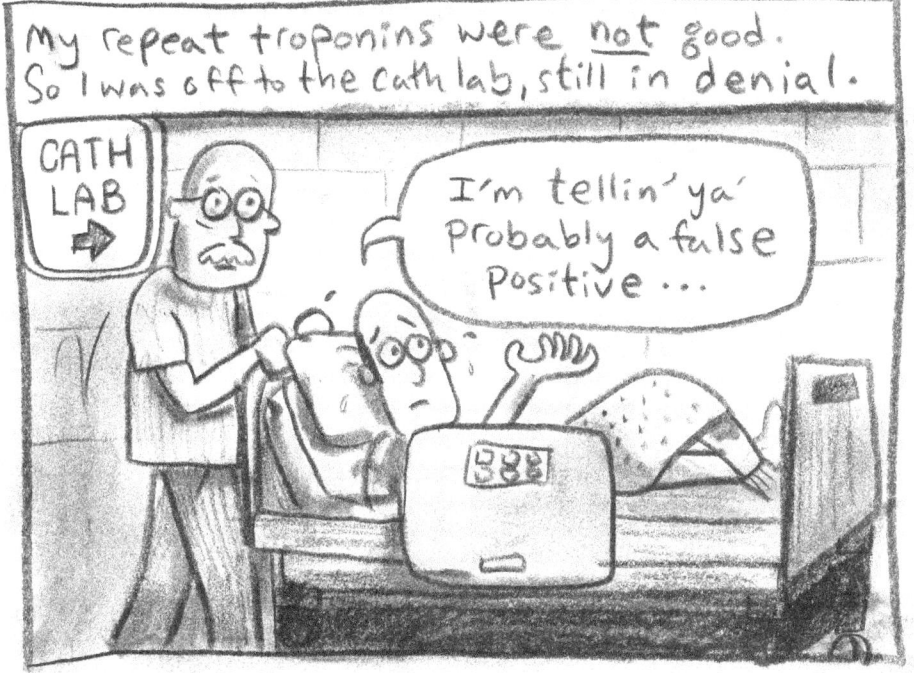

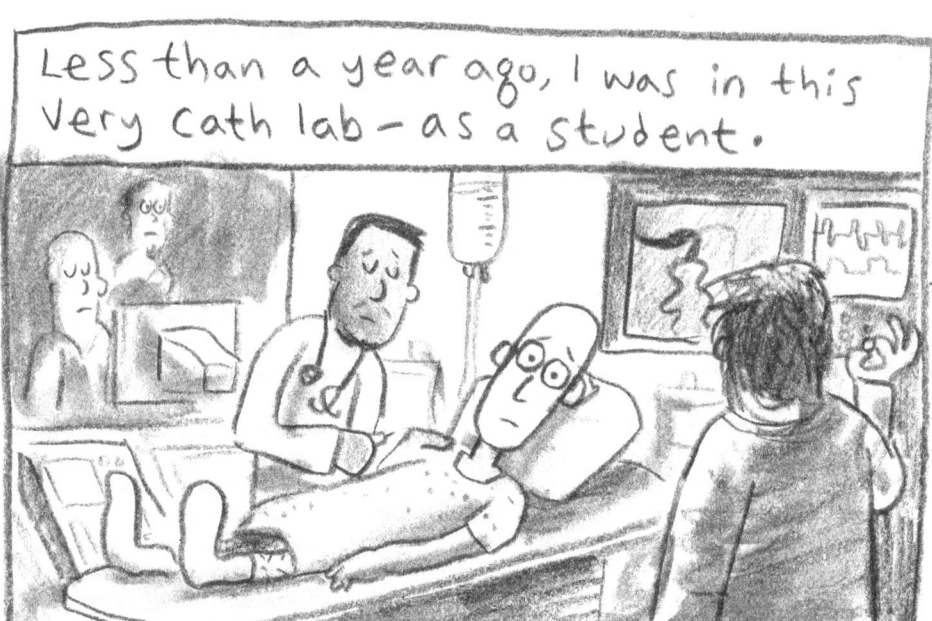

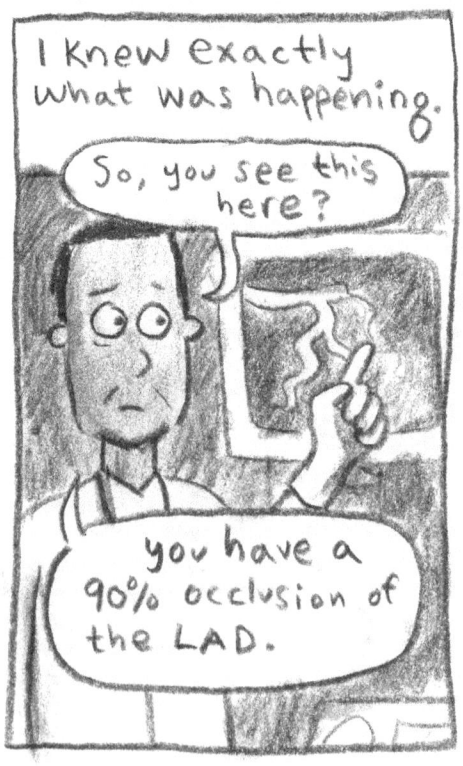

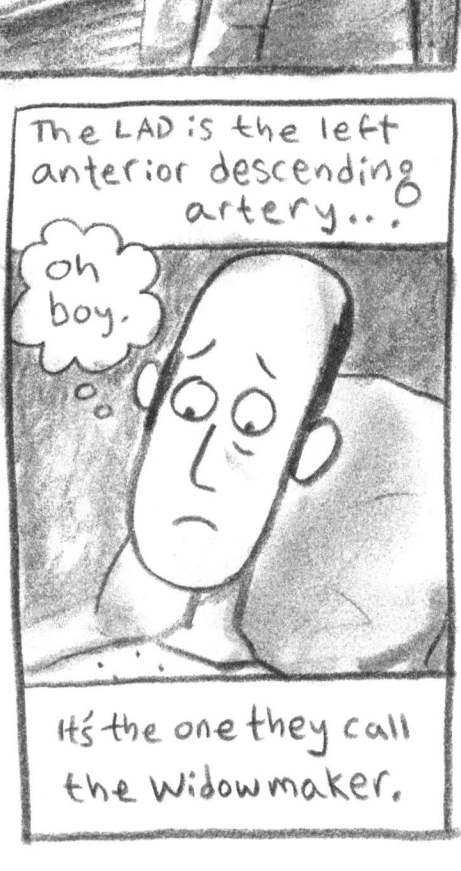

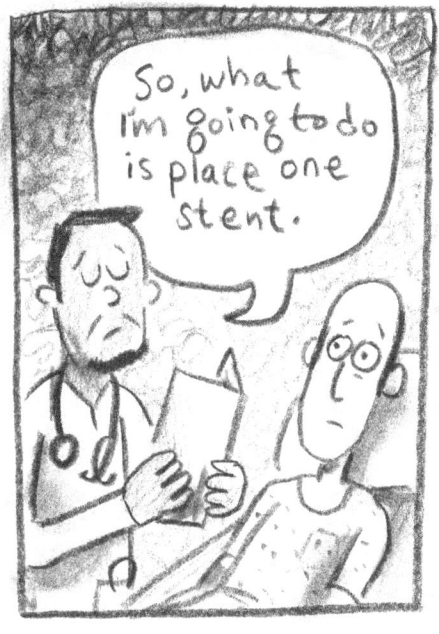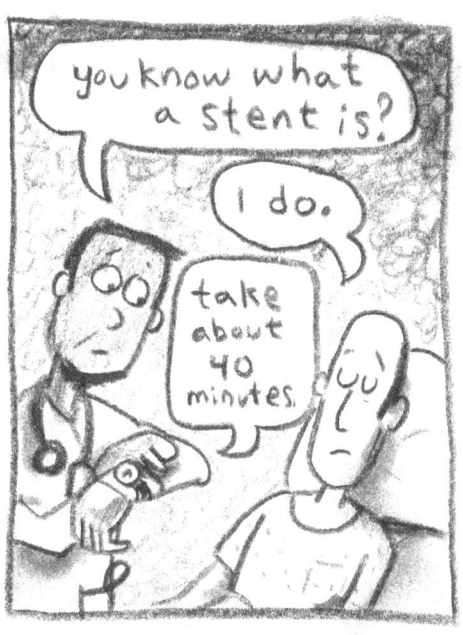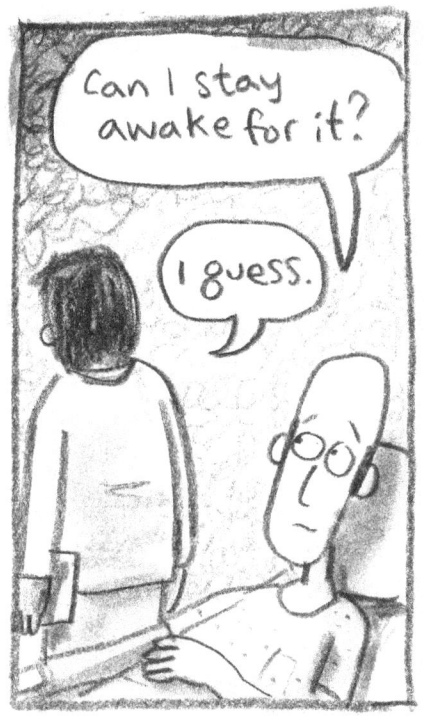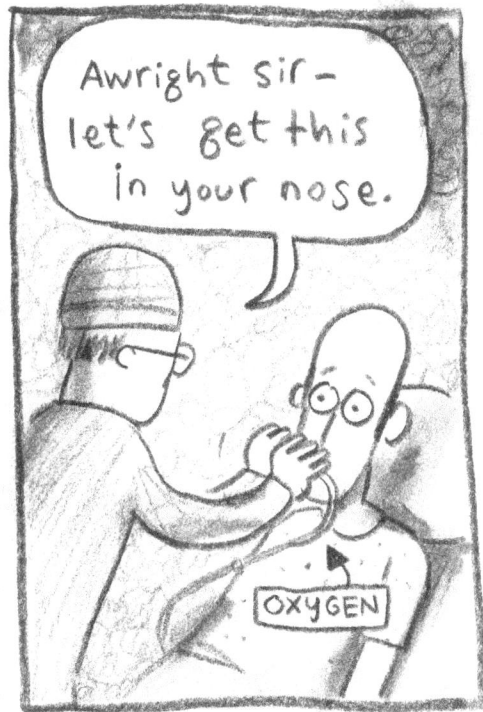

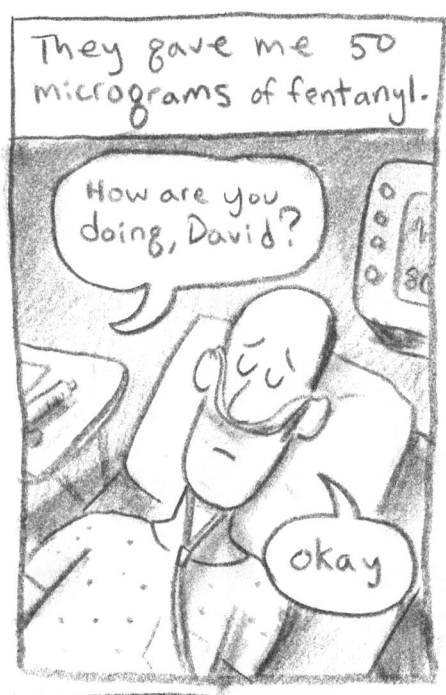
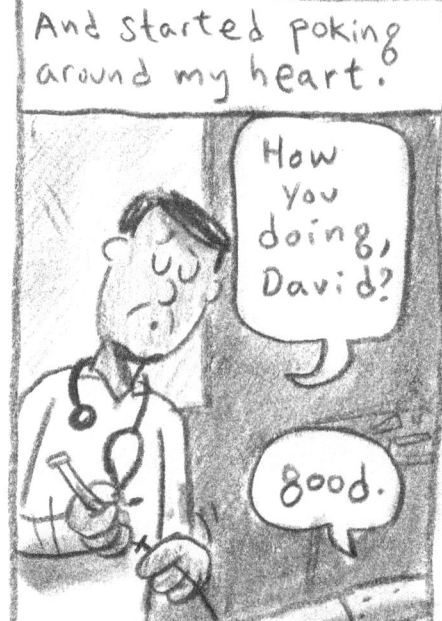
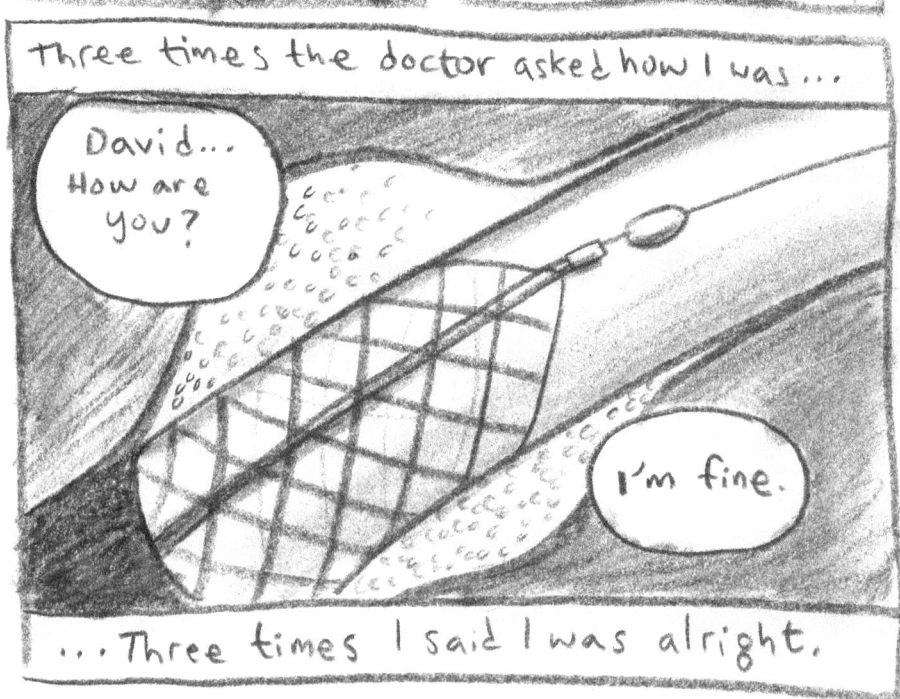

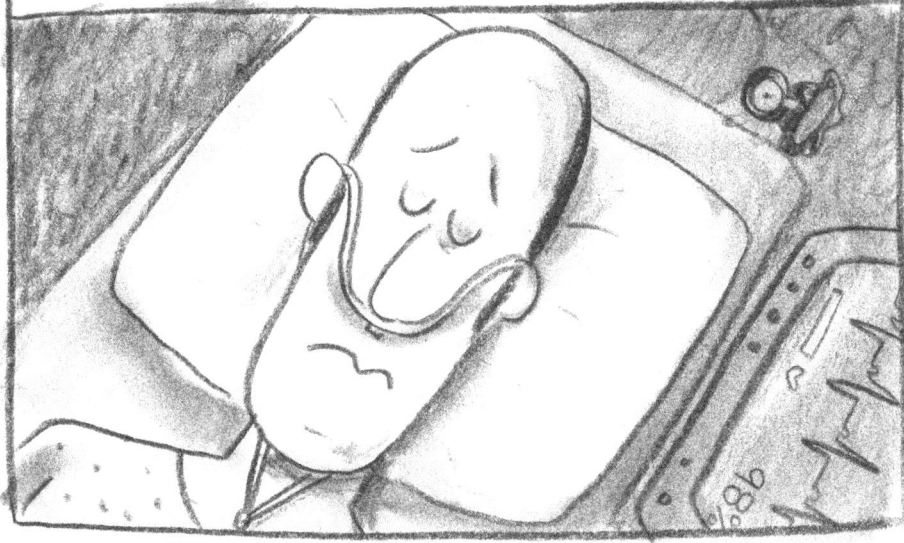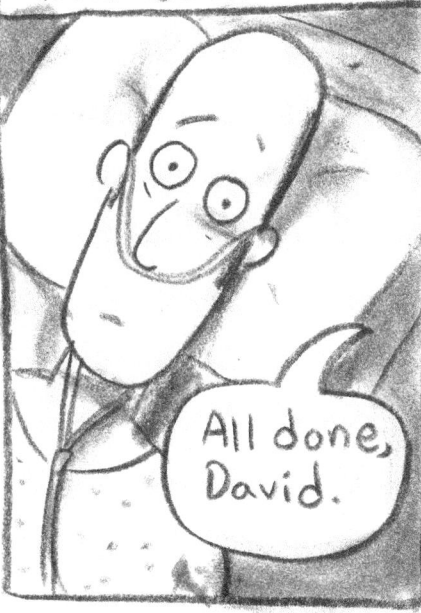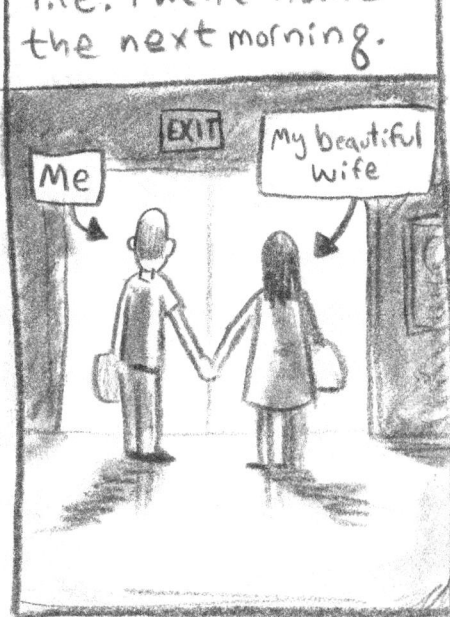

Being Patient

For the next few months, I was a patient. There was a lot of sitting around in waiting rooms.

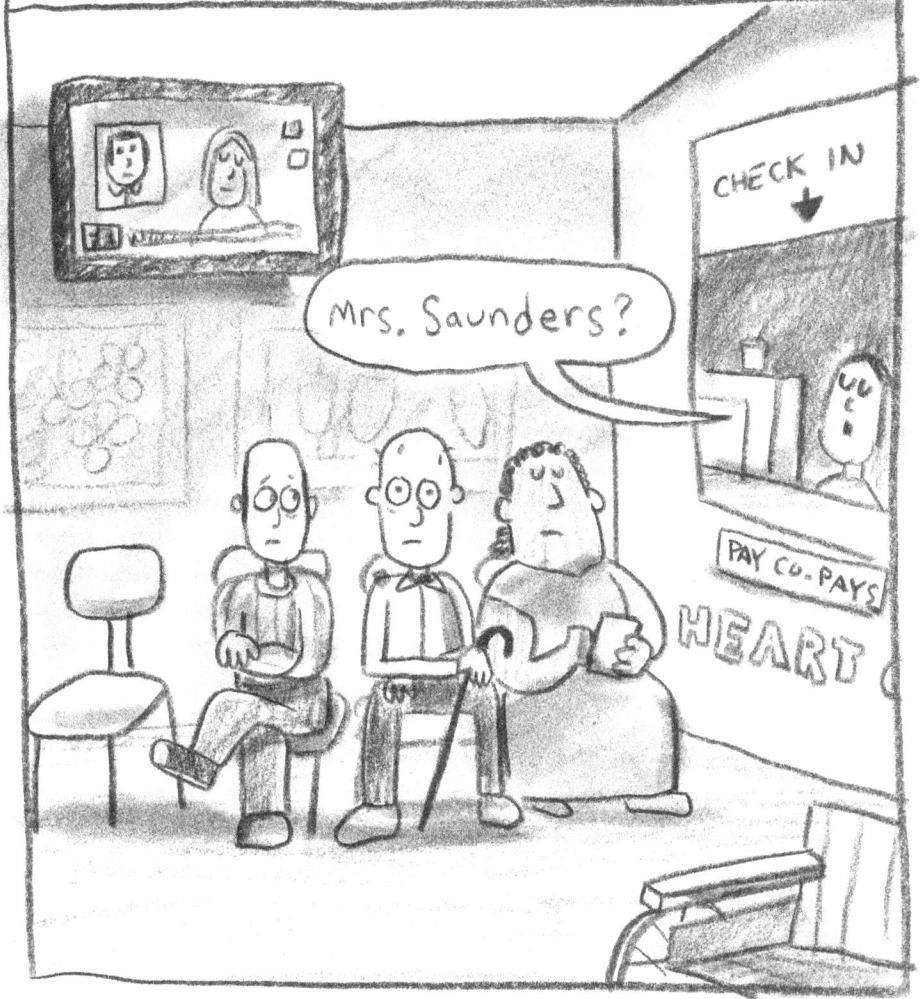

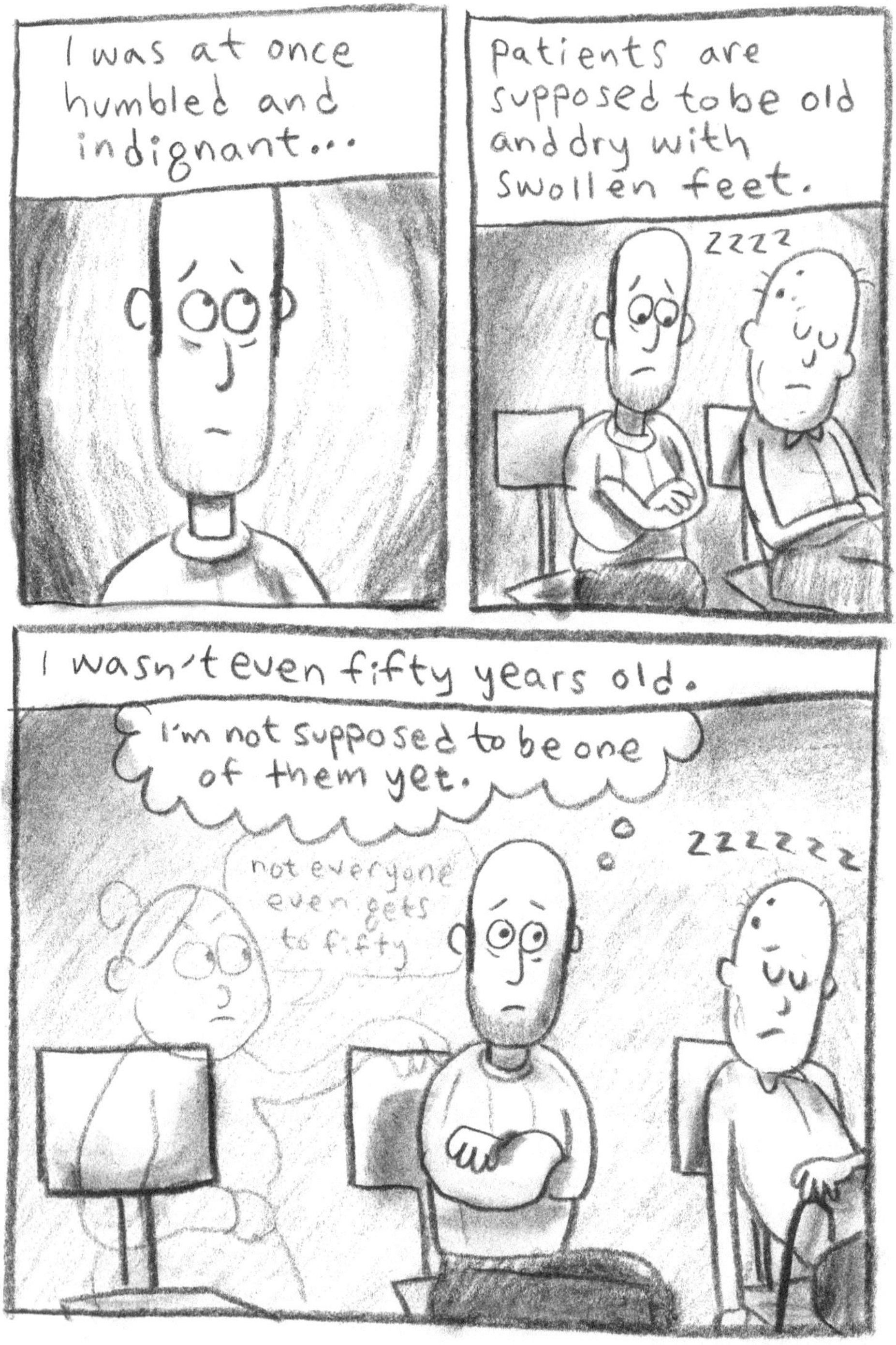

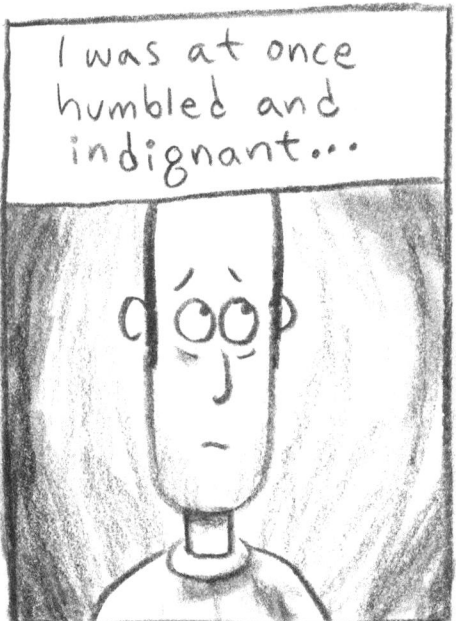

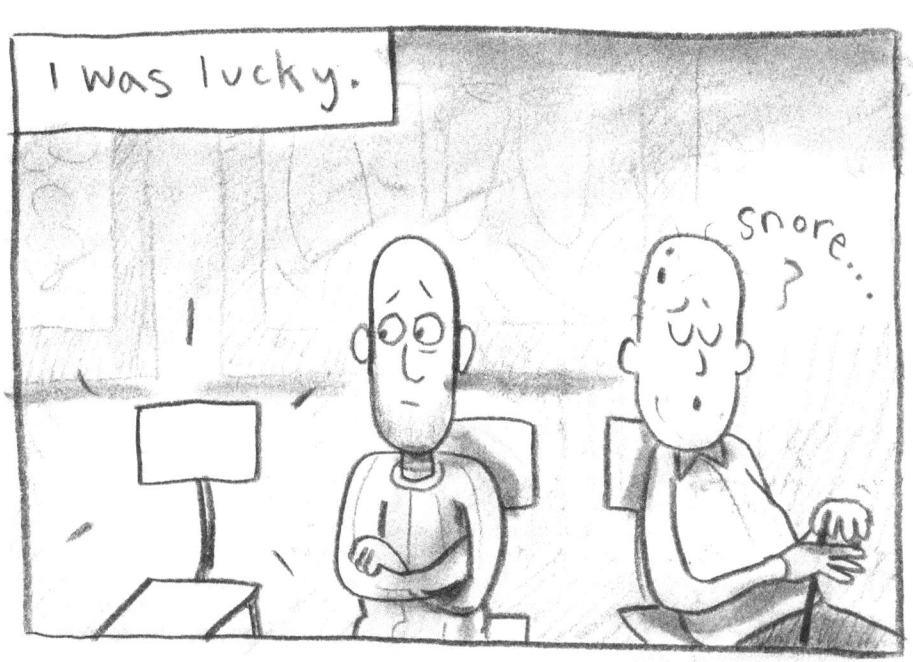
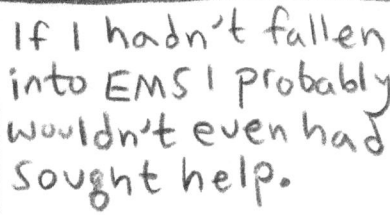
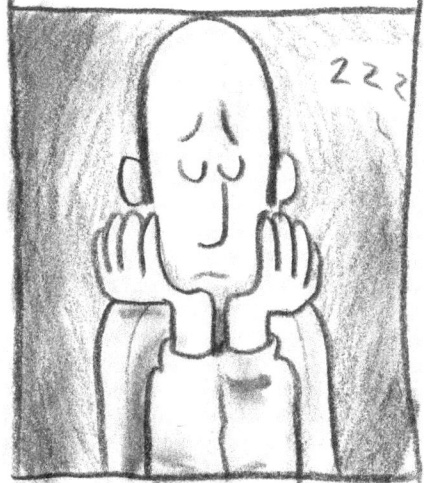
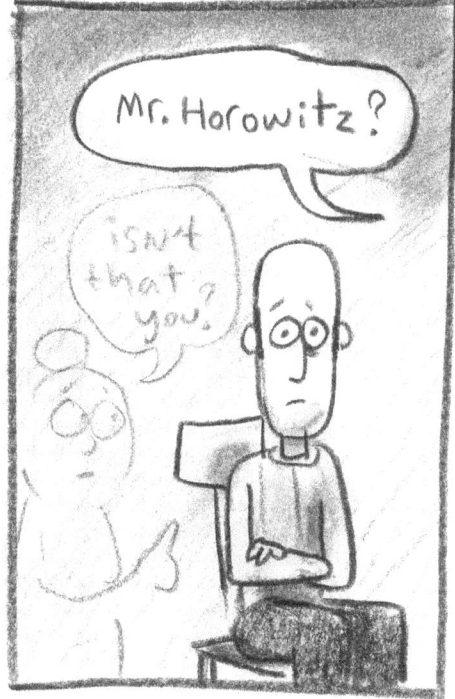

It wasn't long before I was cleared to return to work. I couldn't wait to be on the other side of the stethoscope.

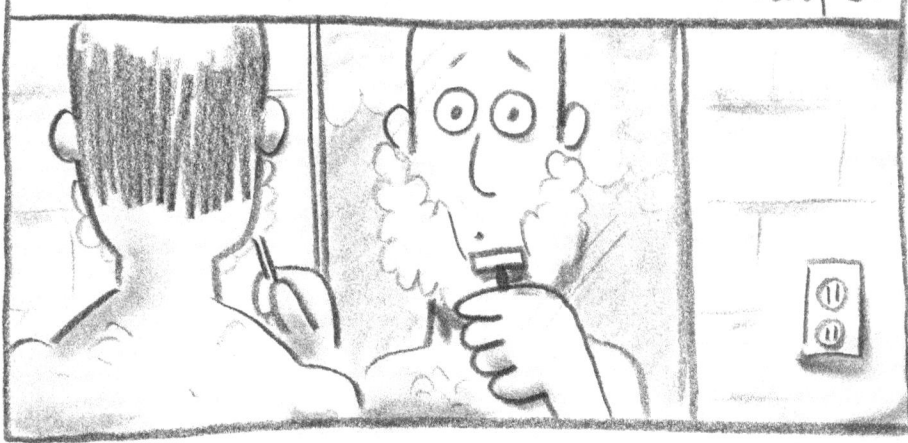

My only hope was that I wouldn't have to do any heavy lifting. At least for a few shifts...

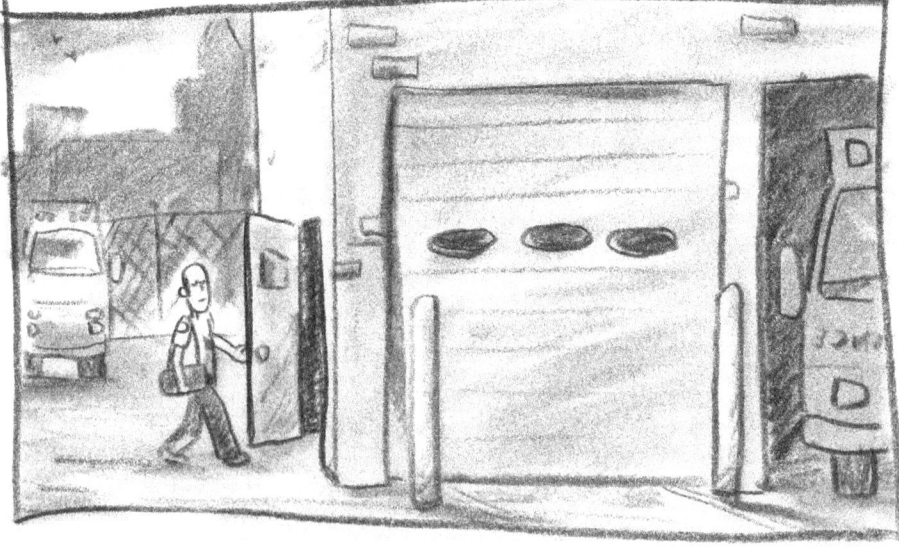

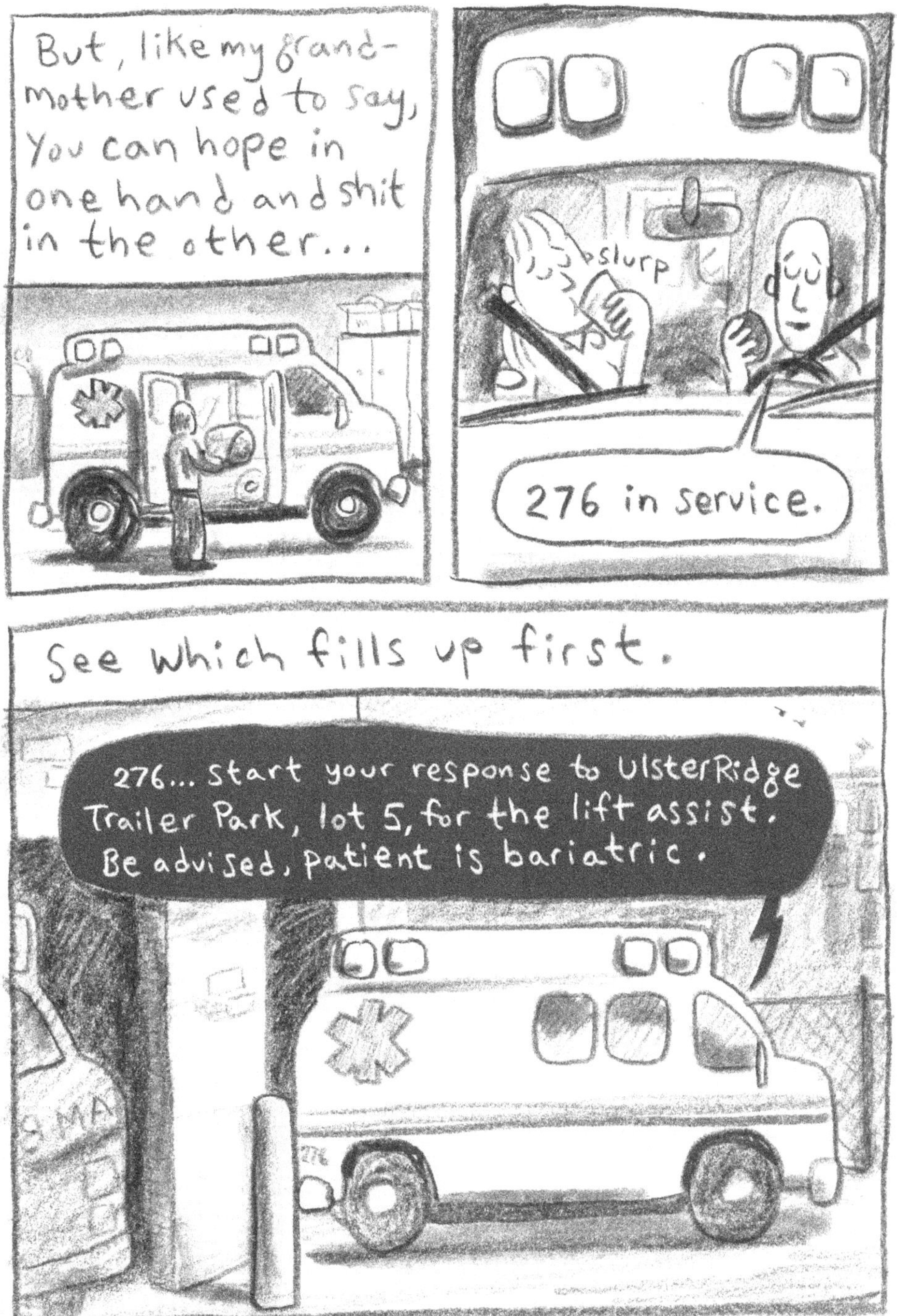

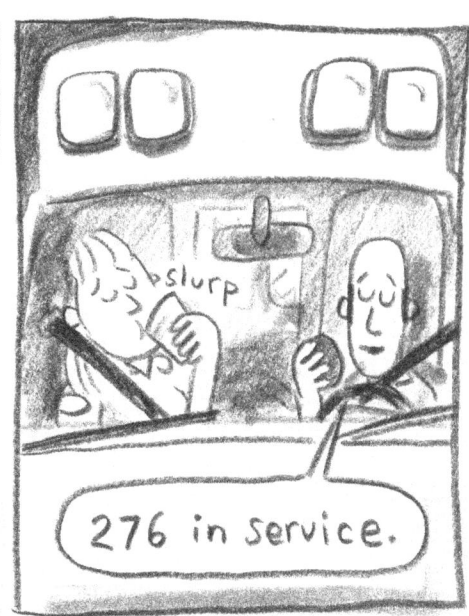

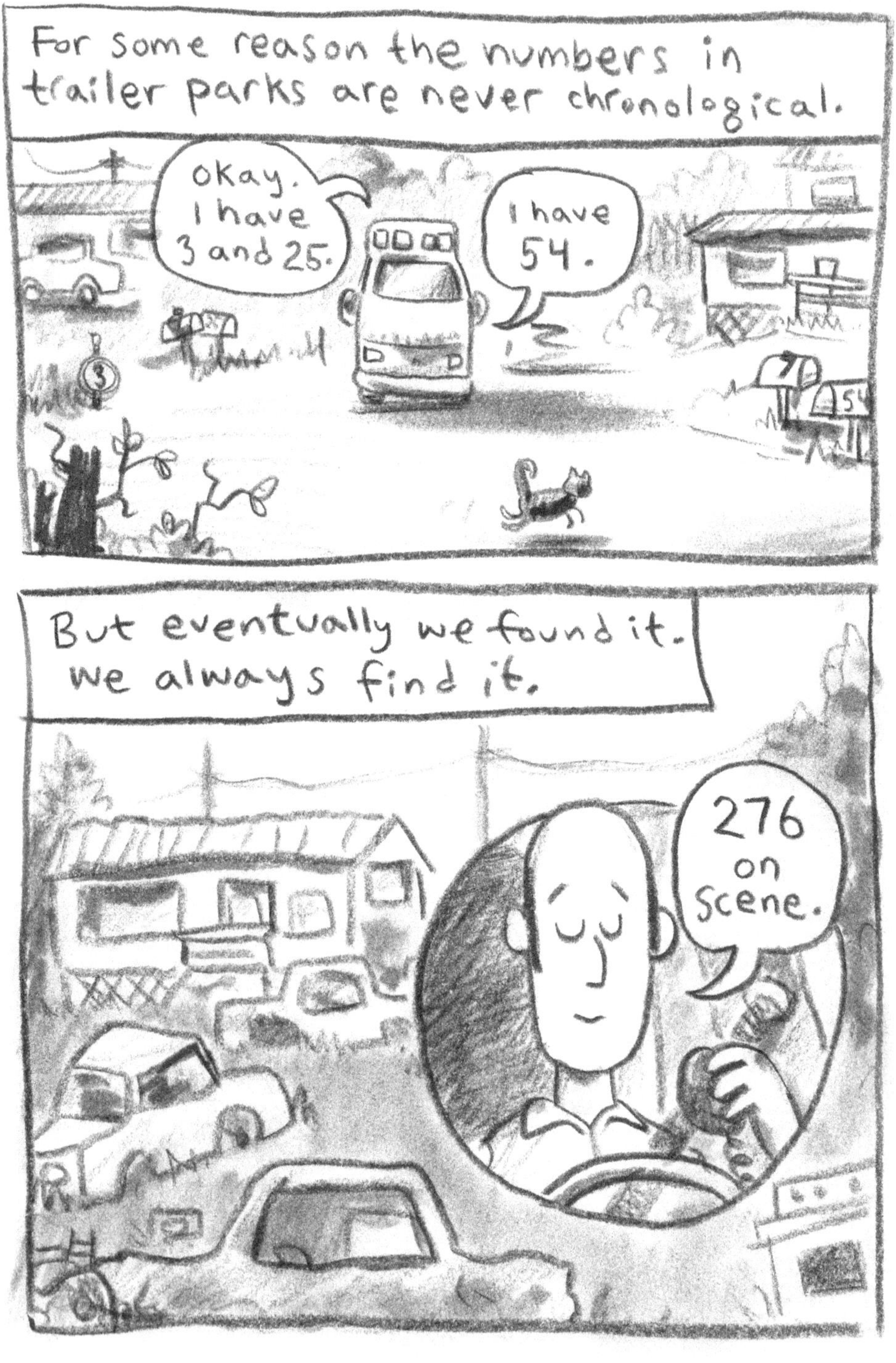

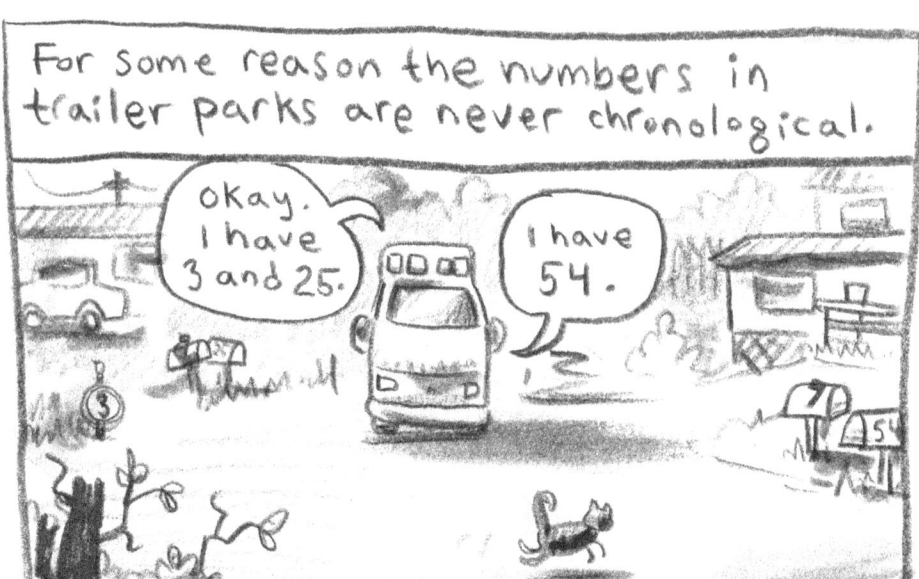

With some effort we got Carolyn back in her chair.

"I'm not going to no hospital!"

...and called back in service.

Dispatch - 276 back in service with a lift assist.

Received 276... Standby

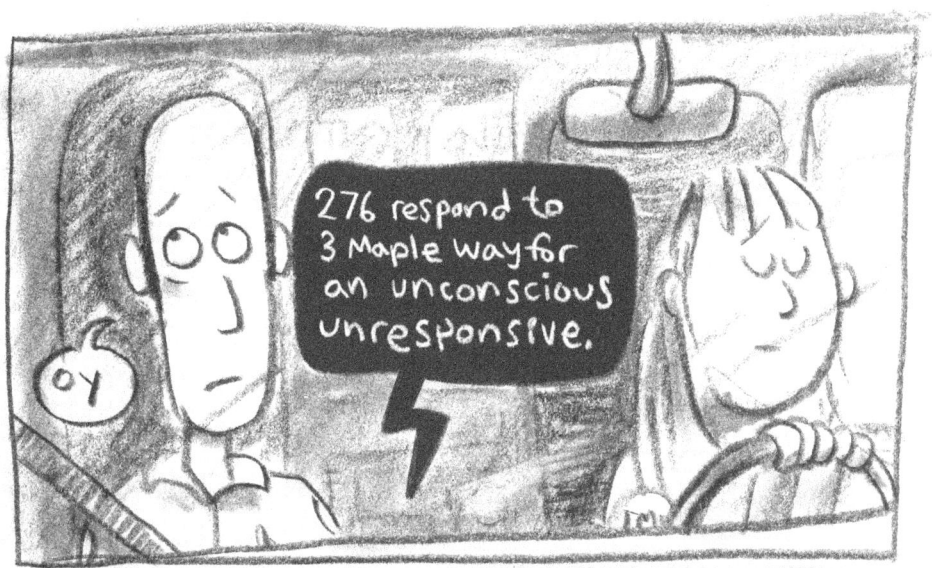

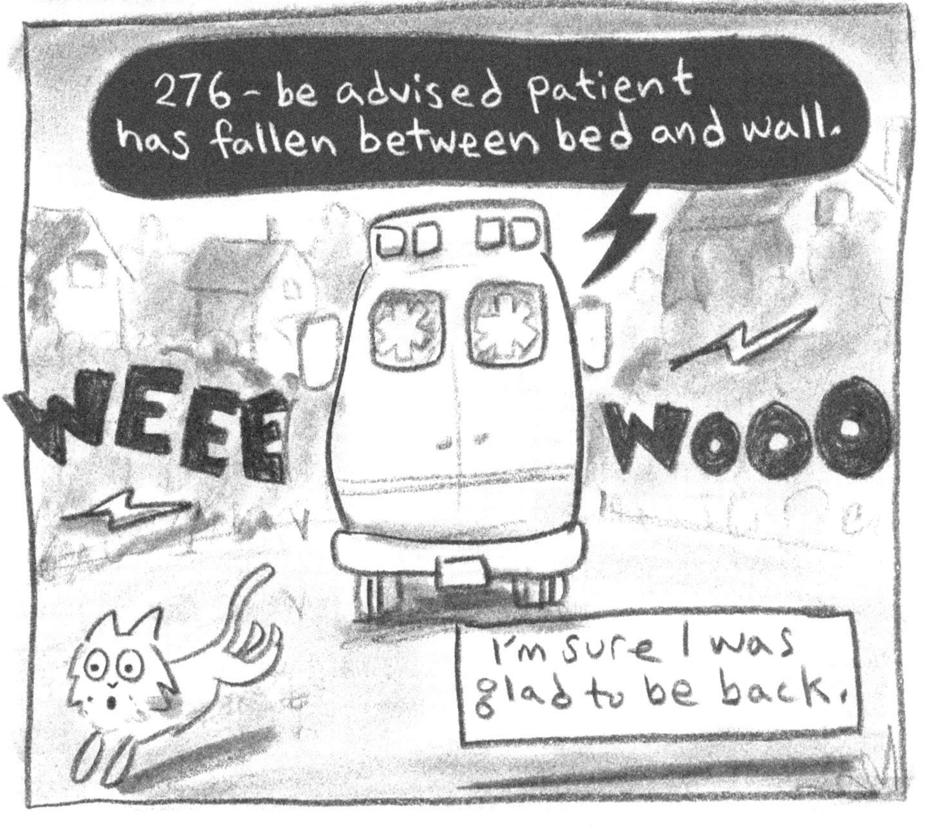

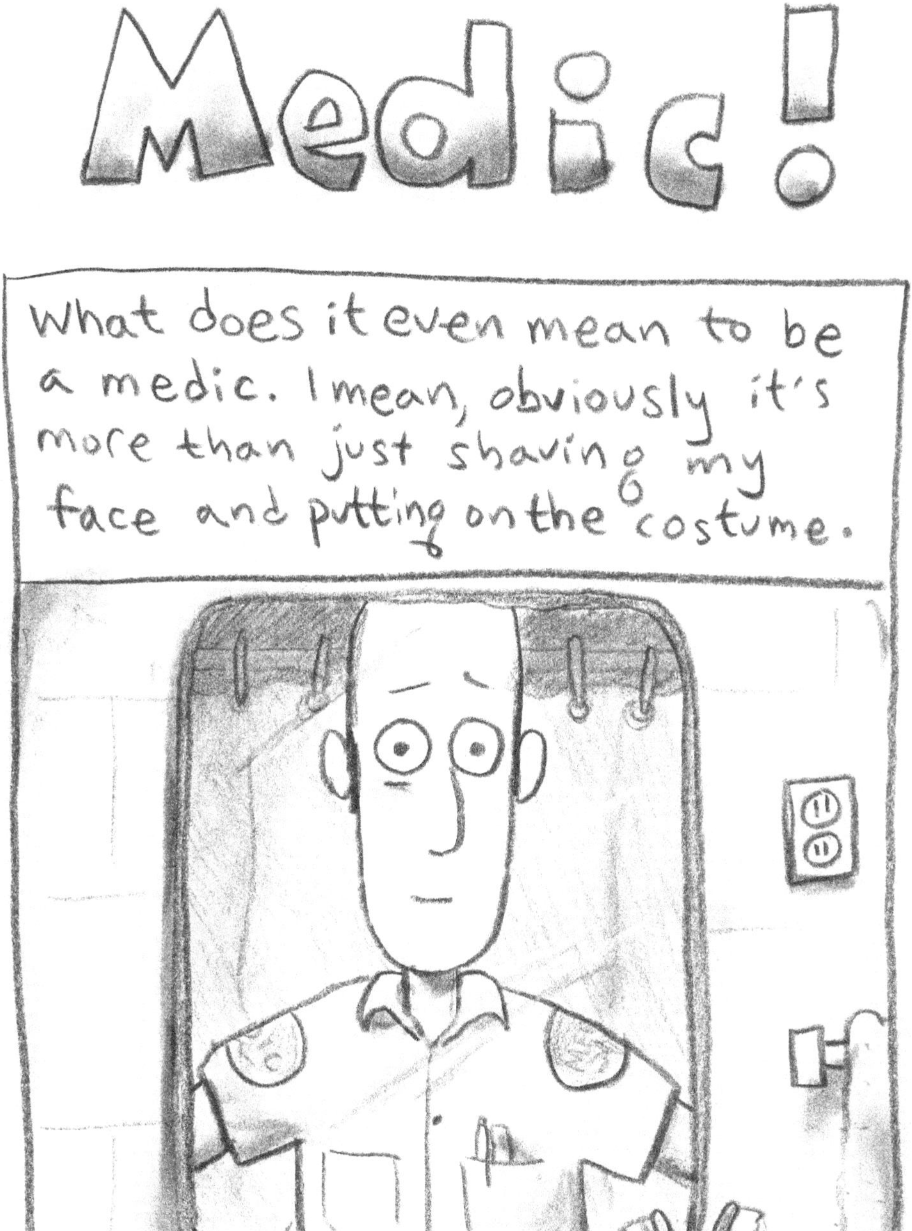

Medic!

What does it even mean to be a medic. I mean, obviously it's more than just shaving my face and putting on the costume.

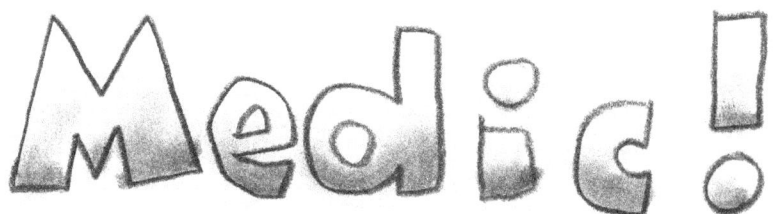

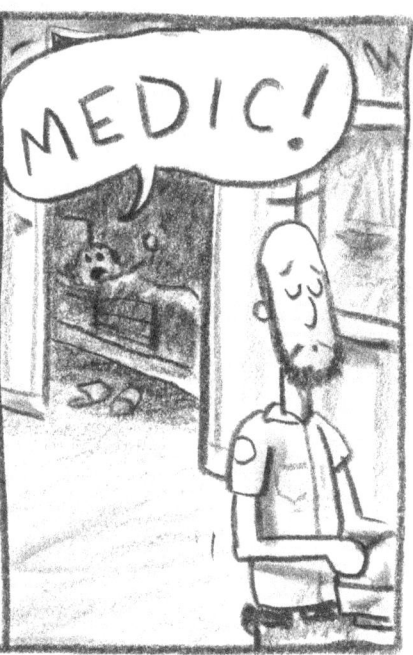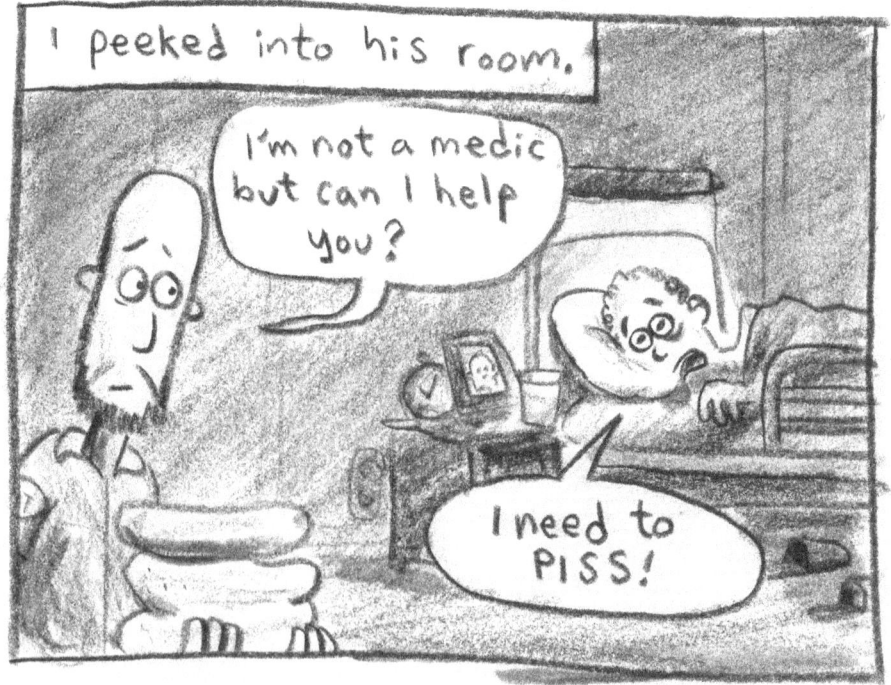

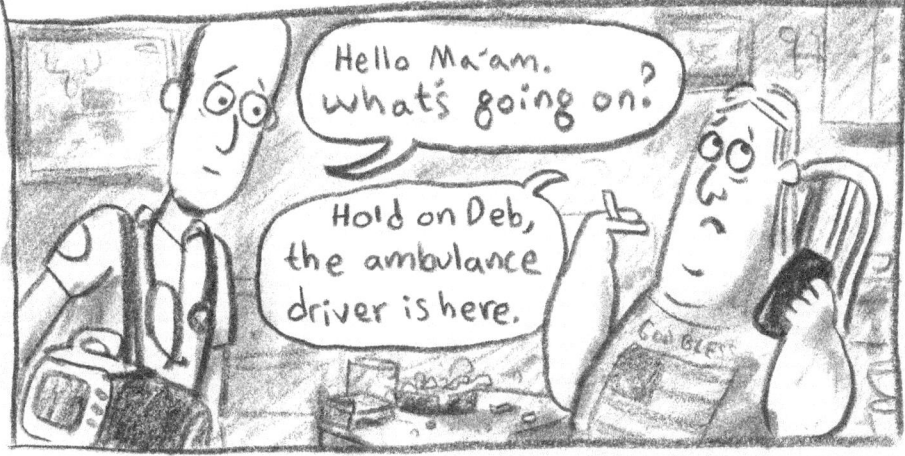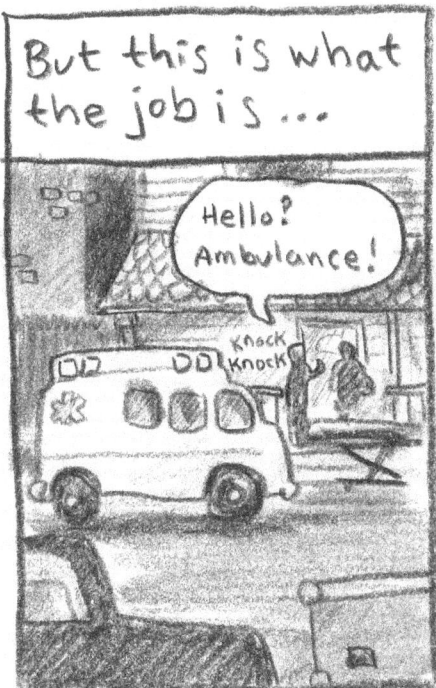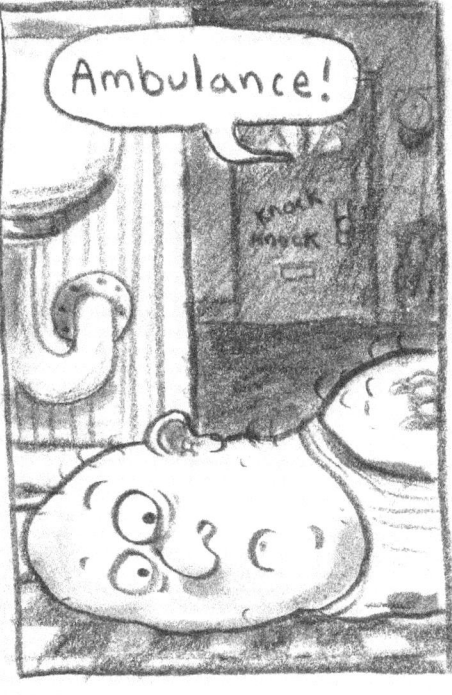

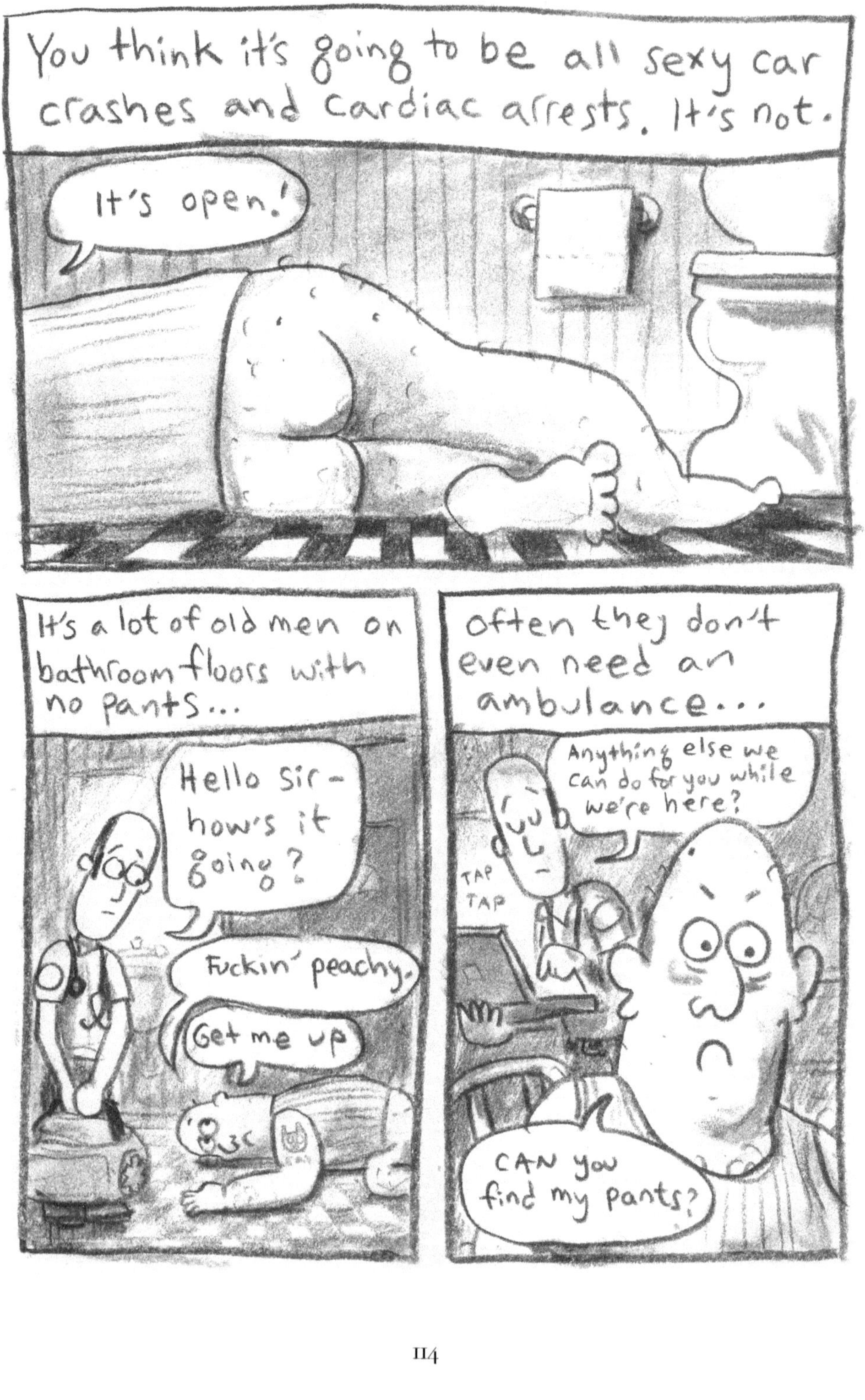

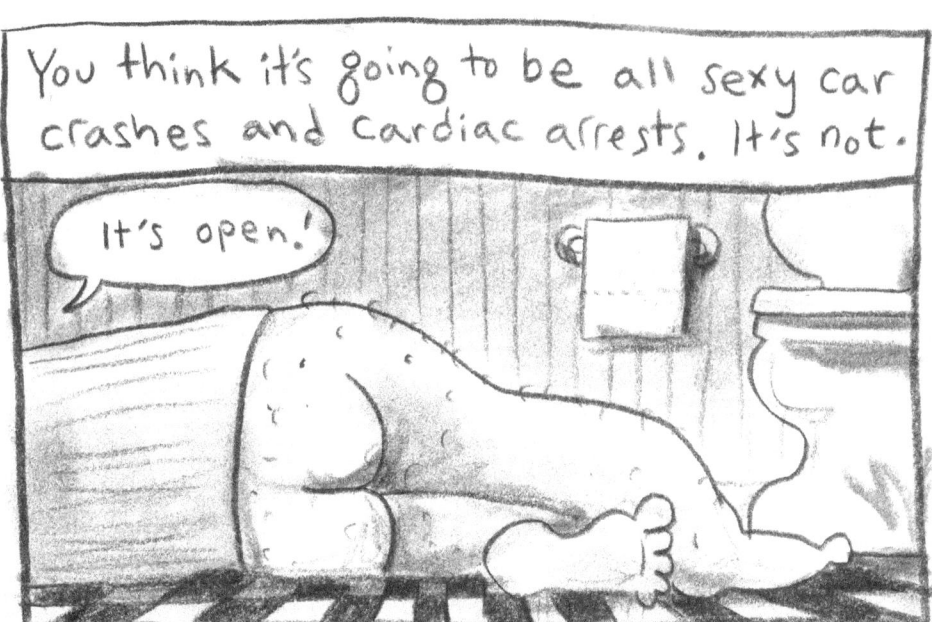

And sometimes you get dispatched to what sounds like nonsense at a nursing home...

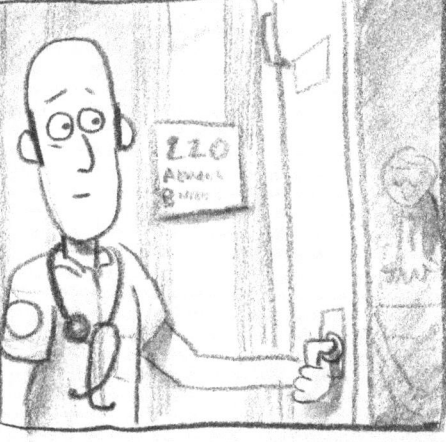

But you walk in on a cardiac arrest.

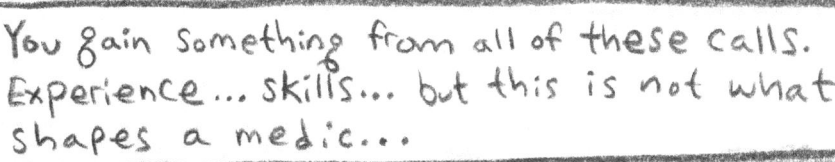

You gain something from all of these calls. Experience... skills... but this is not what shapes a medic...

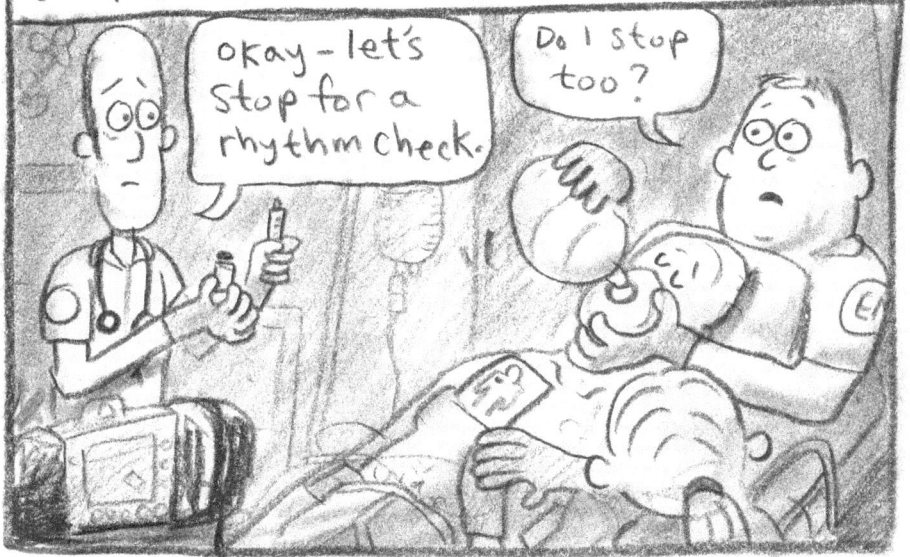

The calls that shaped me into a medic were the ones that went badly.

Dispatch to 244

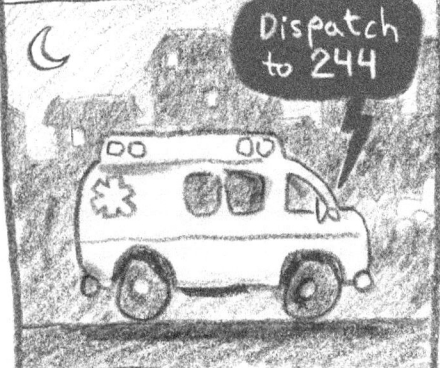

I had been a medic for about a year when I got sent to Polly.

244- Respond to 33 Sunshine Ct... Adult female vomiting blood.

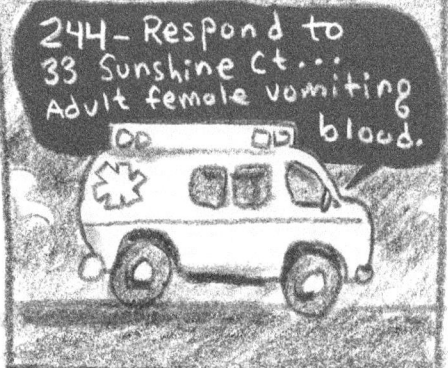

We found Polly on the cold tile laying half-way under a Christmas tree.

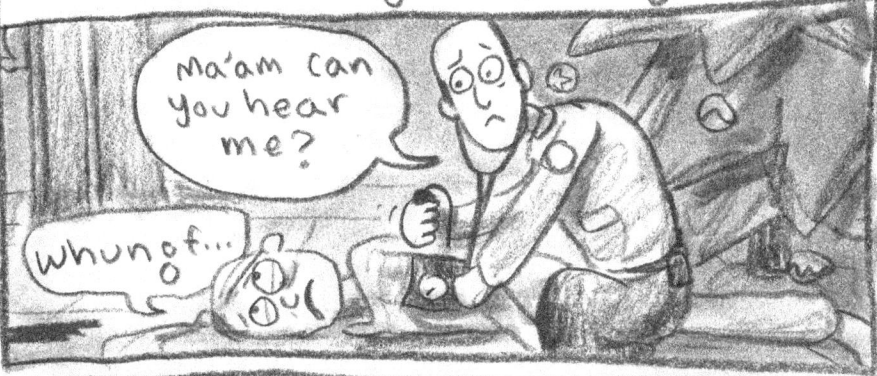
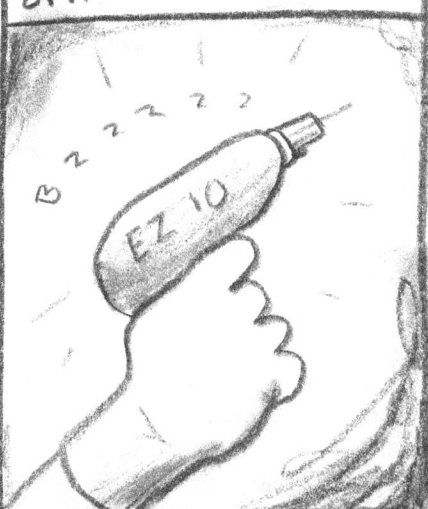

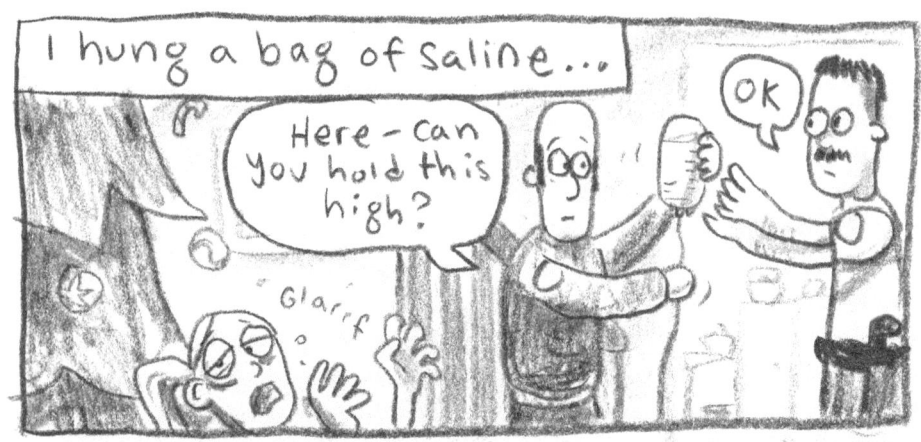

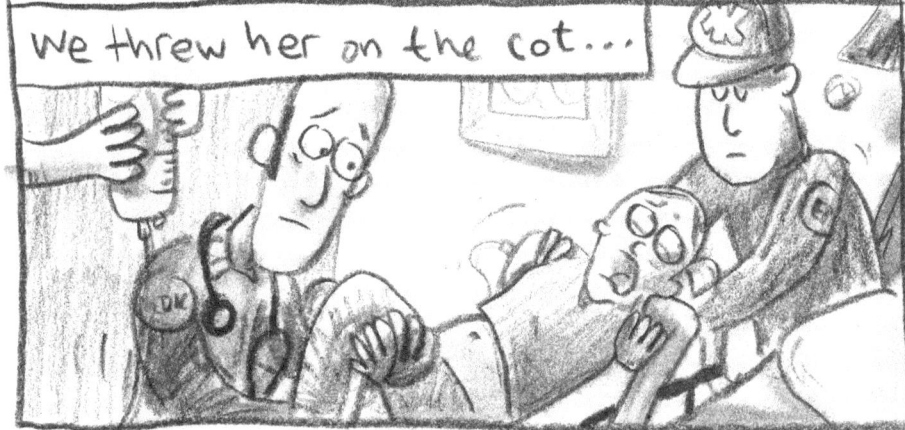

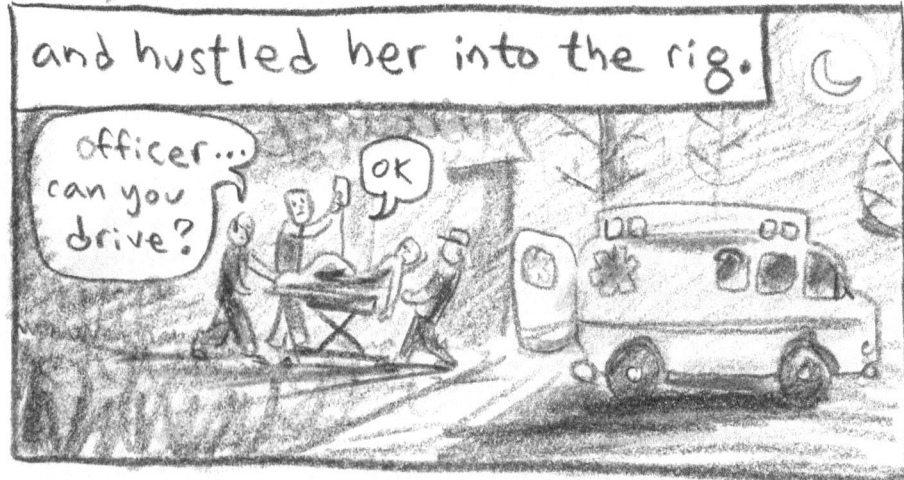

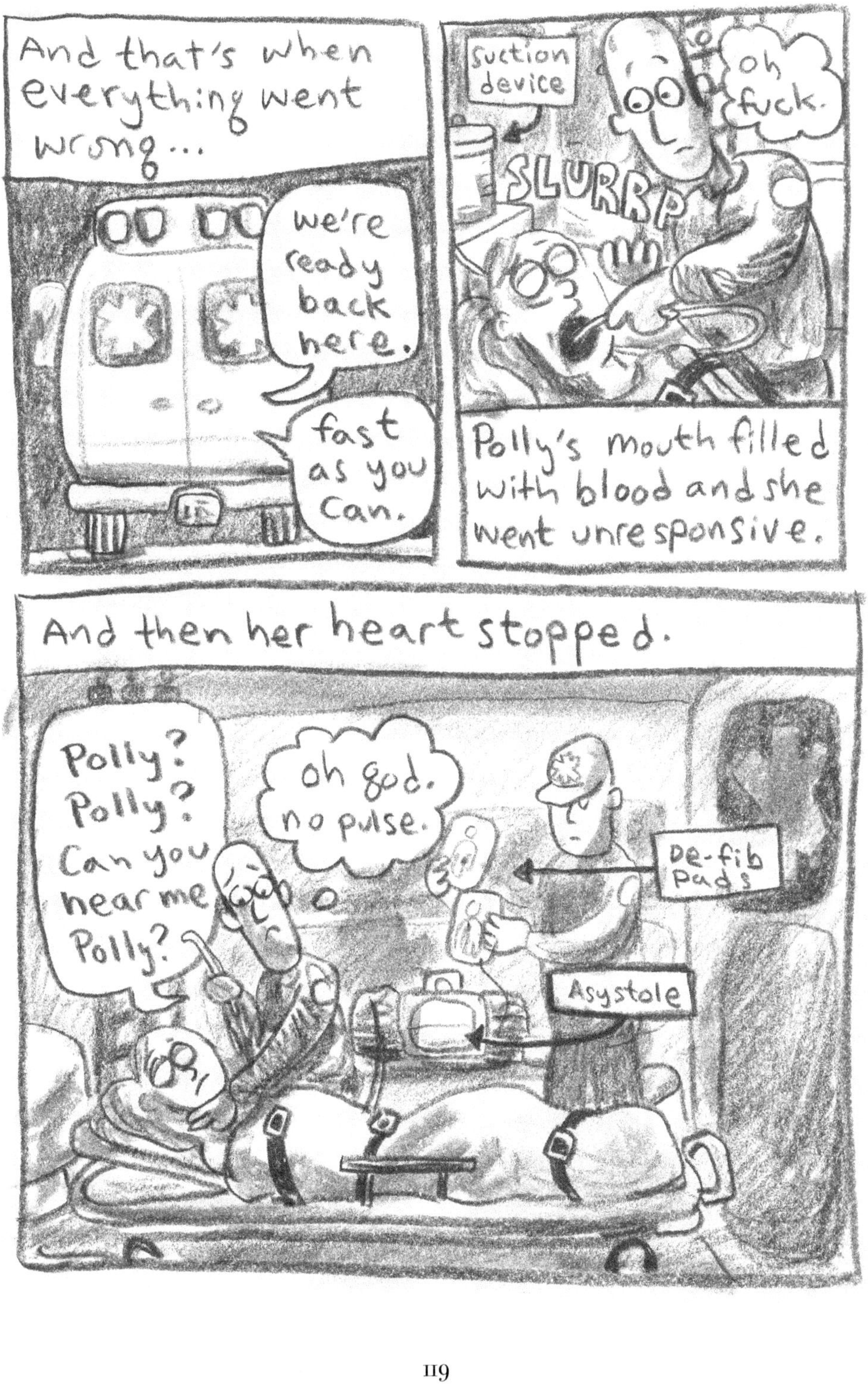

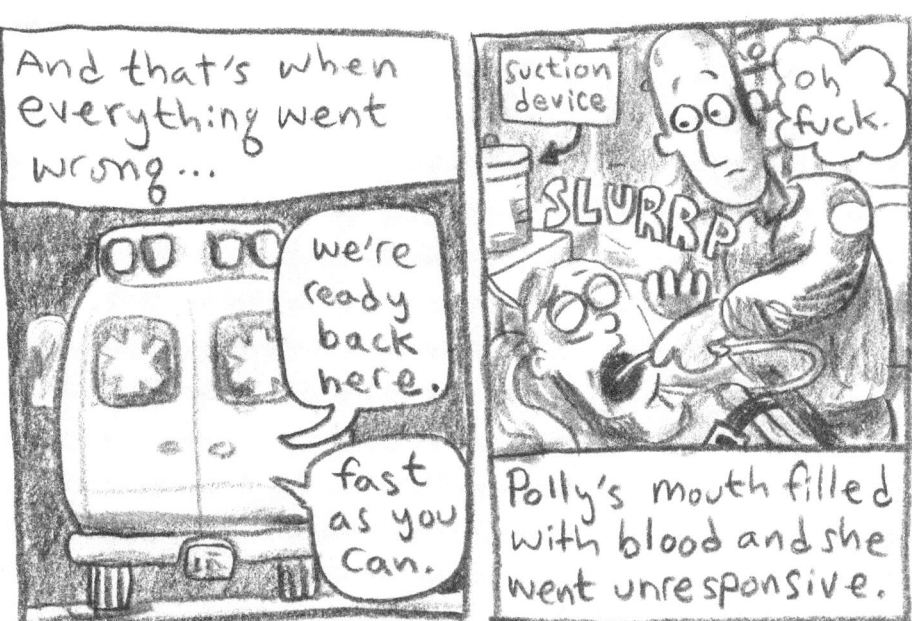

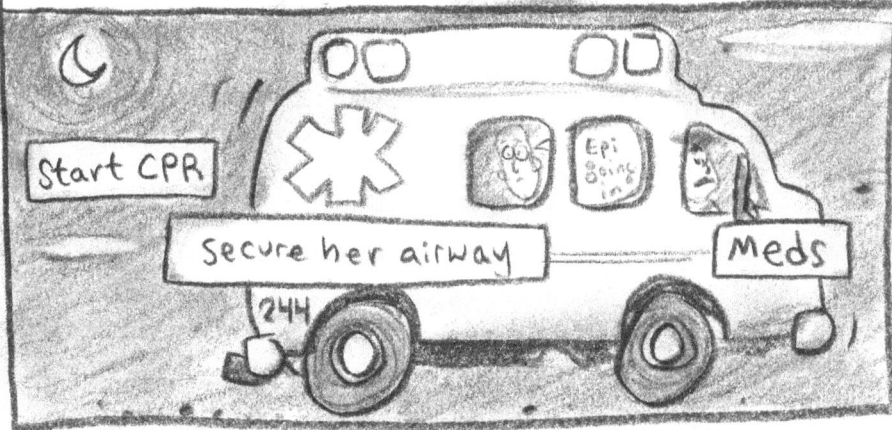

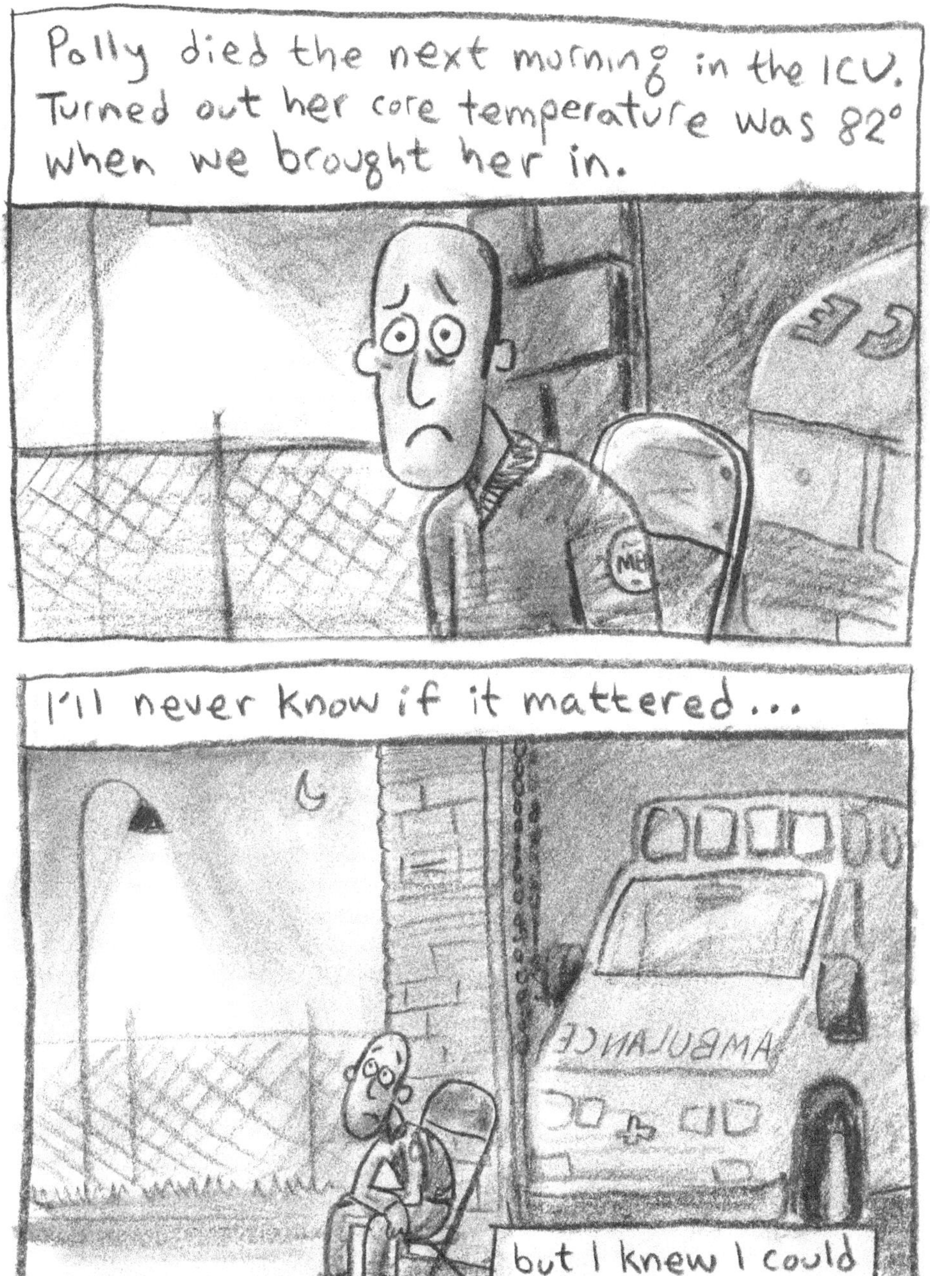

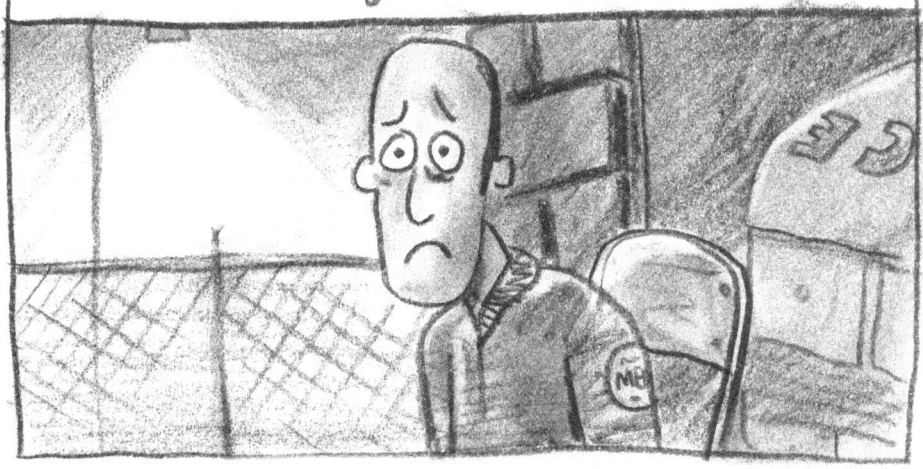

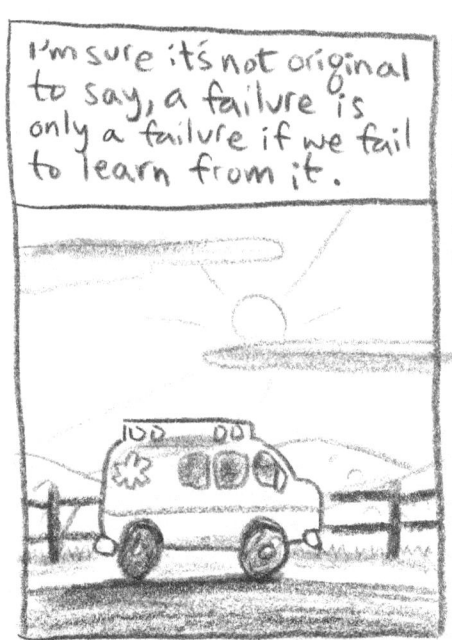

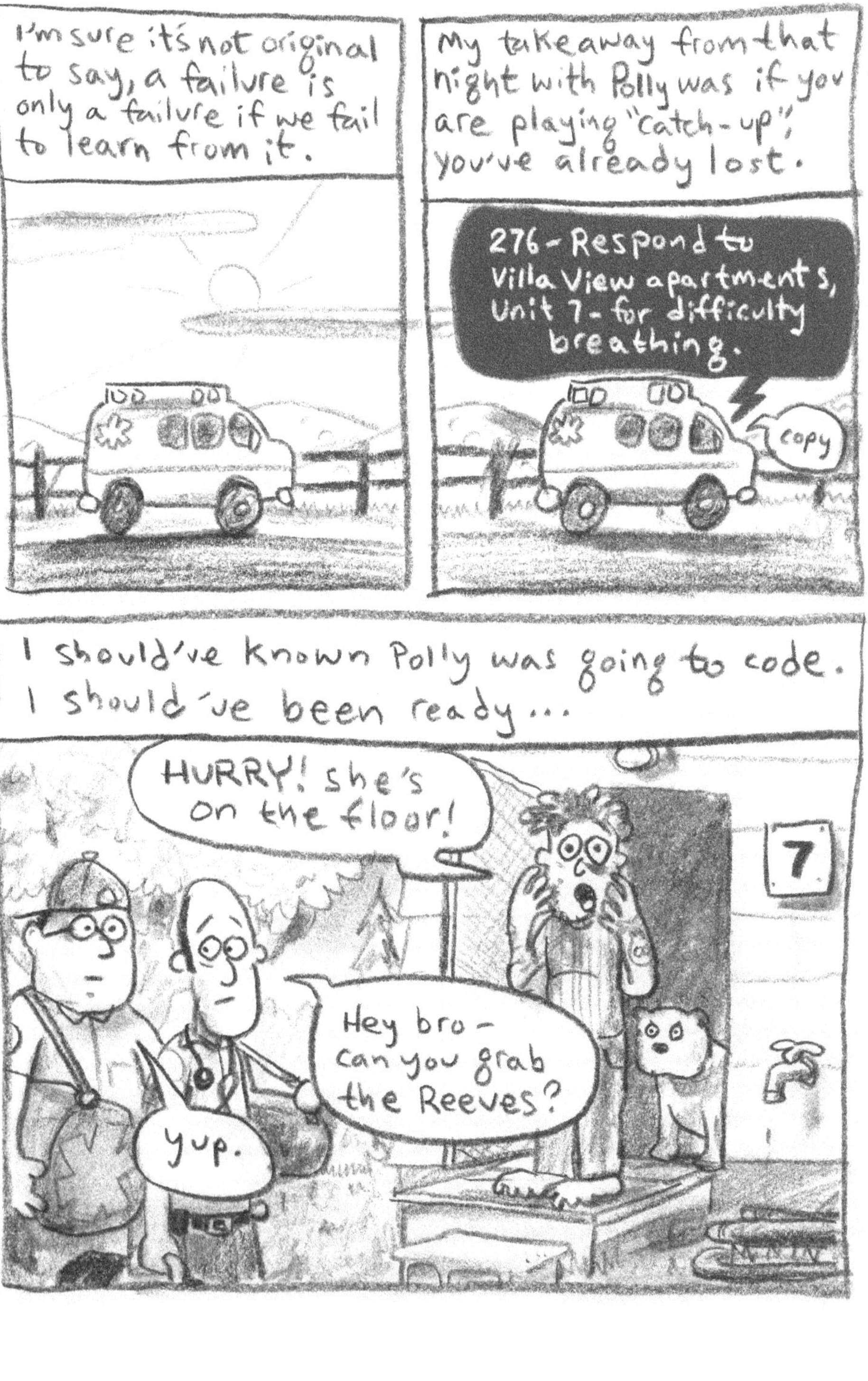

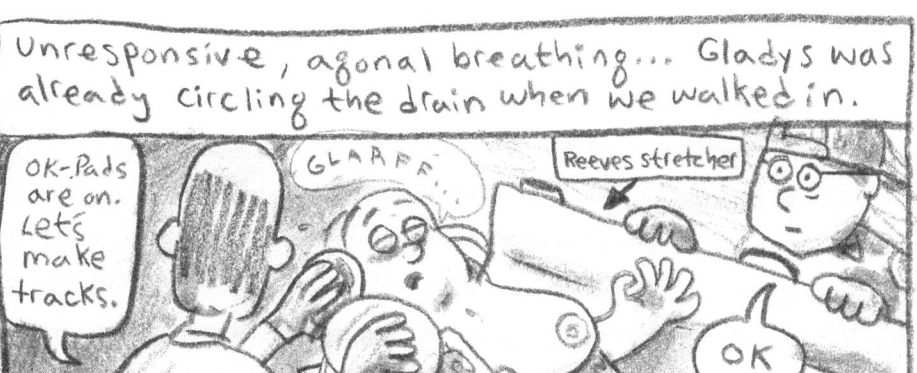

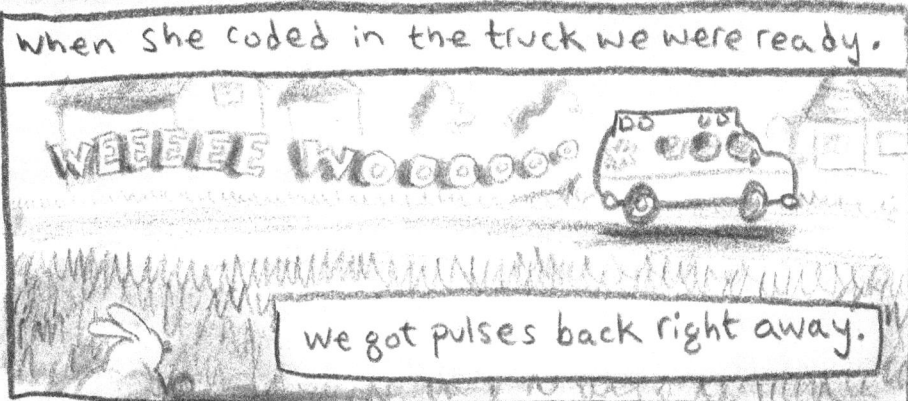

Like Polly, Gladys died the next day in the hospital. Maybe what we did, didn't make much of a difference, but I knew — and her family could be sure — she got the best possible chance she was going to get.

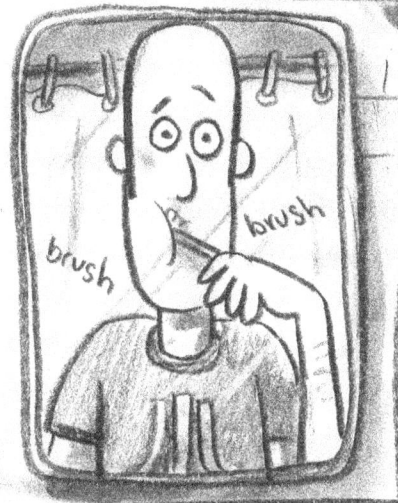

The Worst Thing

An unwritten rule, when writing on the subject of EMS, is that you must address the question everyone asks: What's the worst thing you've seen?

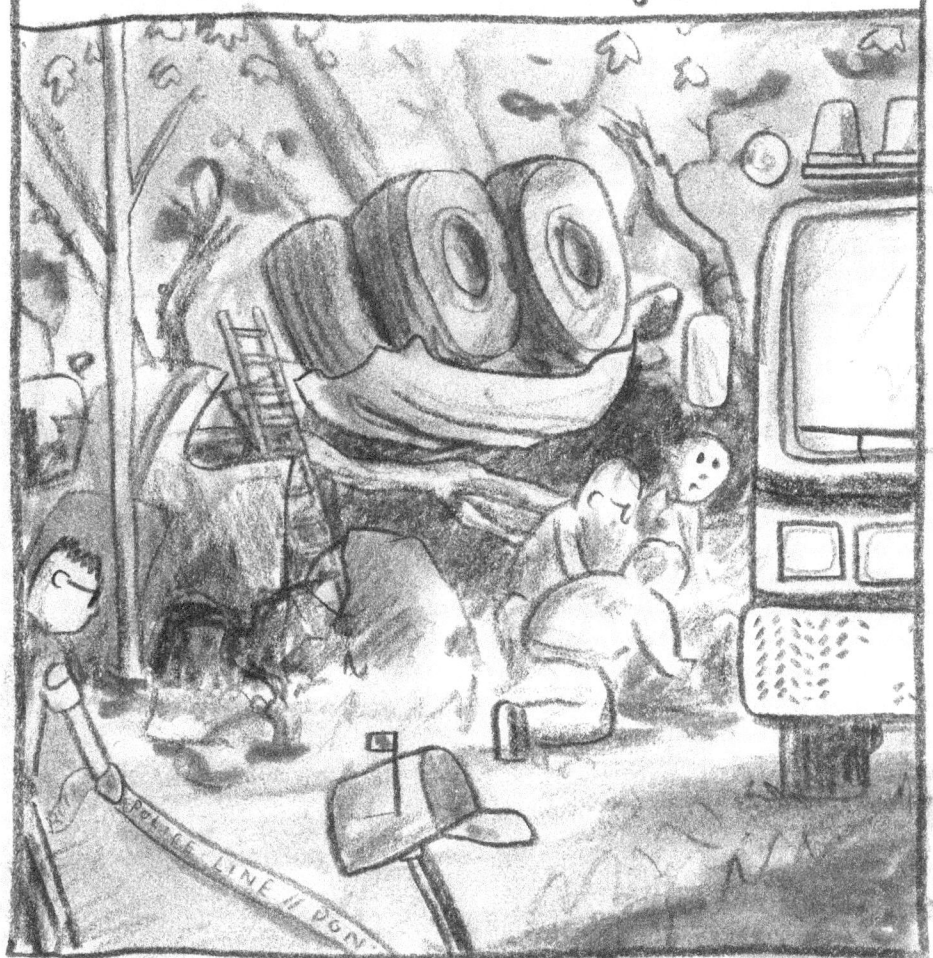

I'm sure when people ask they want to hear about the gore.

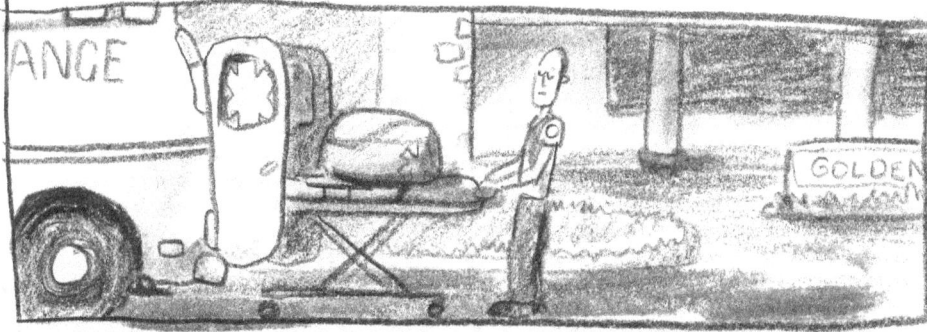

They want to hear about the teenager who got shot in the head and was still breathing.

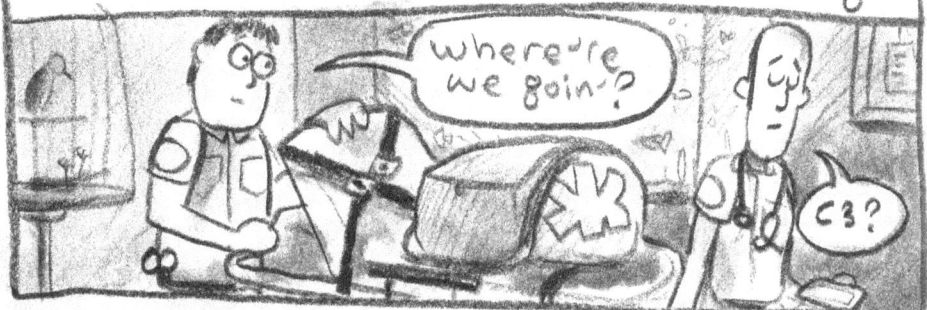

Where're we goin'?

C3?

They want to hear about the person whose head got caved in by a tree and their eye was hanging out.

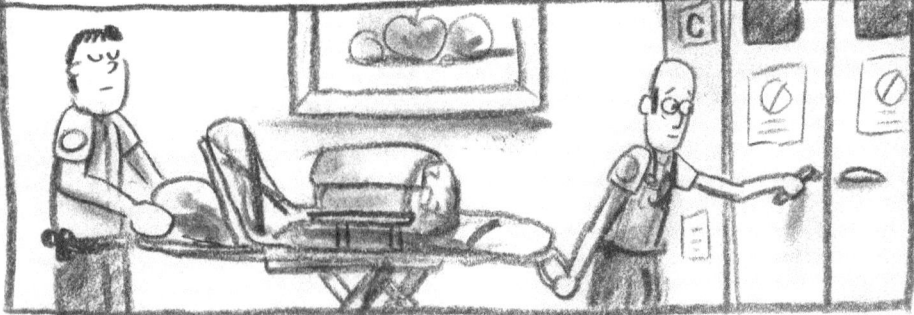

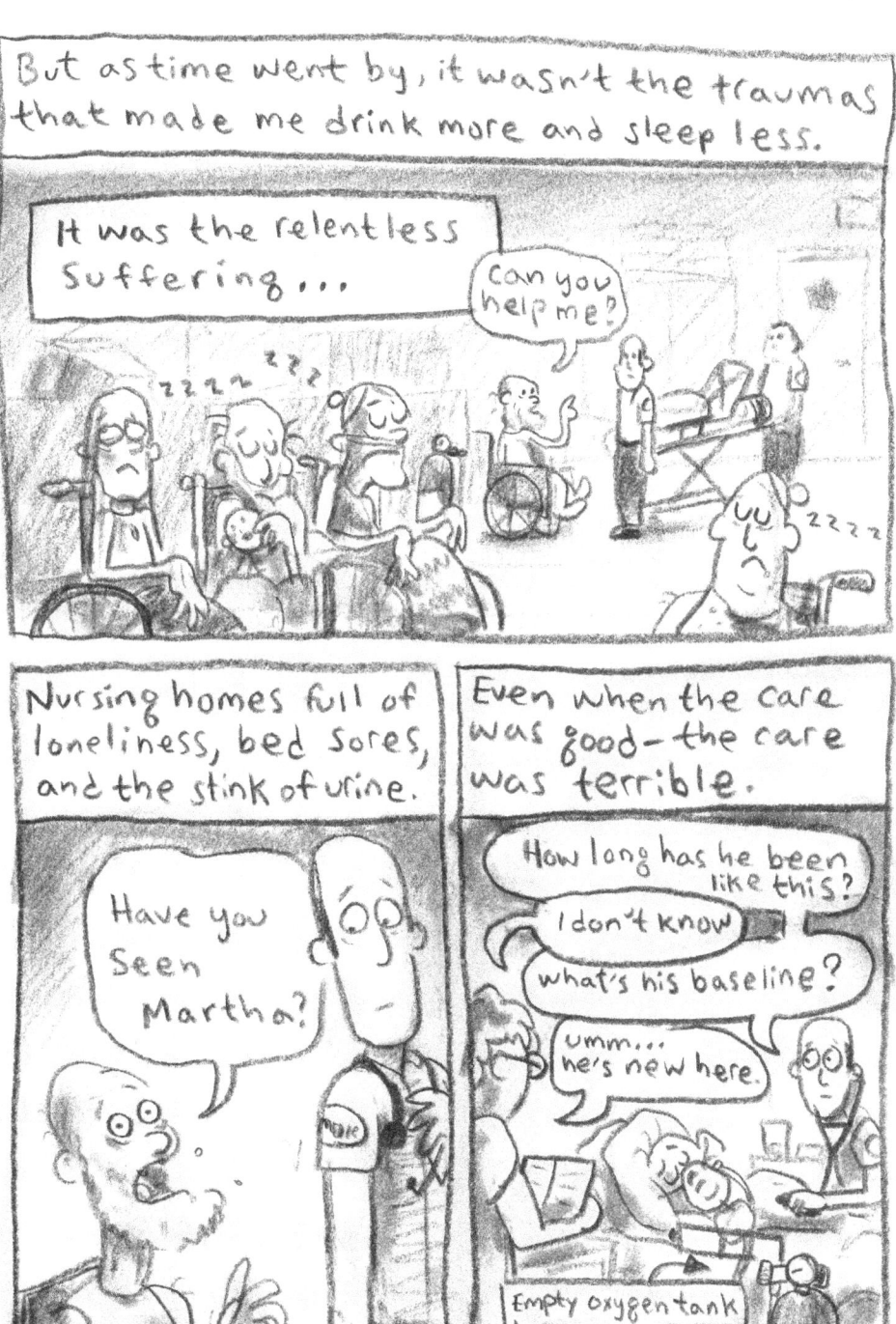

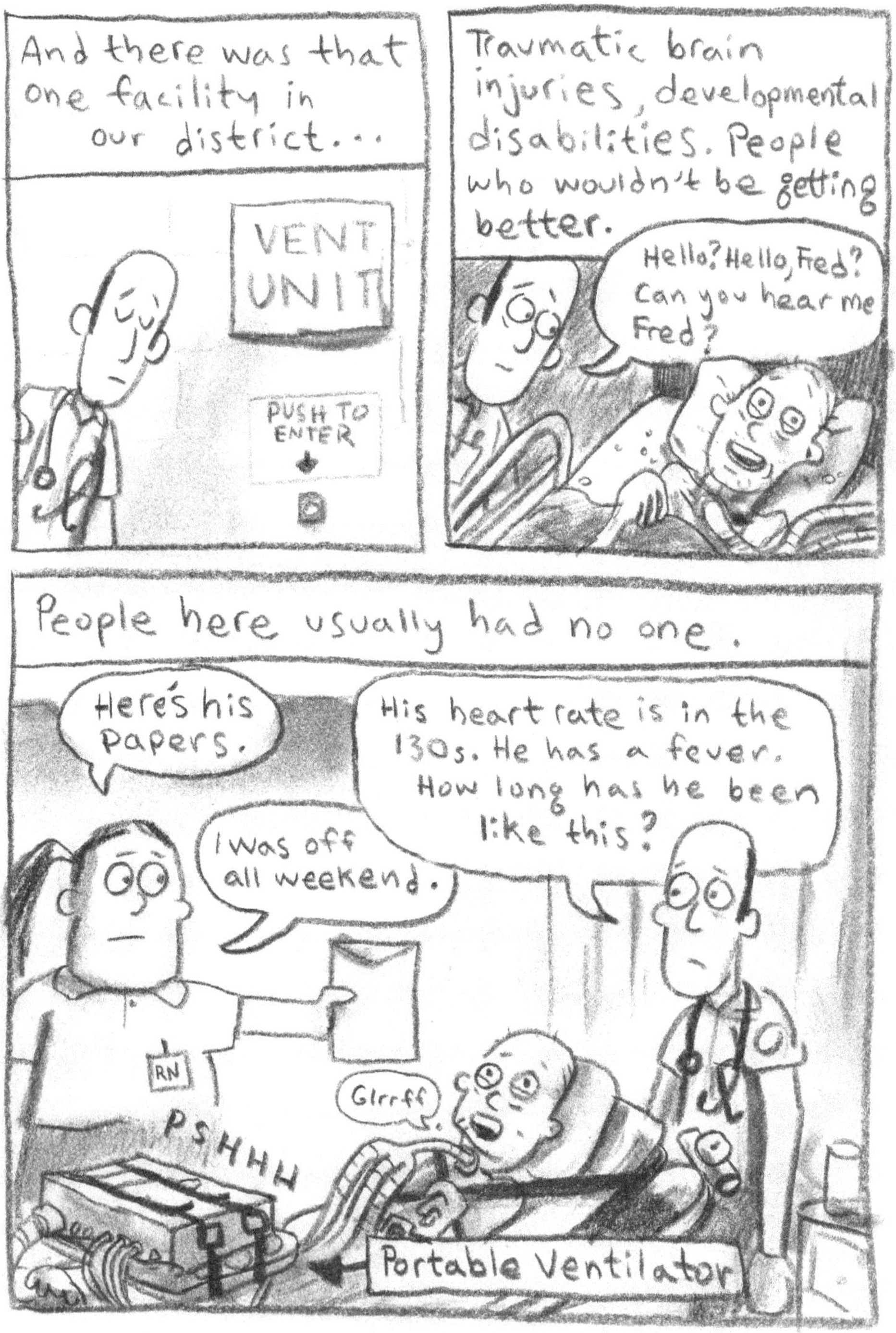

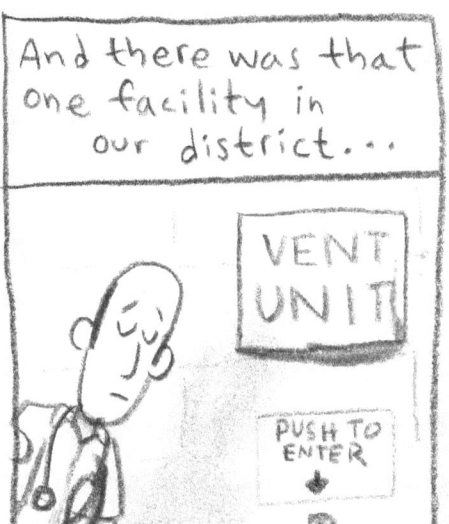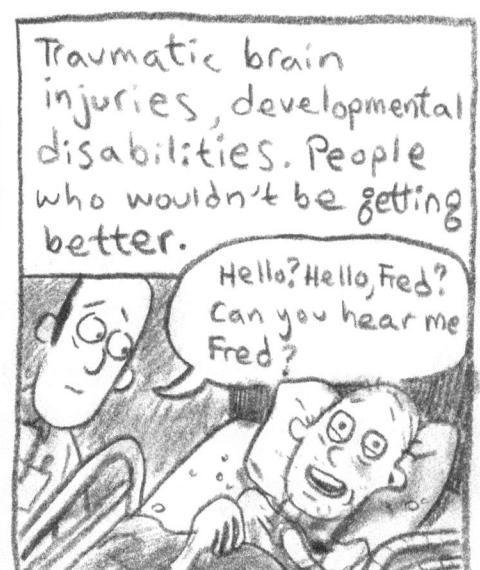

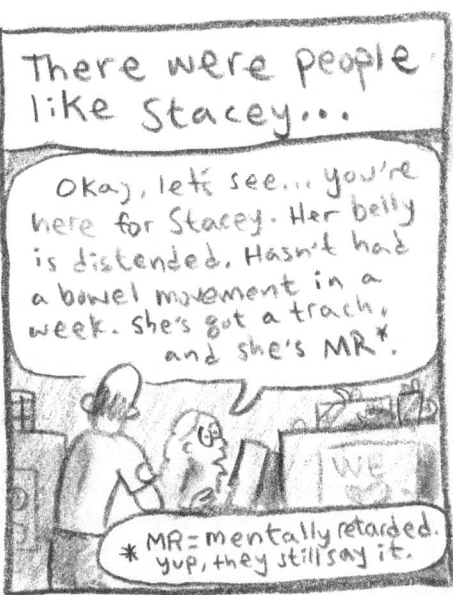
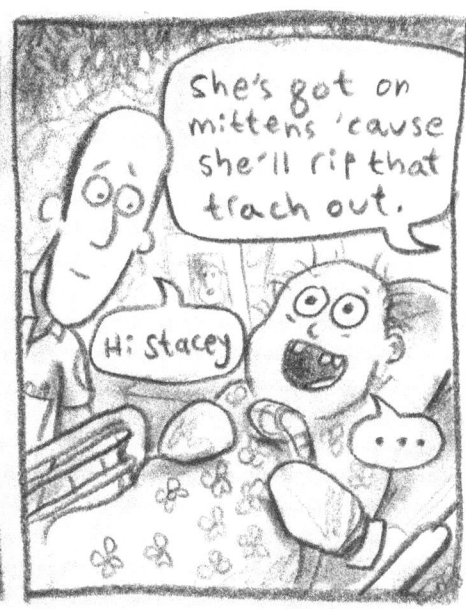
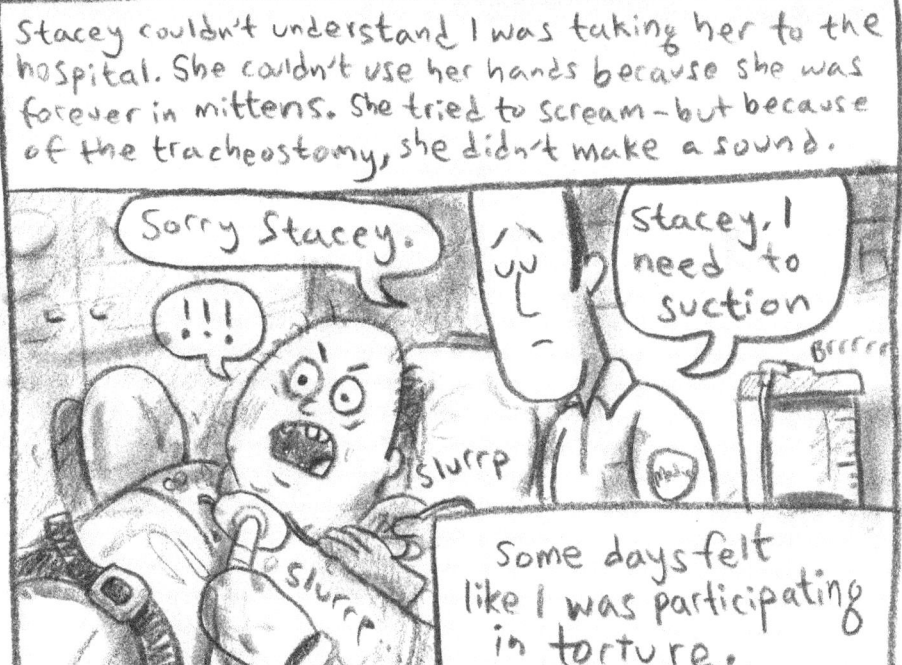

And then there was Harry. Harry was an autistic man who broke his neck diving into the shallow side of a pool. He would constantly rip off his oxygen. He would become hypoxic. He would fight.

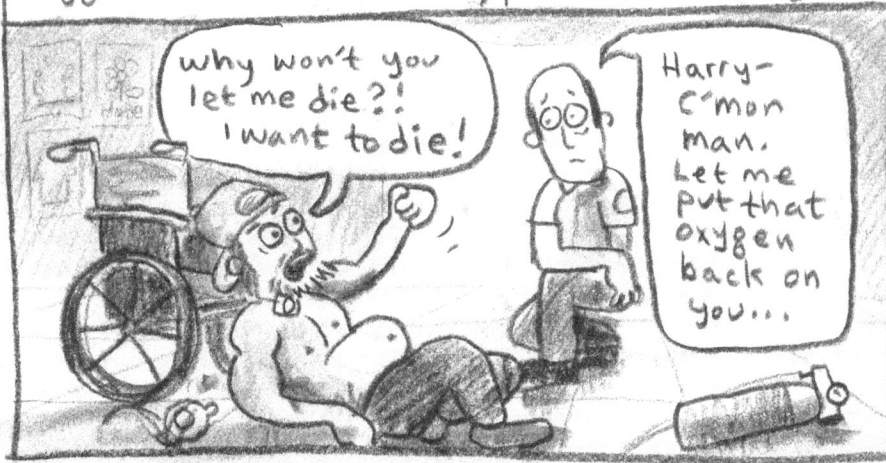

We would take Harry to the hospital where he would be medicated enough to keep his oxygen on.

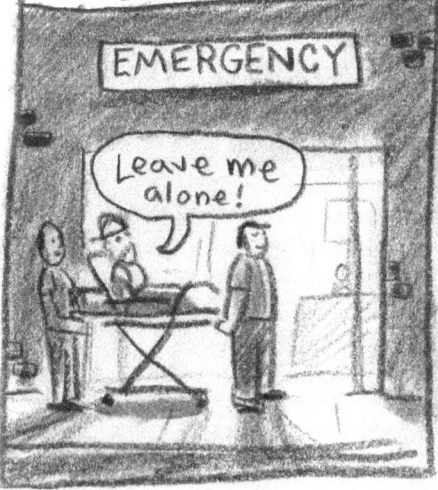

He'd then go back to the nursing home and do it all again.

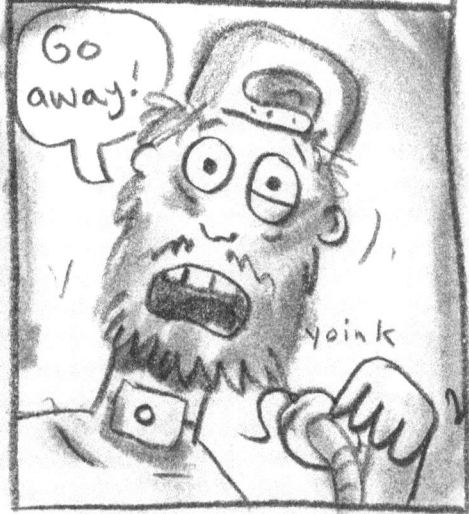

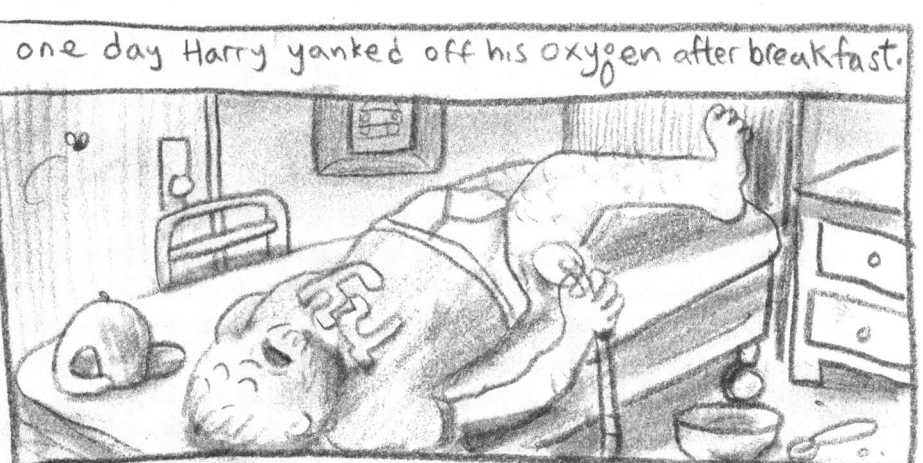

one day Harry yanked off his oxygen after breakfast.

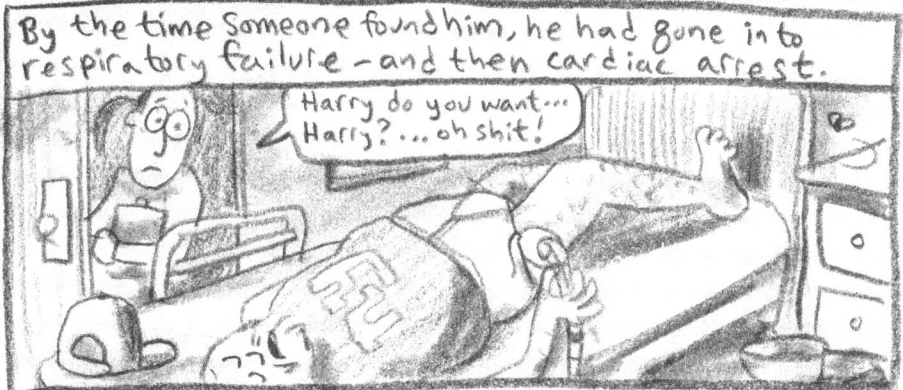

By the time someone found him, he had gone into respiratory failure — and then cardiac arrest.

"Harry do you want... Harry?... oh shit!"

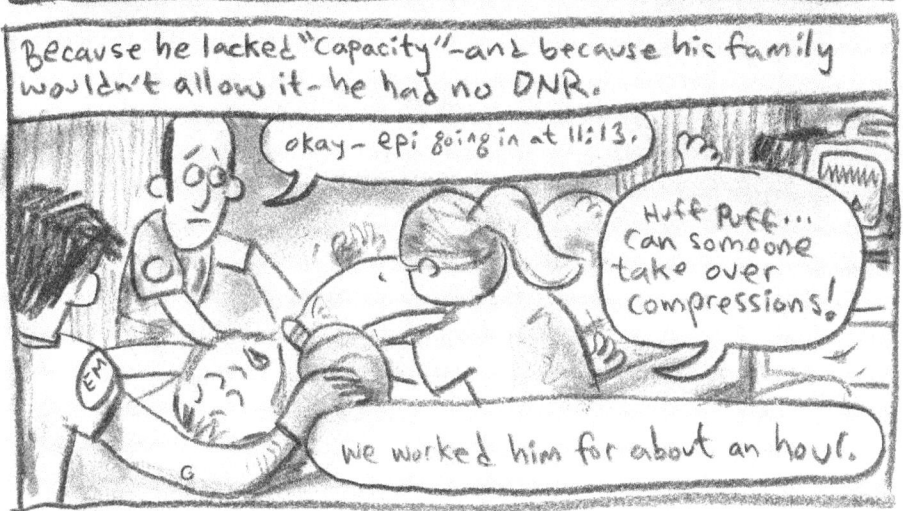

Because he lacked "capacity" — and because his family wouldn't allow it — he had no DNR.

"okay — epi going in at 11:13."

"Huff puff... can someone take over compressions!"

We worked him for about an hour.

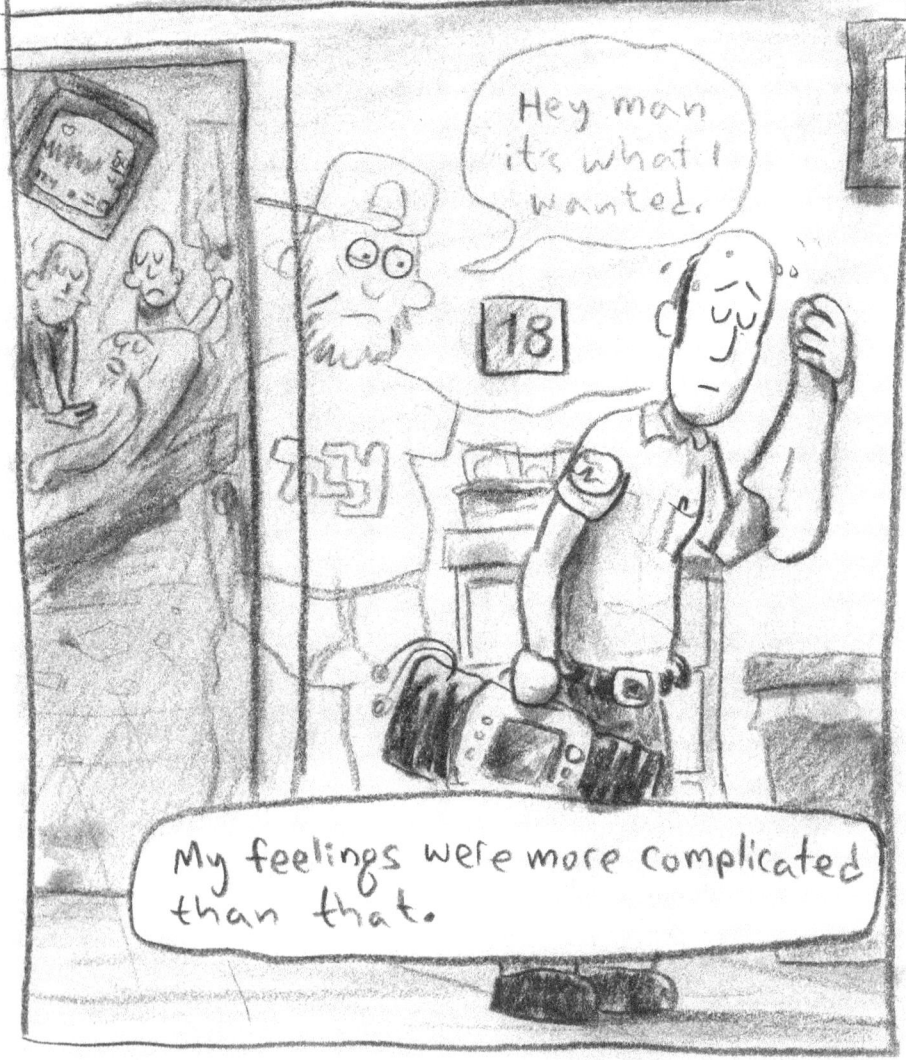

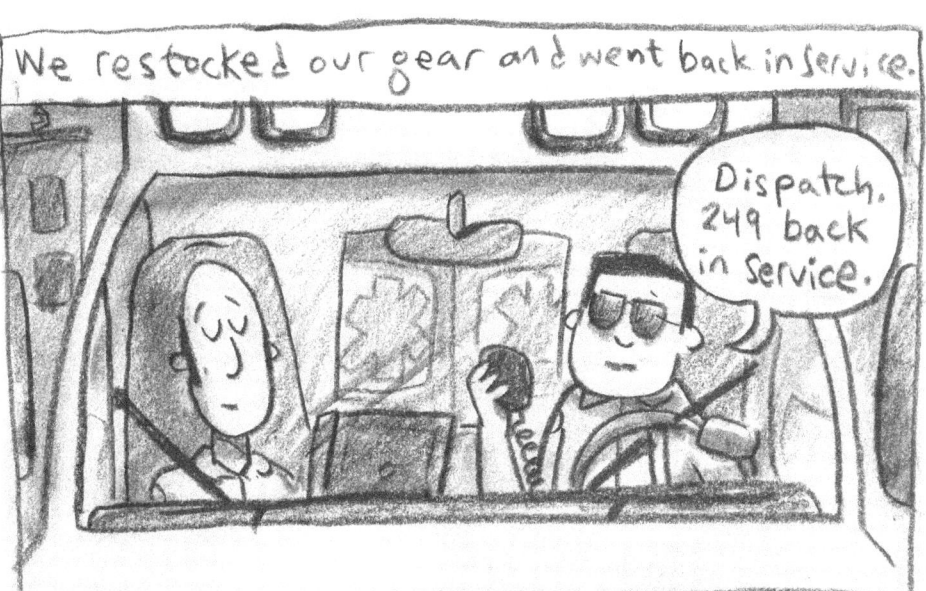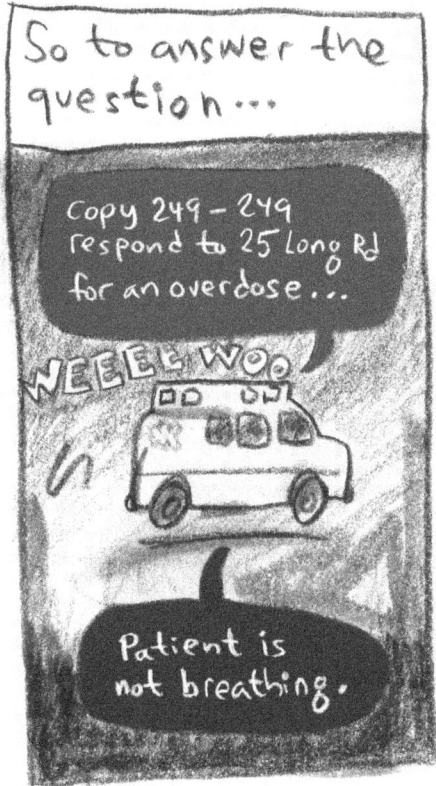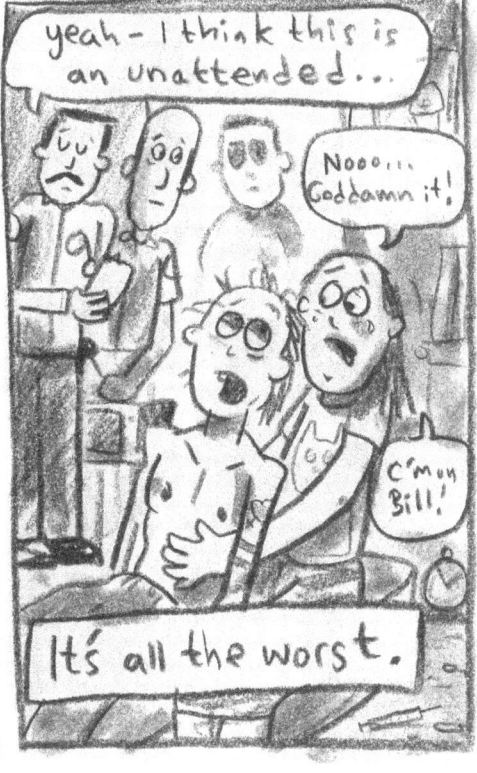

Oh Shit!

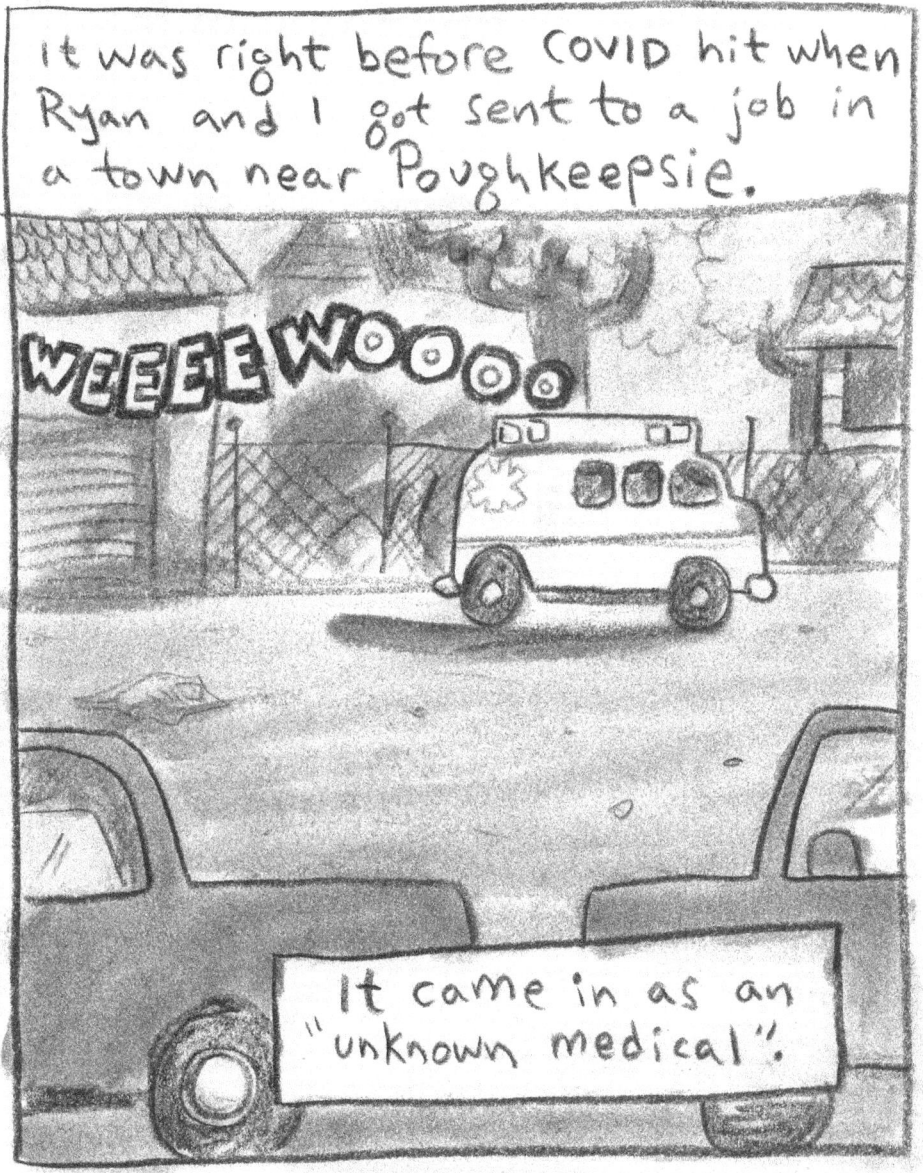

It was right before COVID hit when Ryan and I got sent to a job in a town near Poughkeepsie.

WEEEEWOOOO

It came in as an "unknown medical".

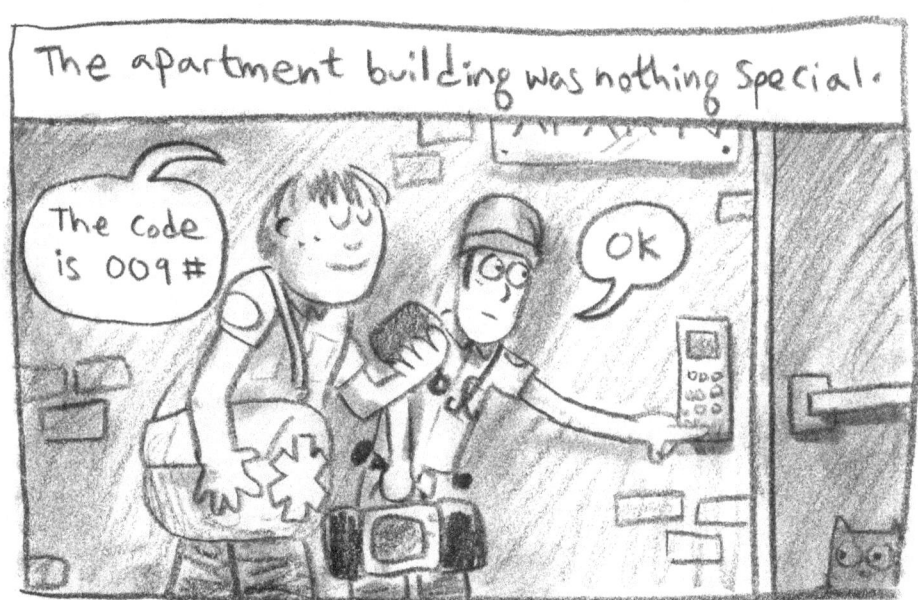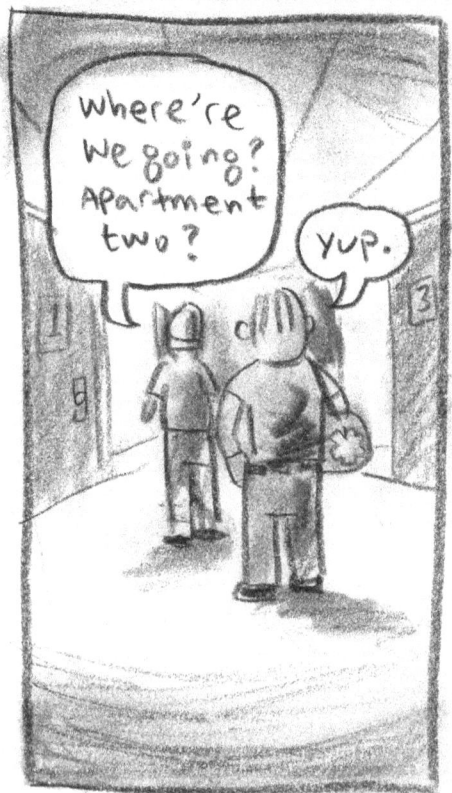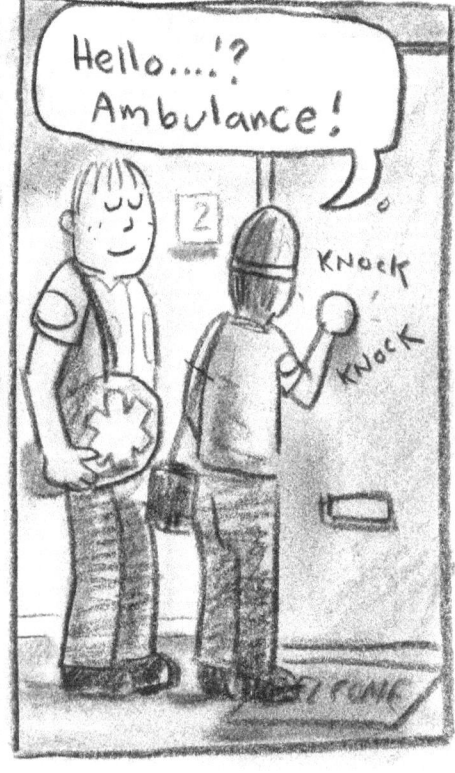

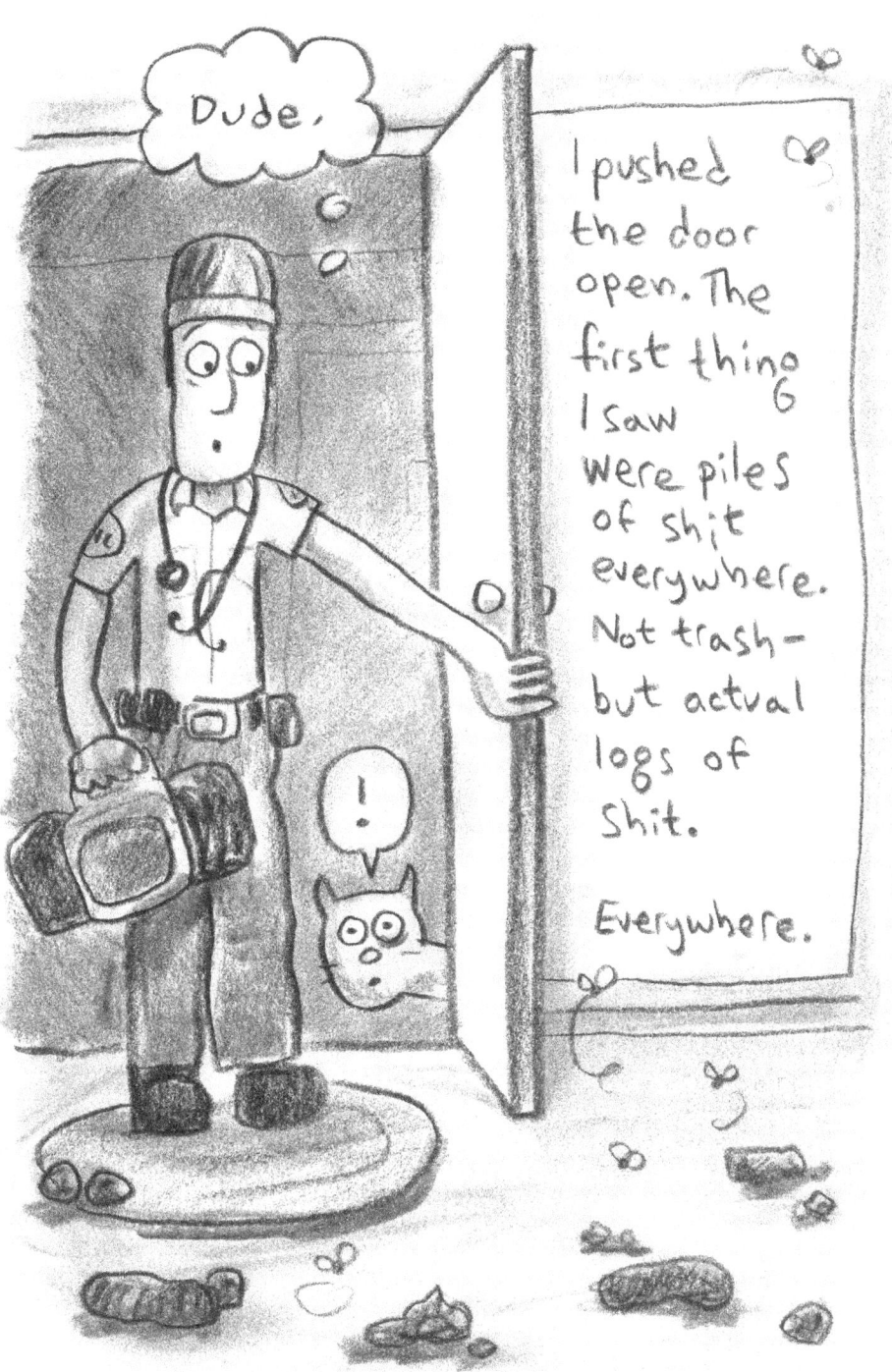

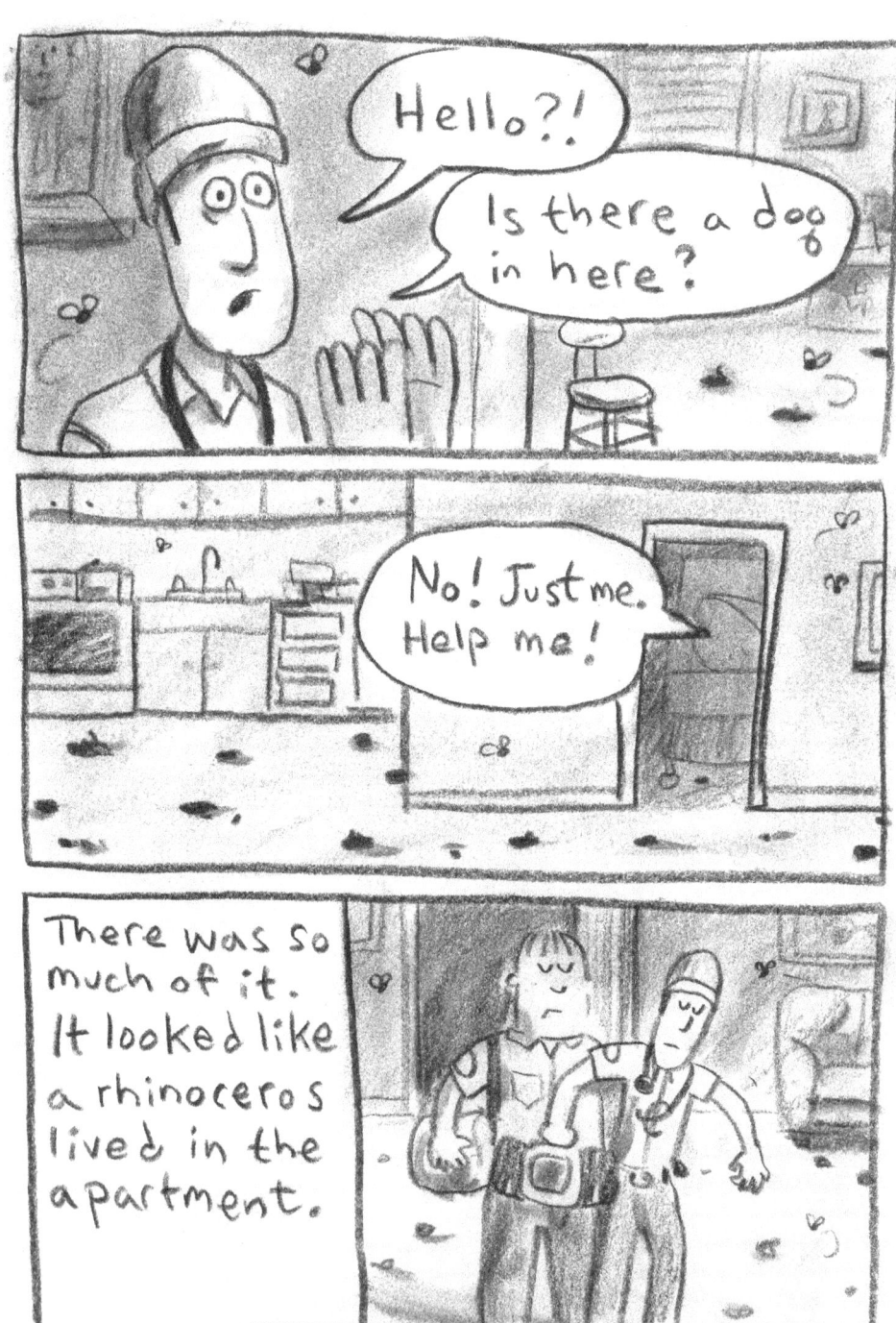

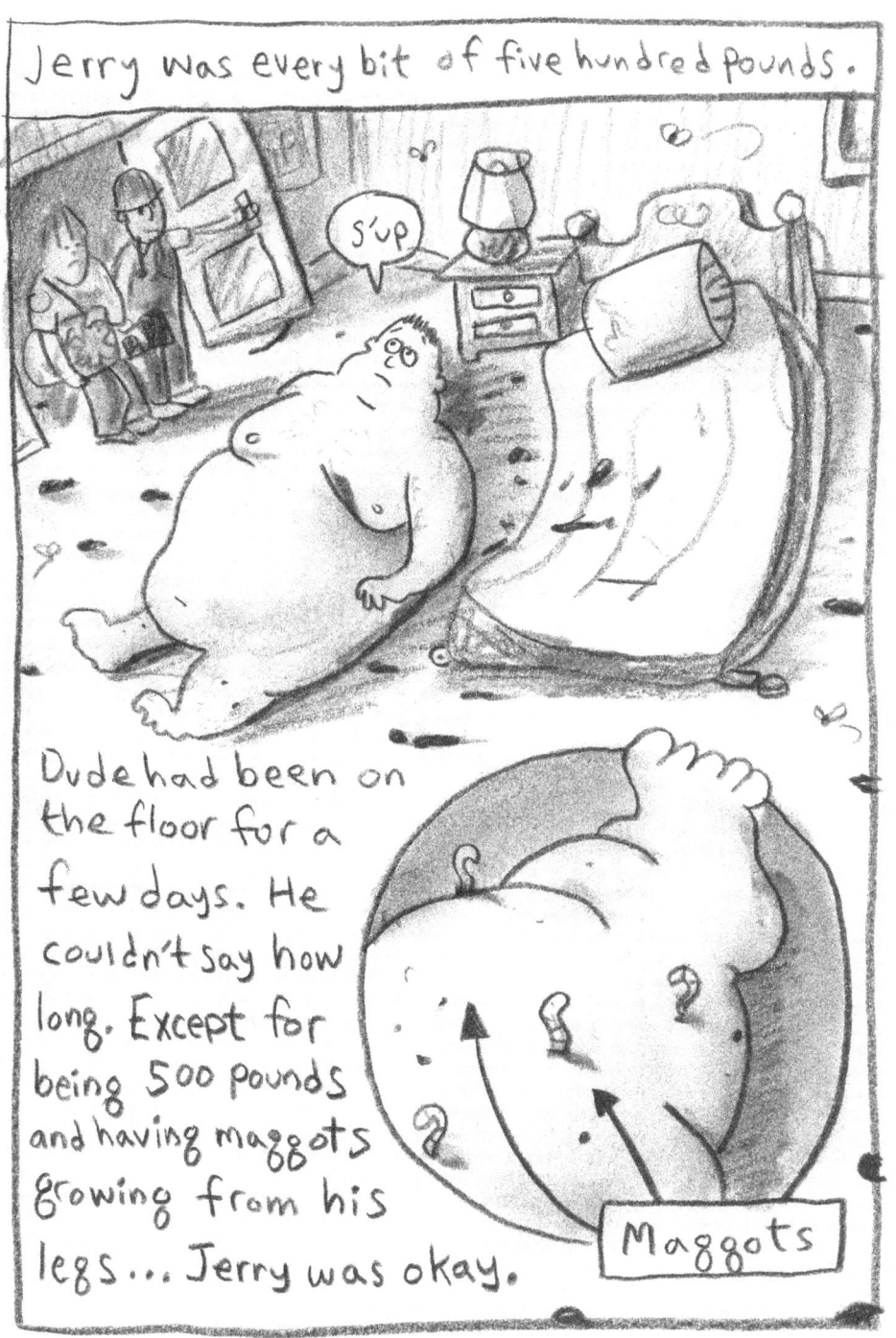

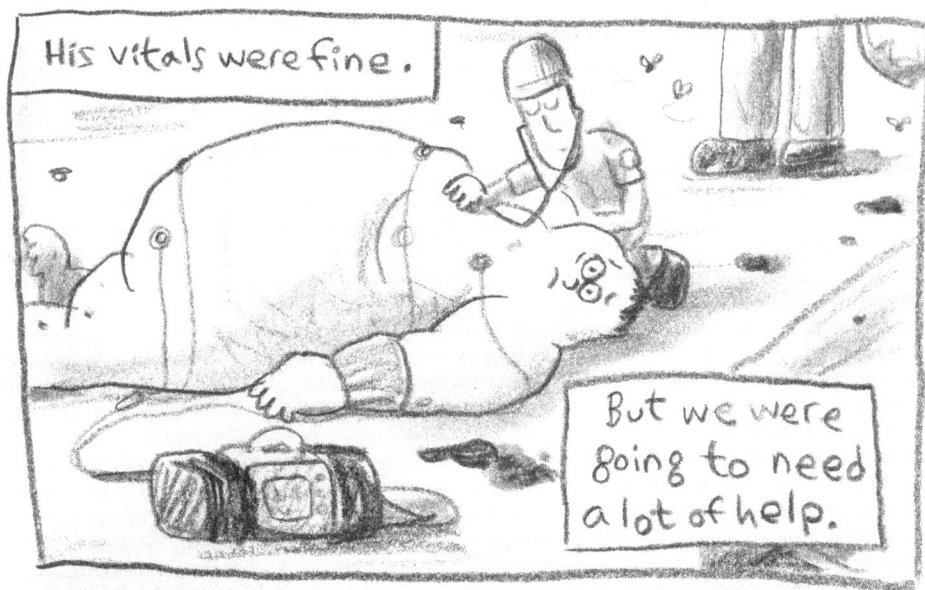

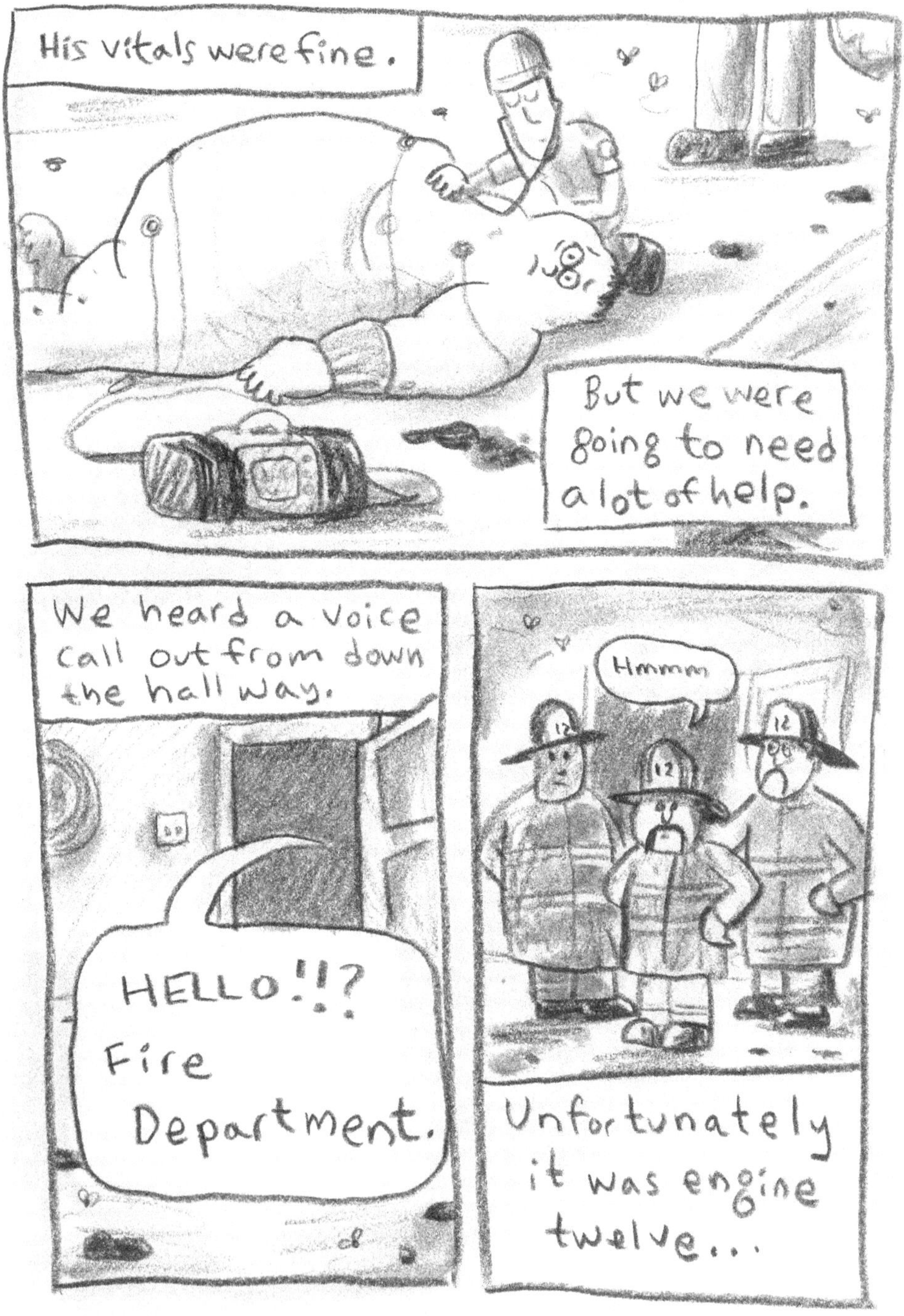

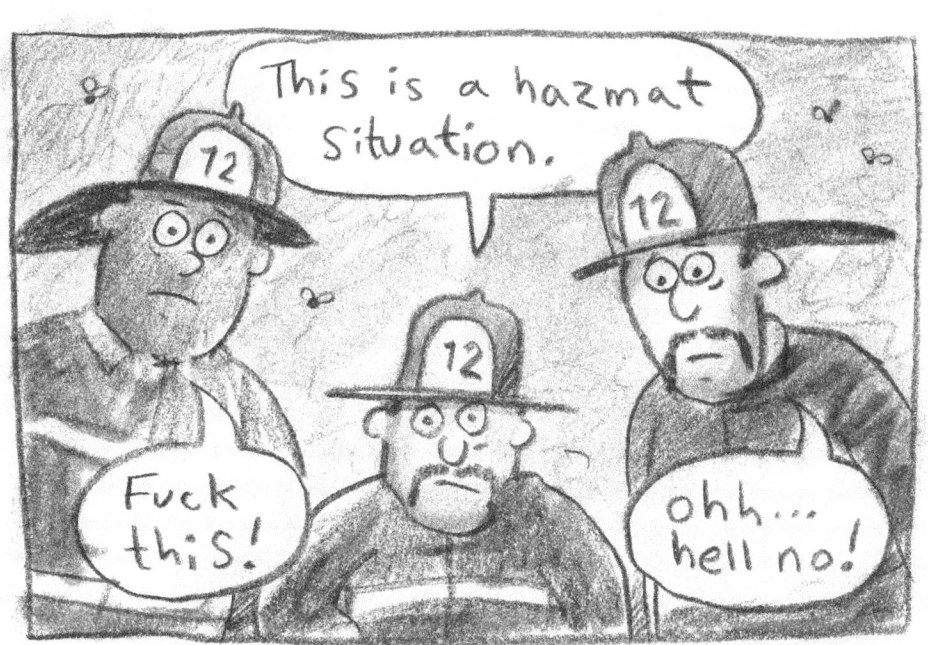

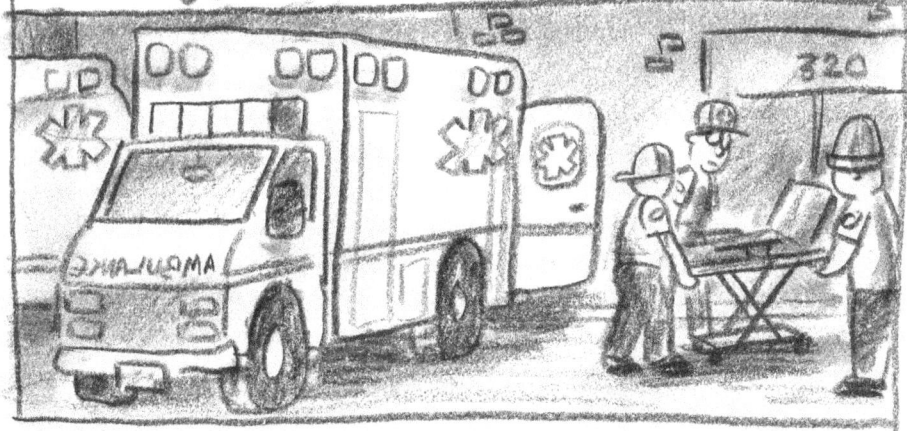

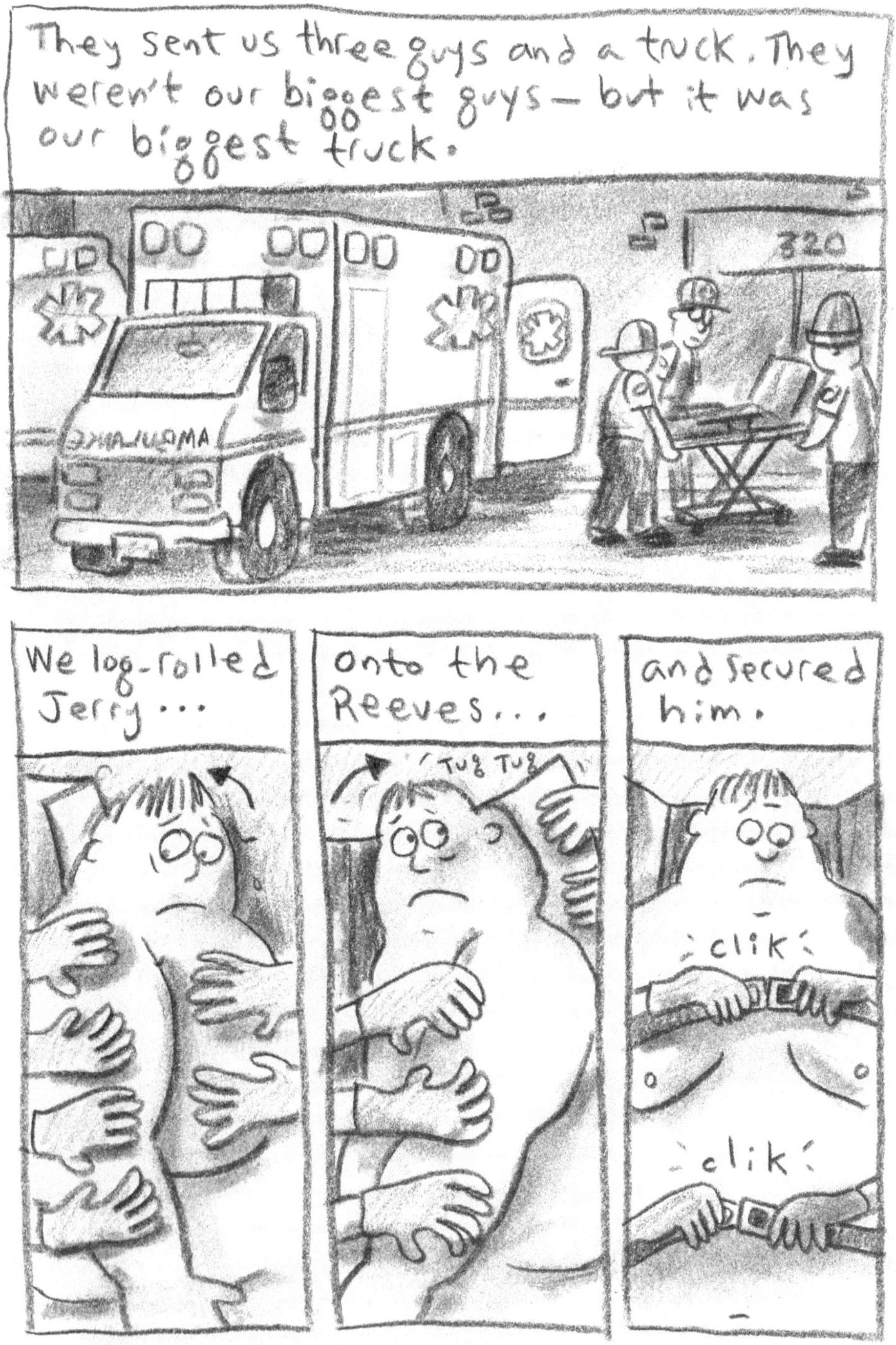

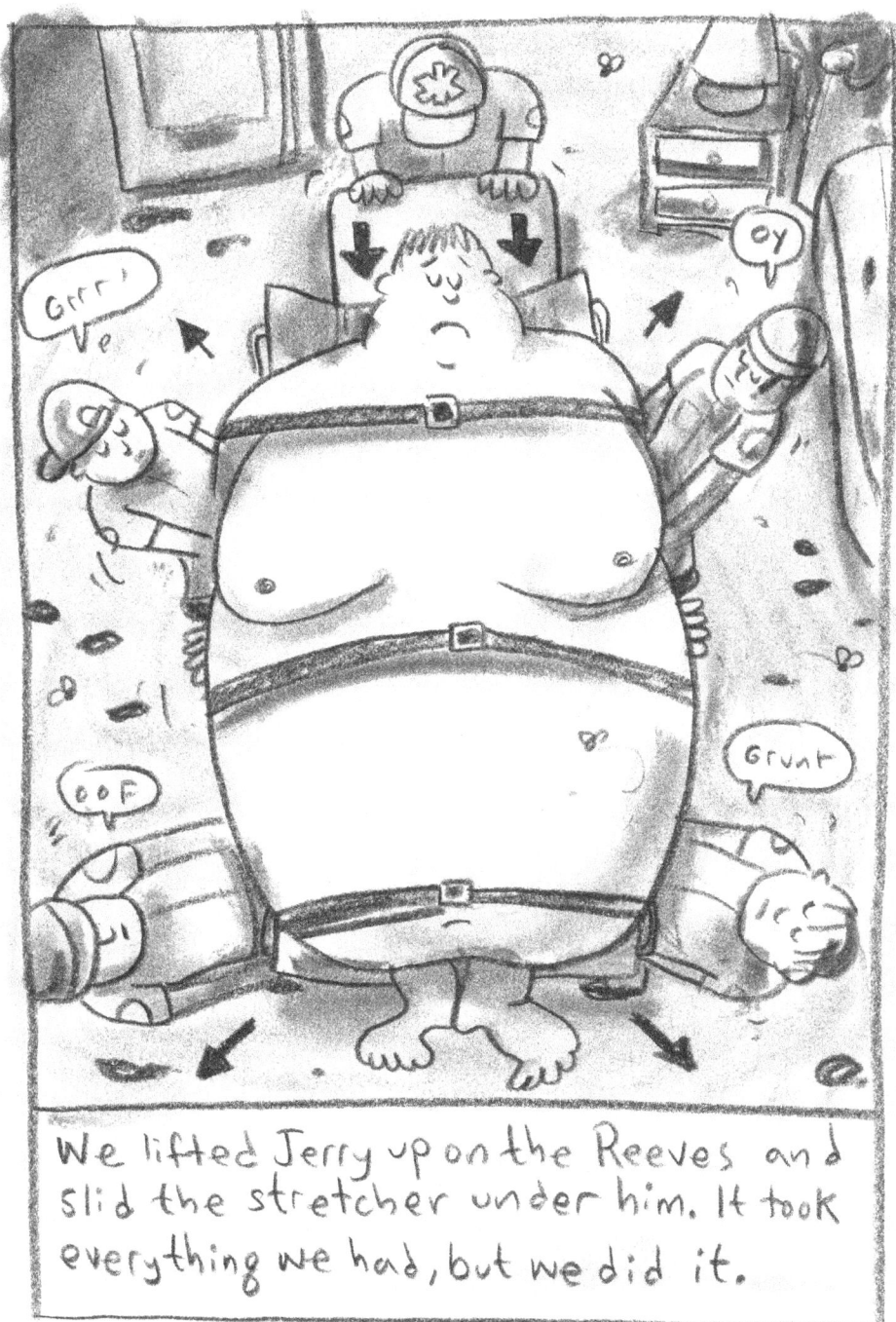

We lifted Jerry up on the Reeves and slid the stretcher under him. It took everything we had, but we did it.

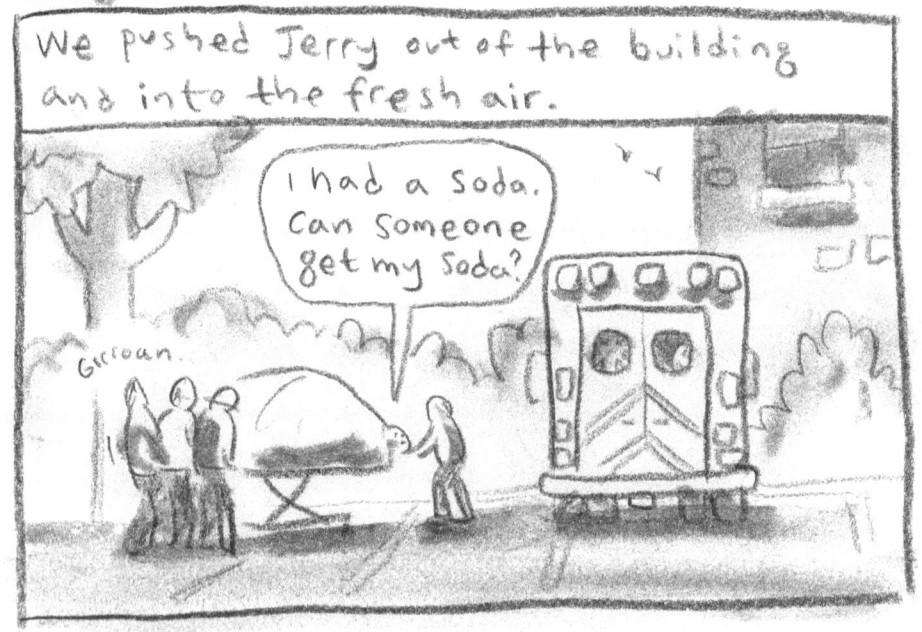

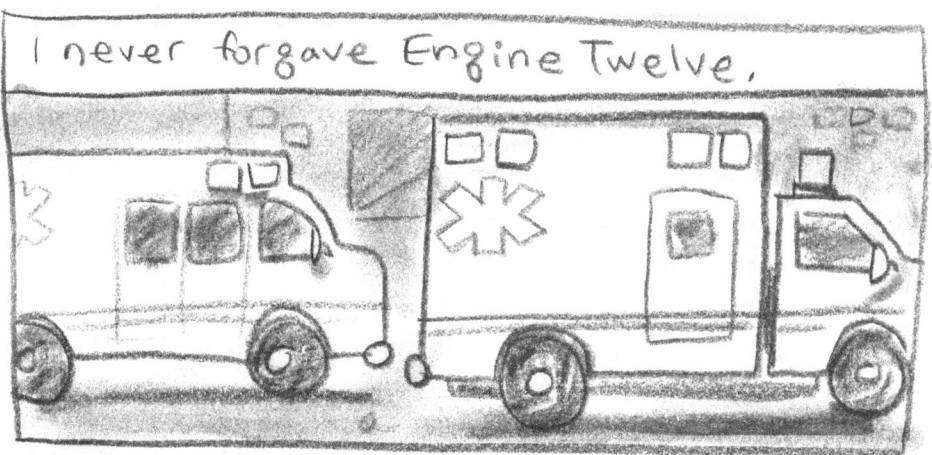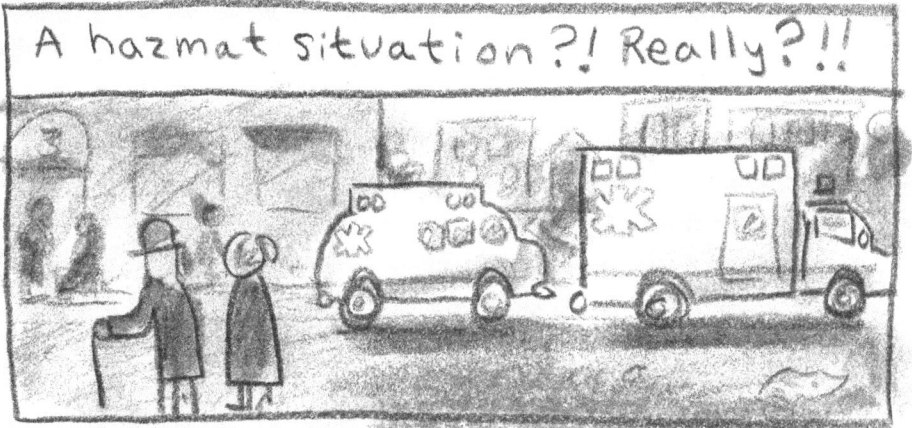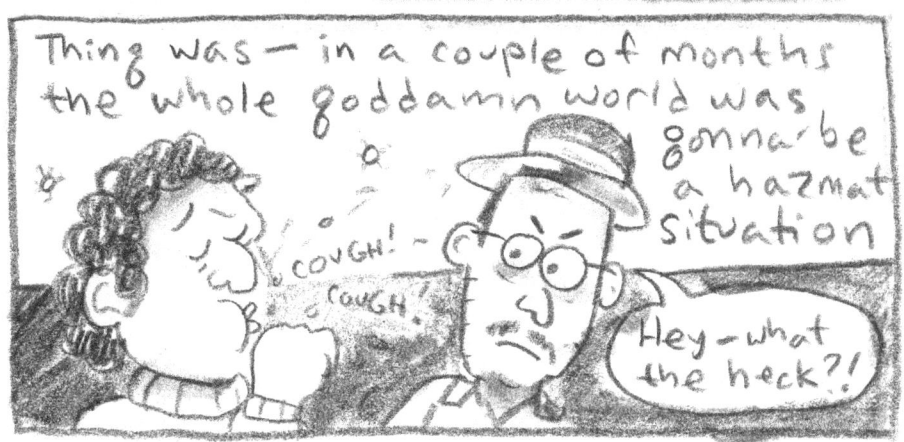

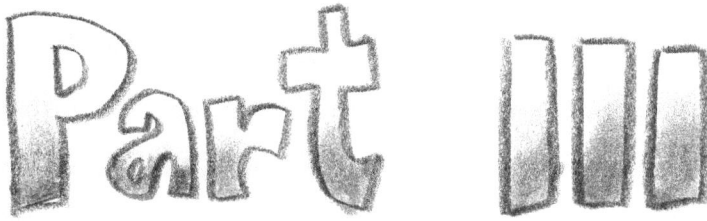

Part III

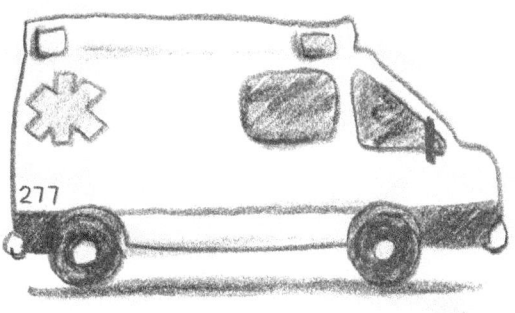

A New Normal

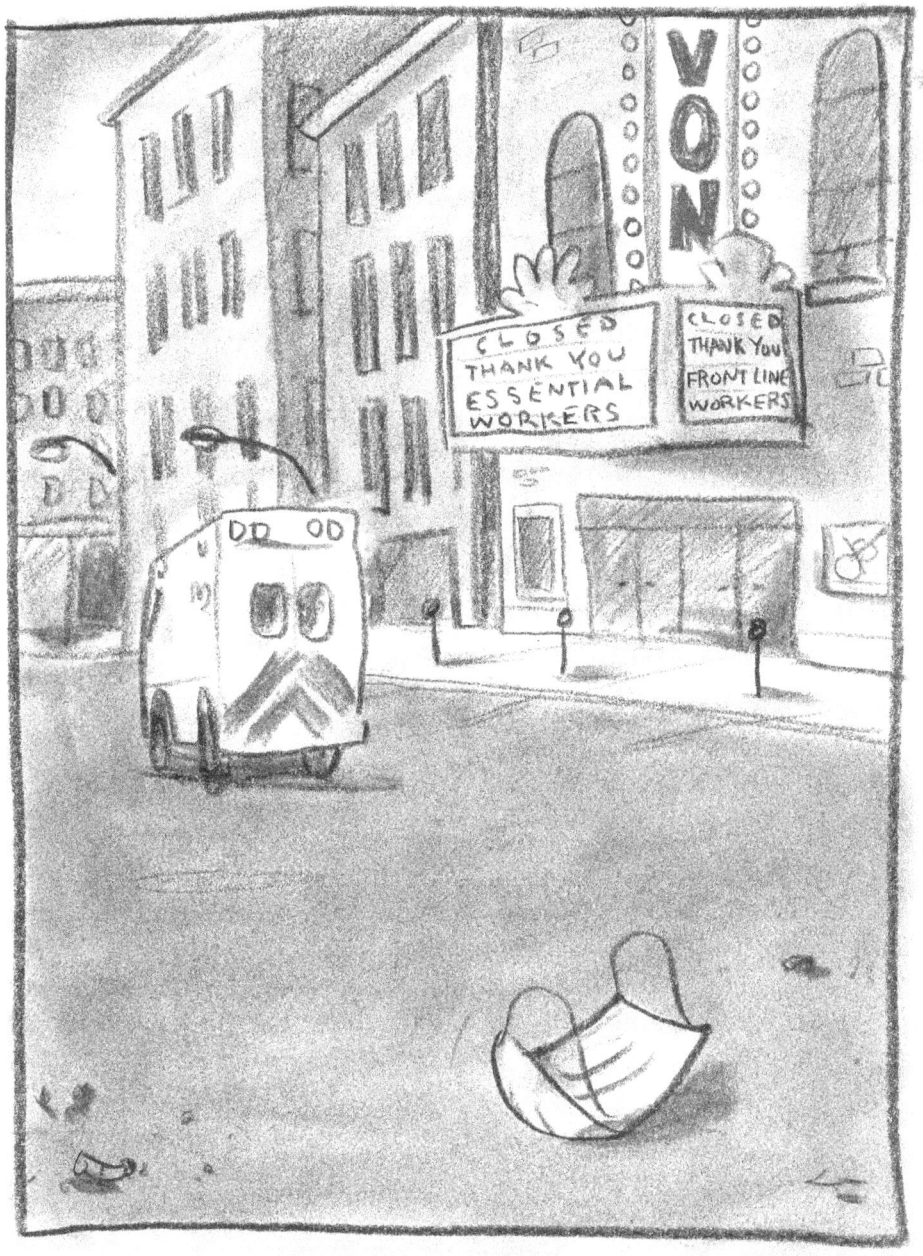

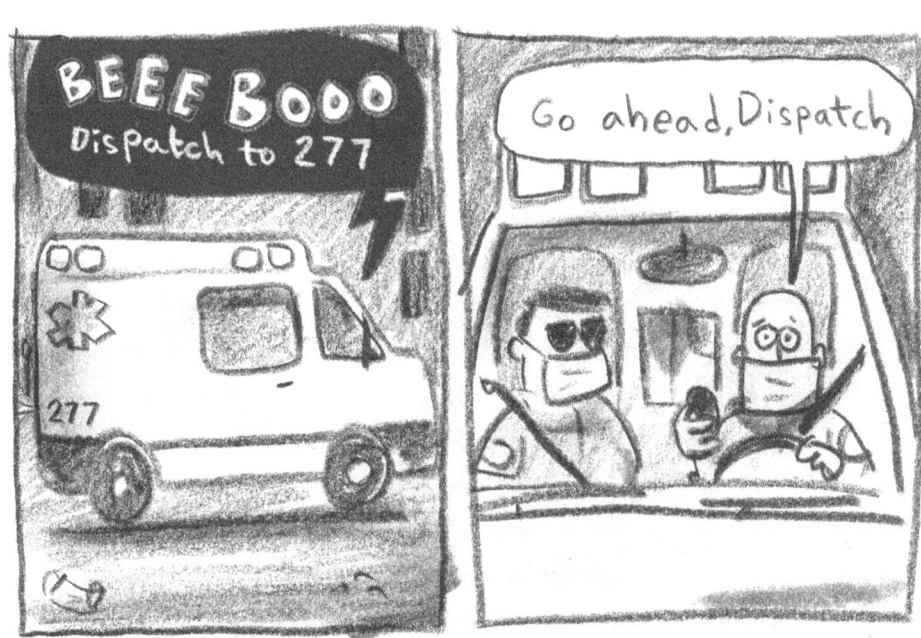

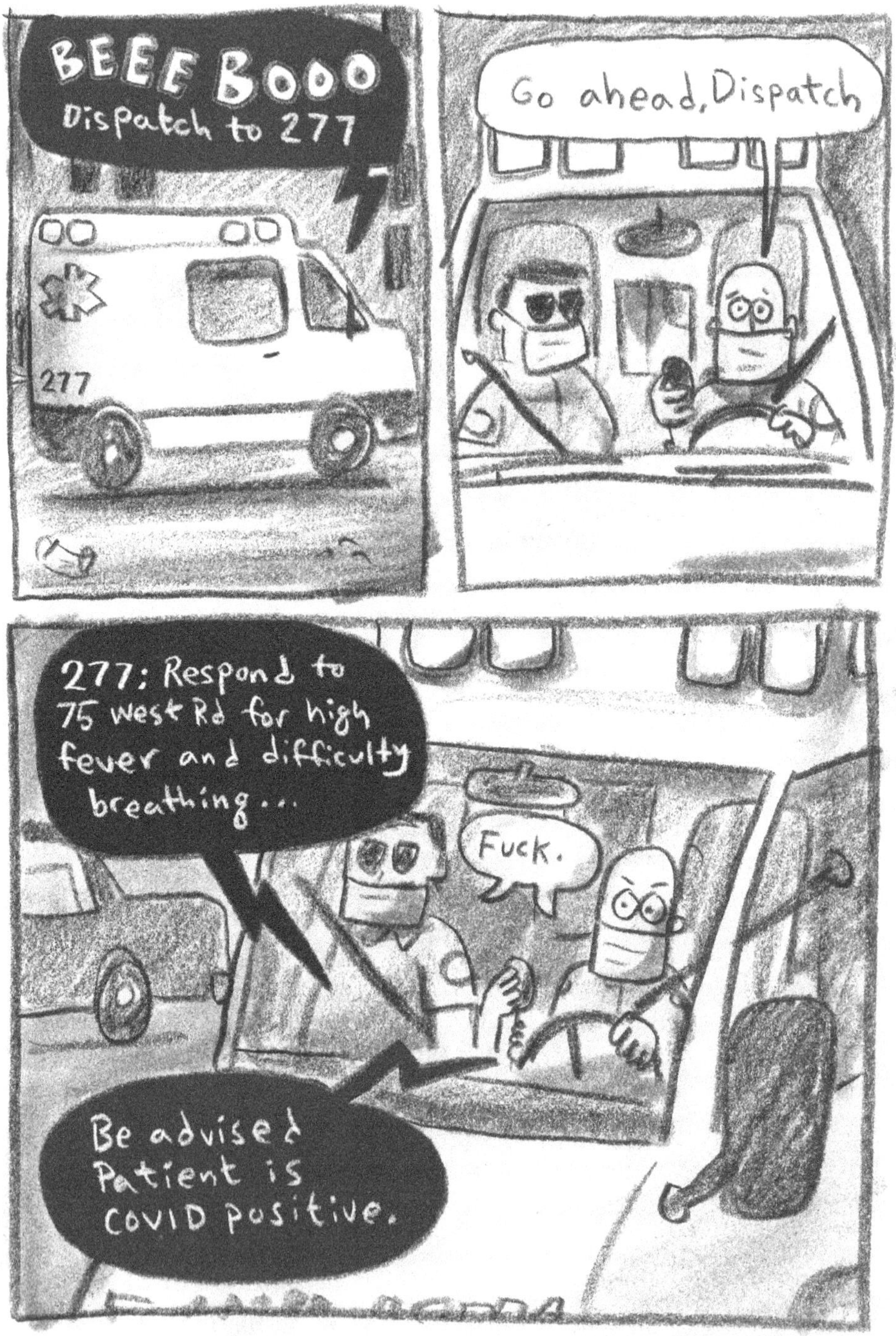

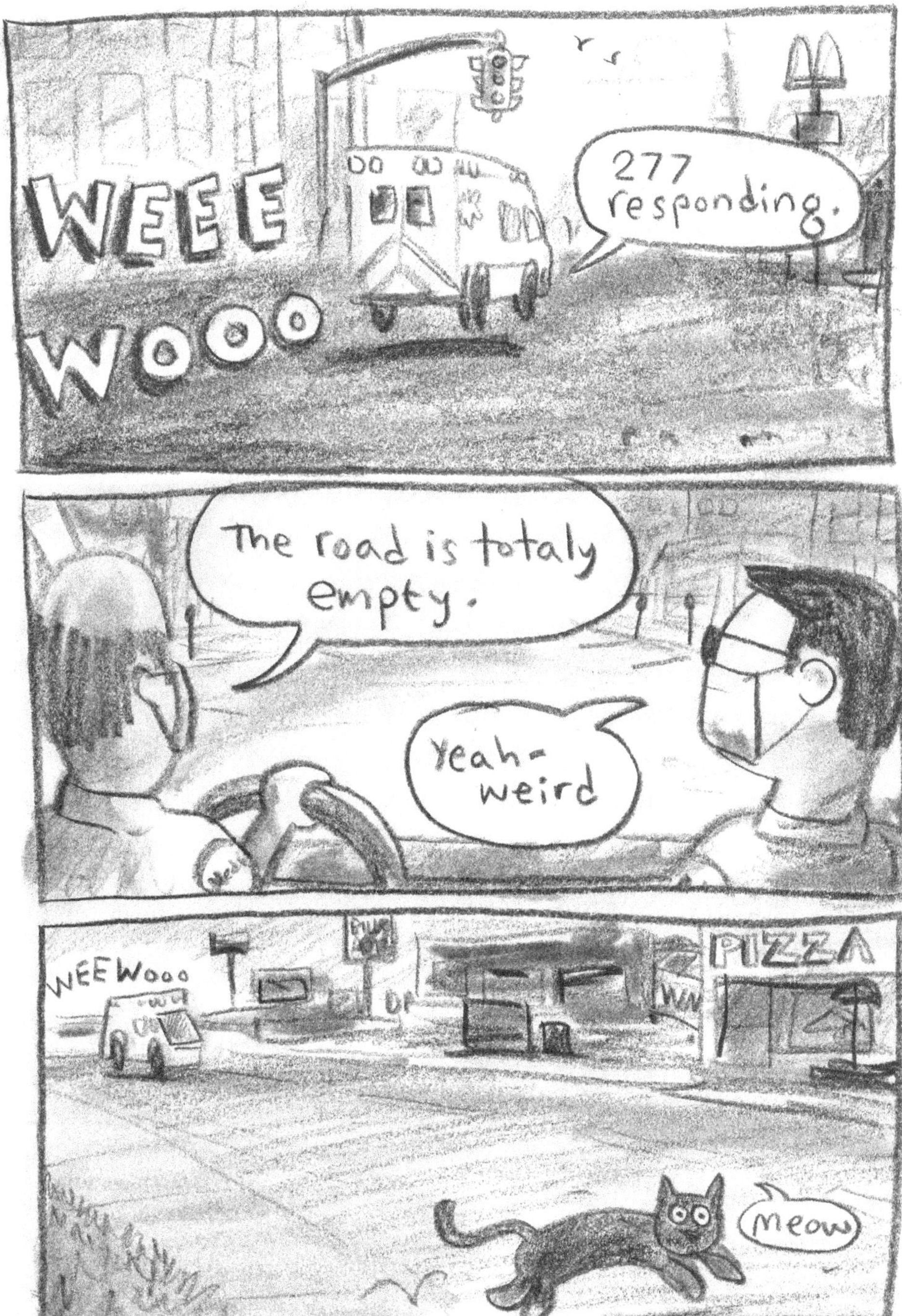

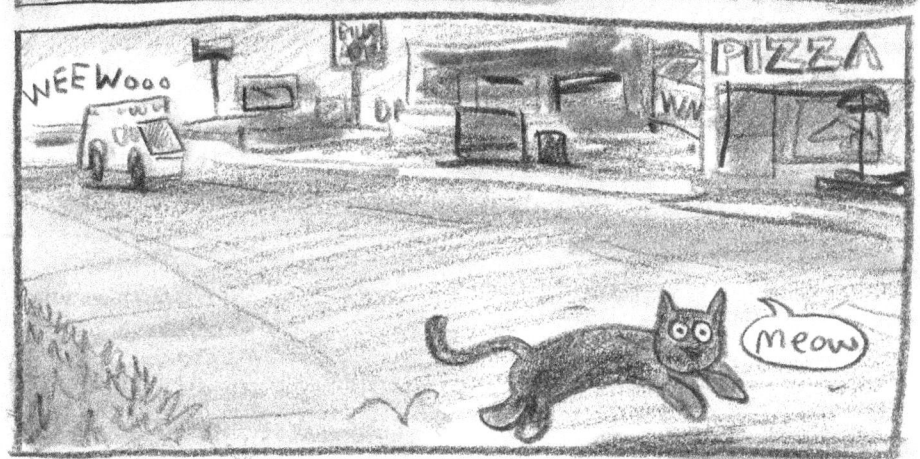

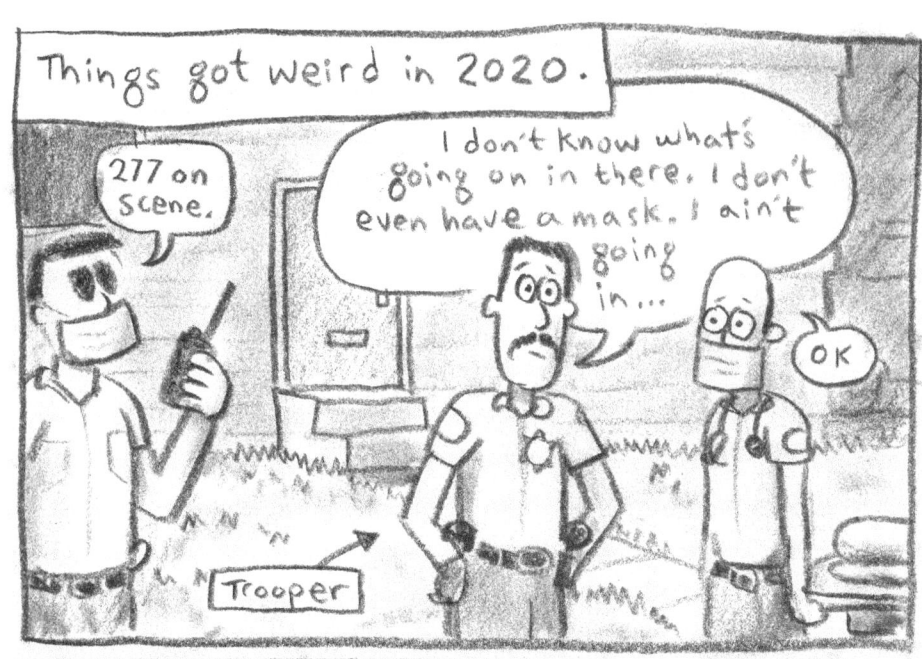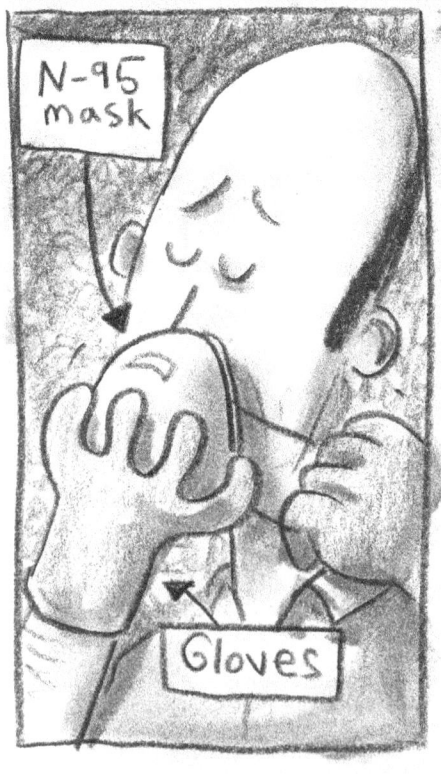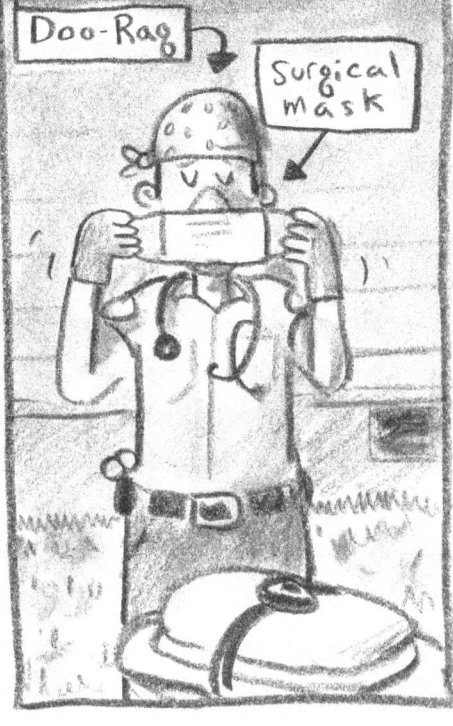

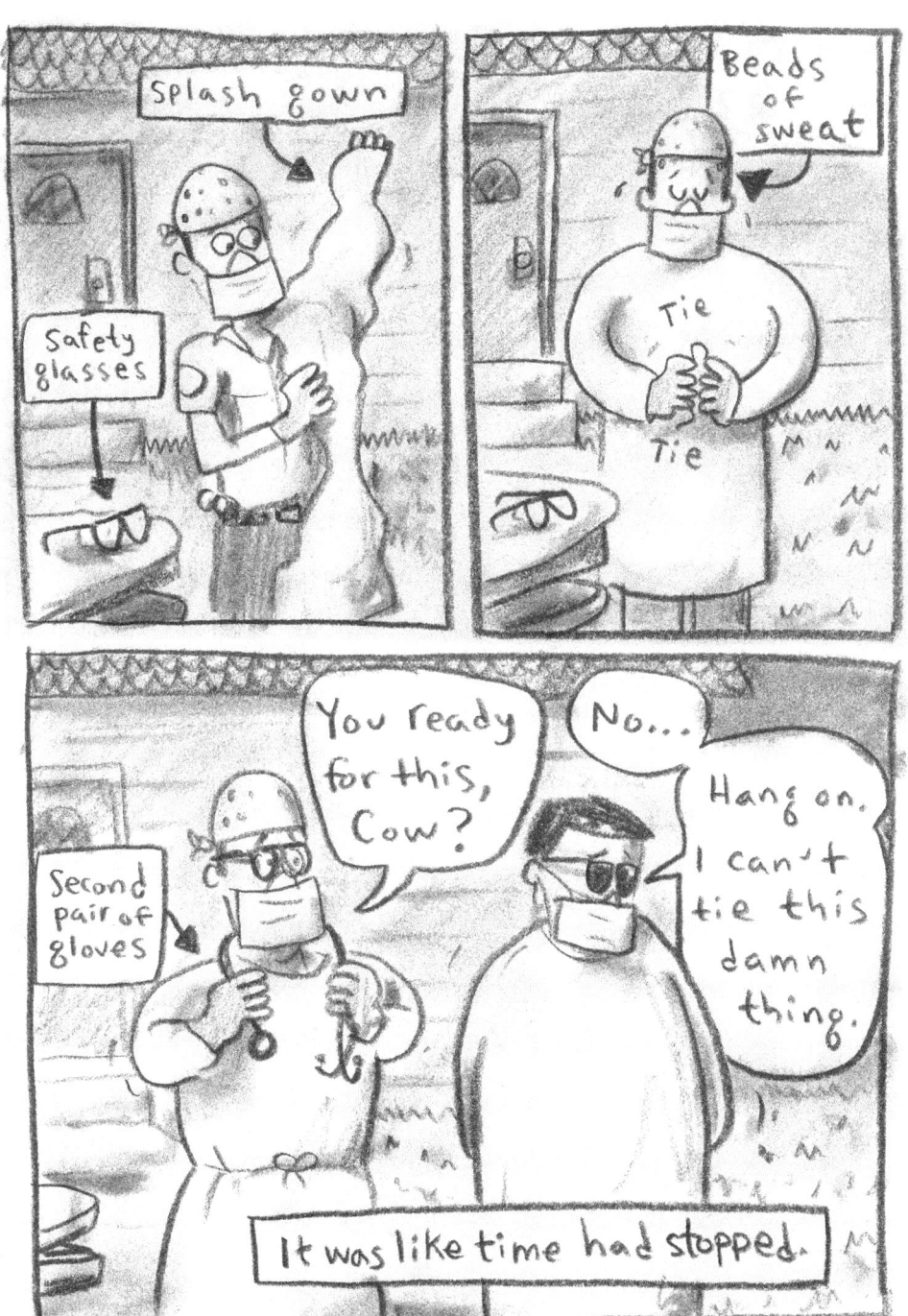

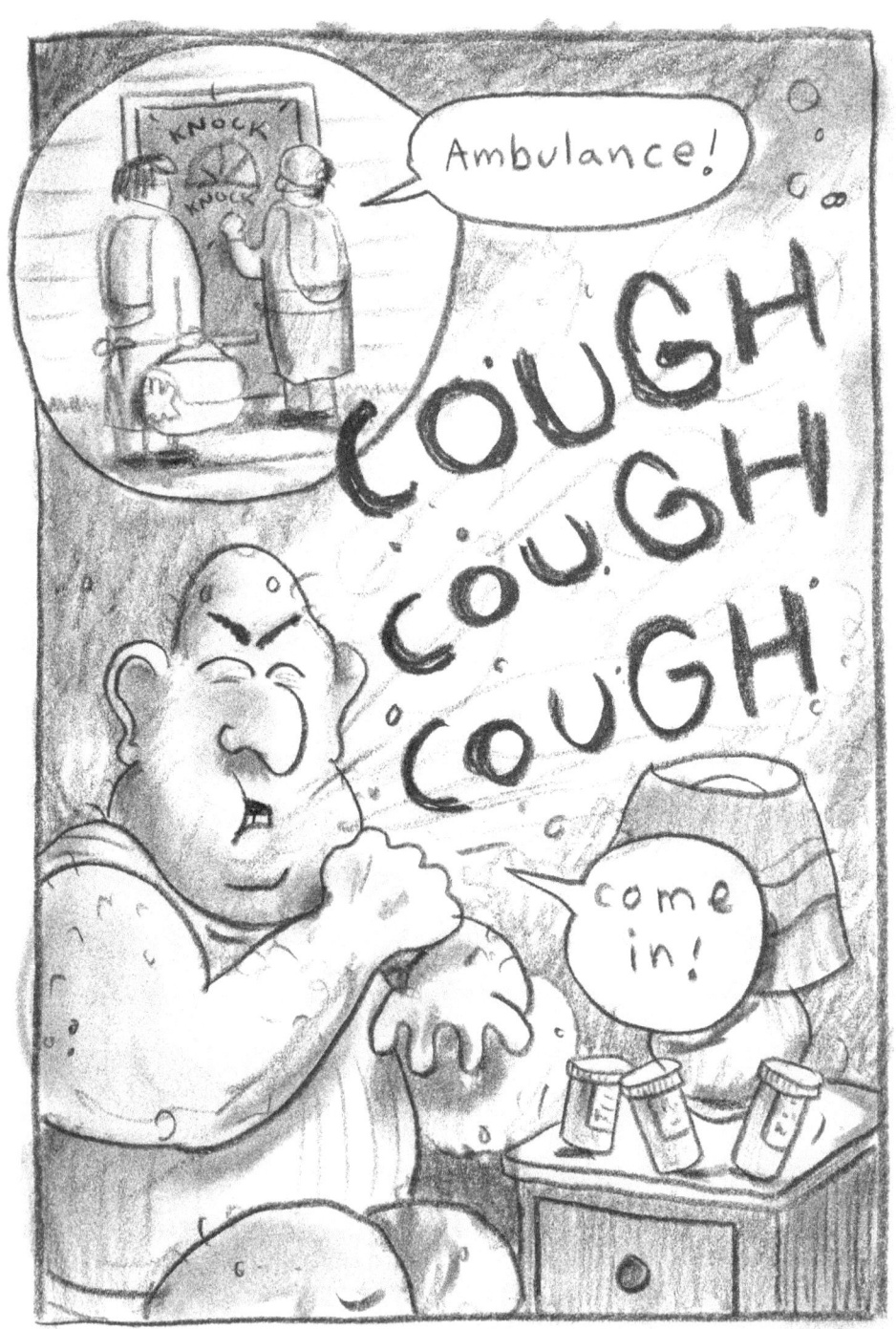

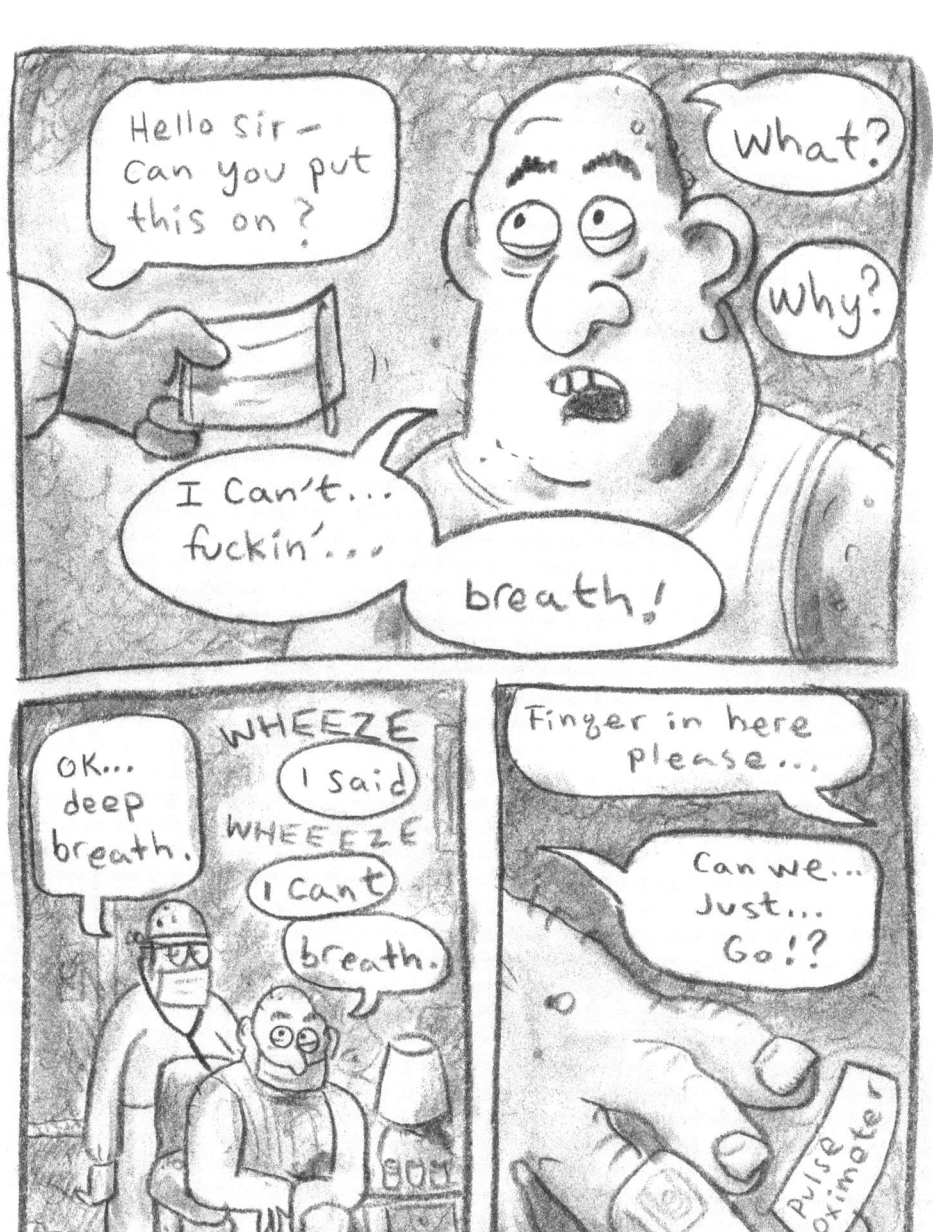

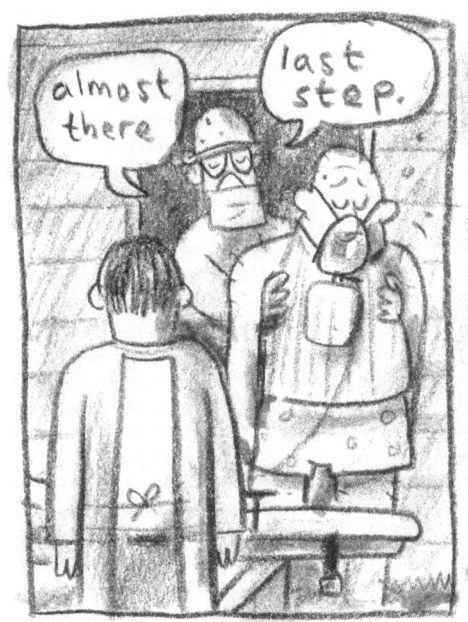
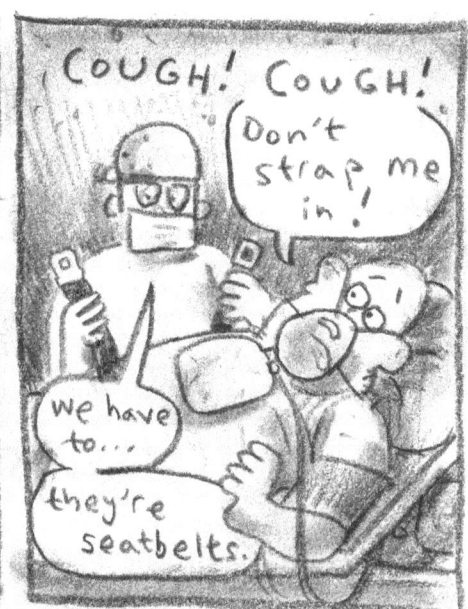

COVID made everything slightly harder.

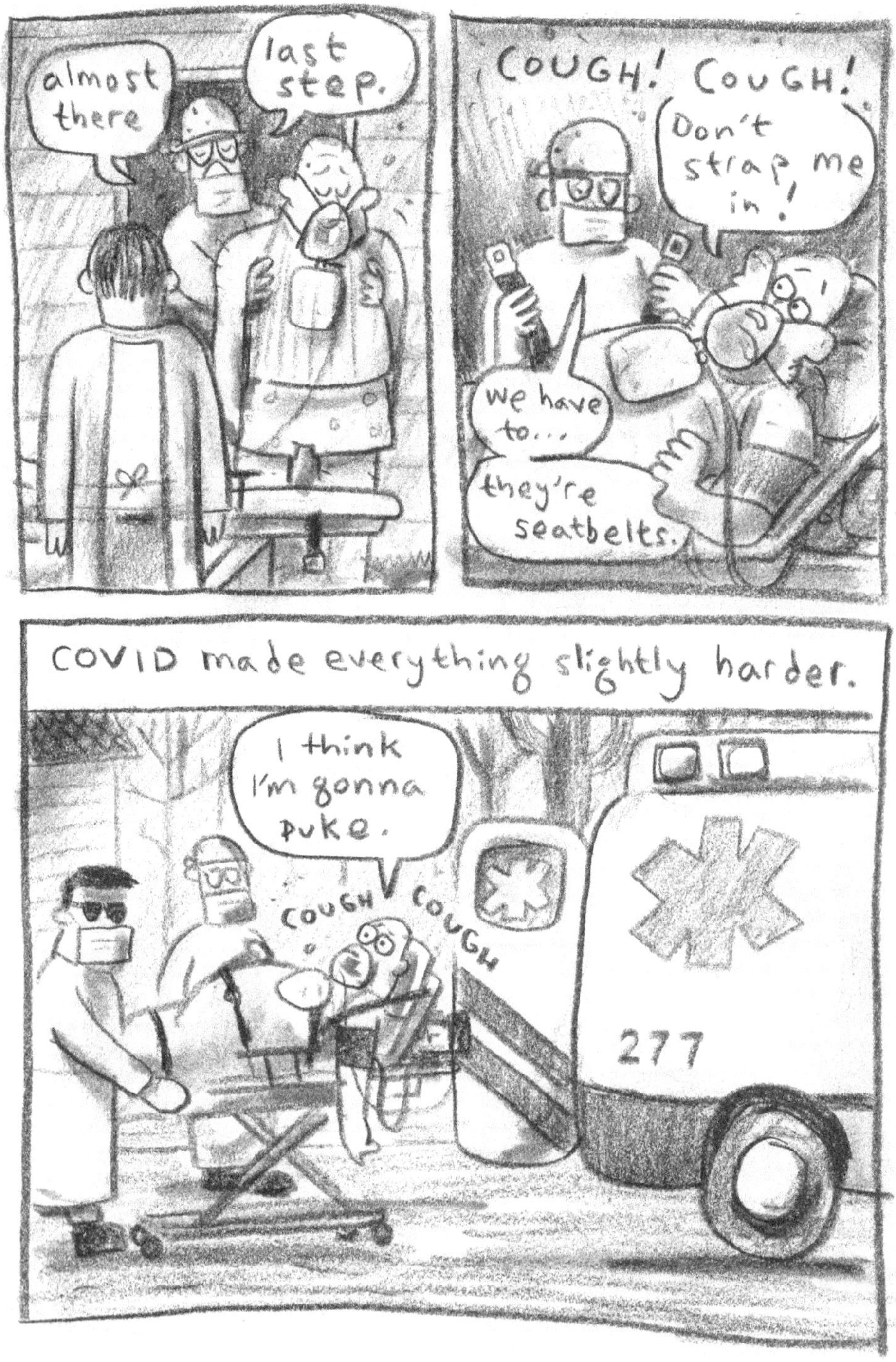

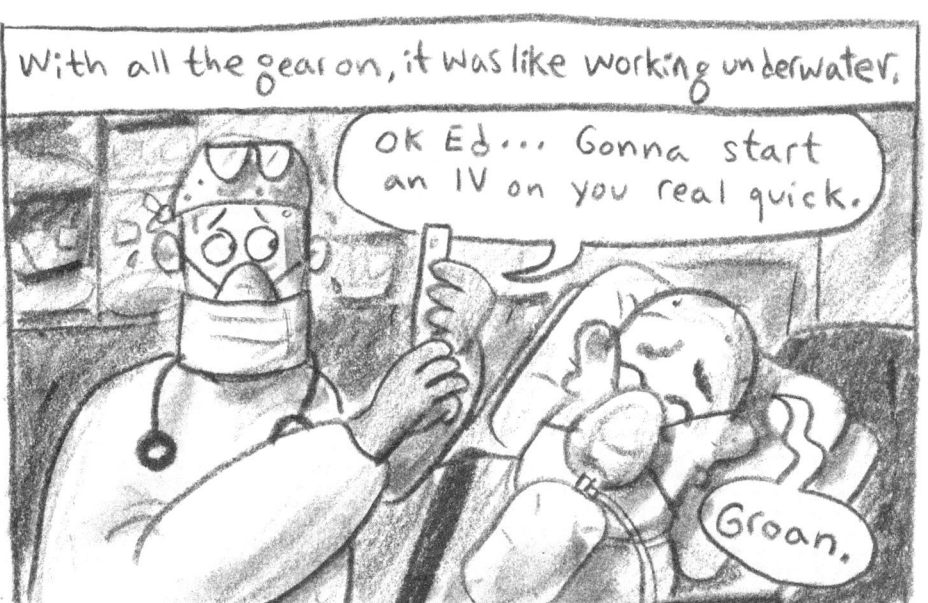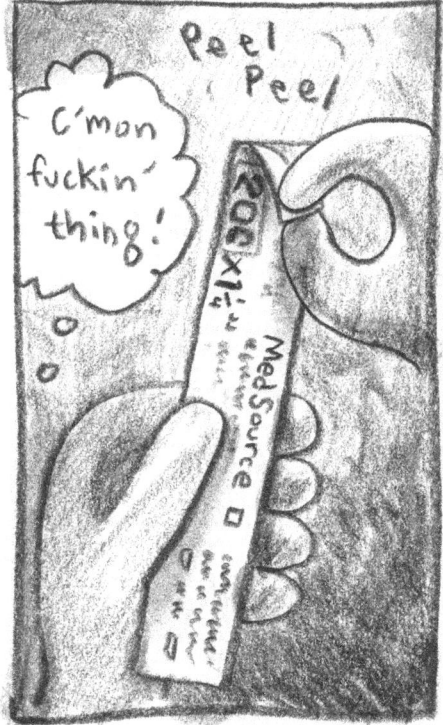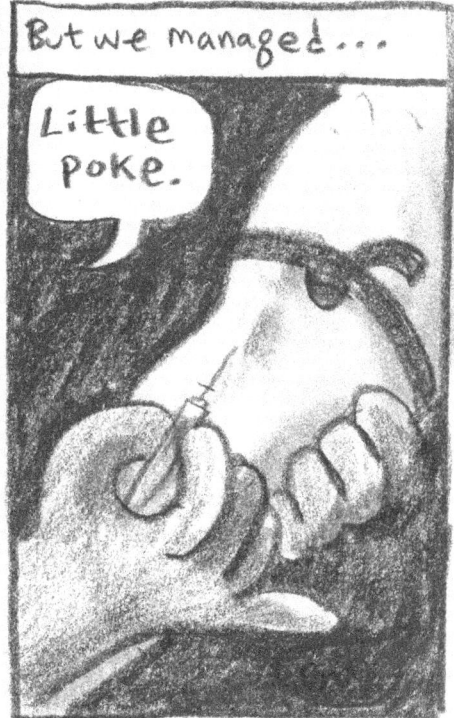

Excess Death

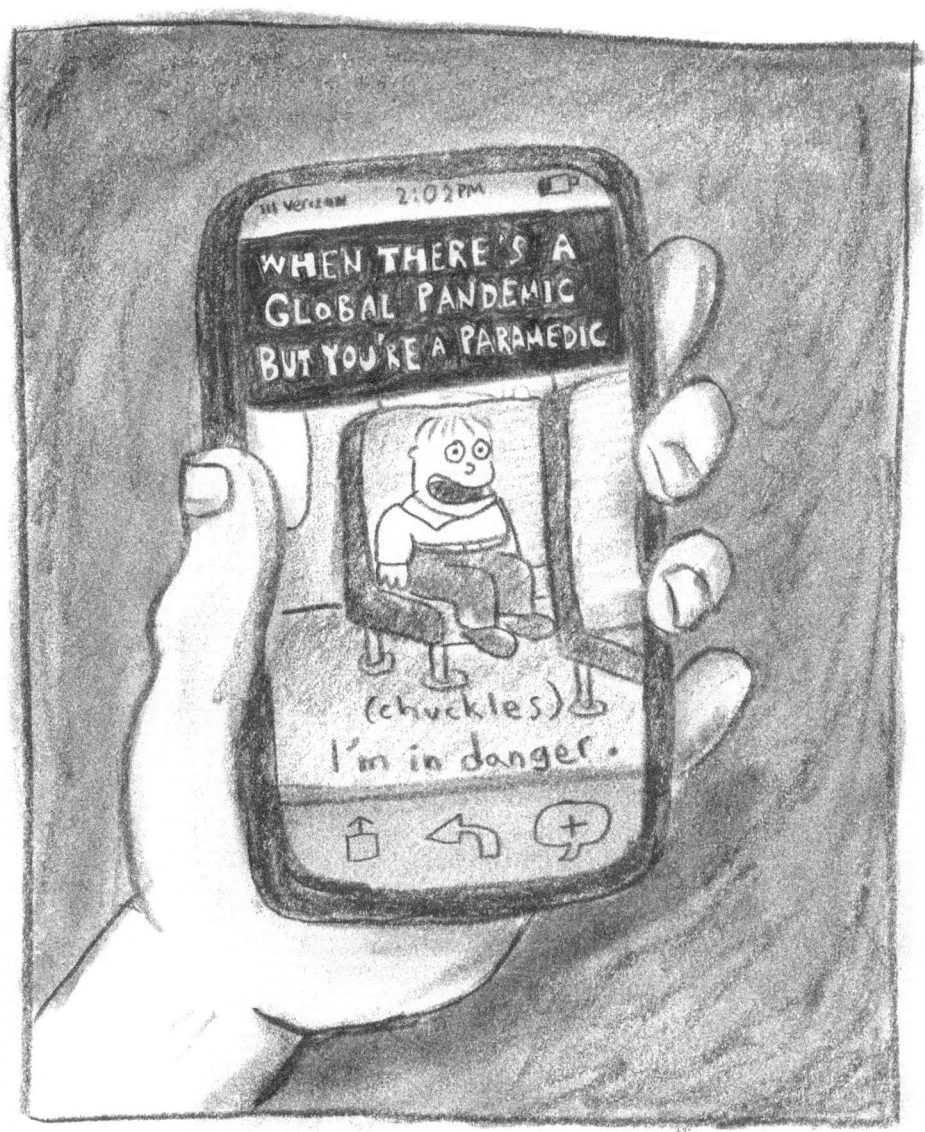

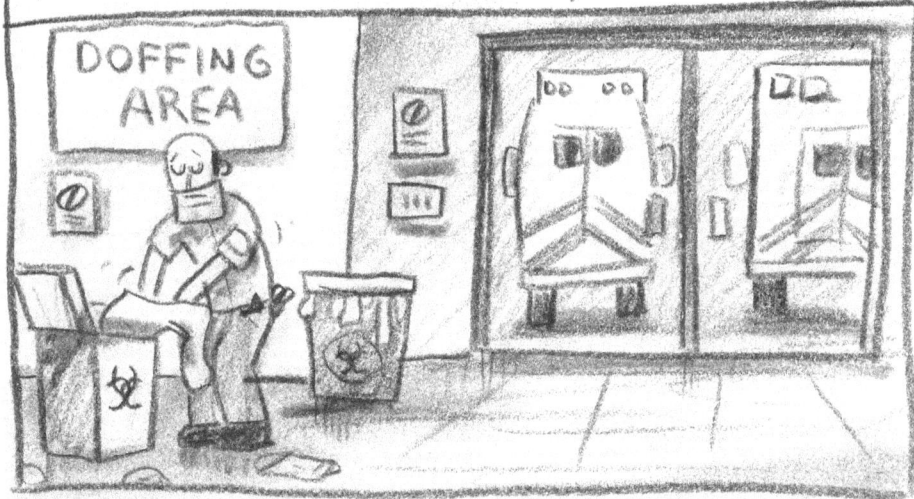

COVID calls did not end with turning over patient care at the hospital.

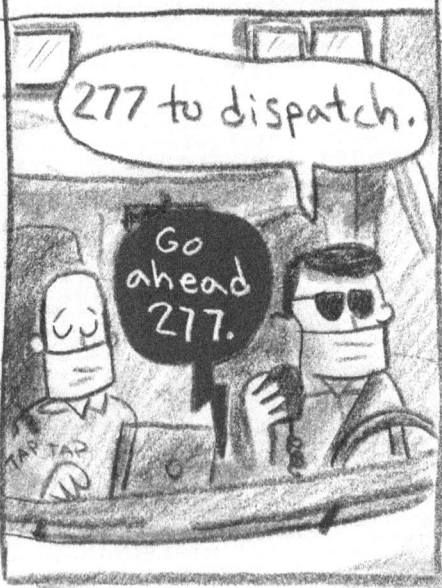

Everything on the rig was considered contaminated.

"277 to dispatch."

"Go ahead 277."

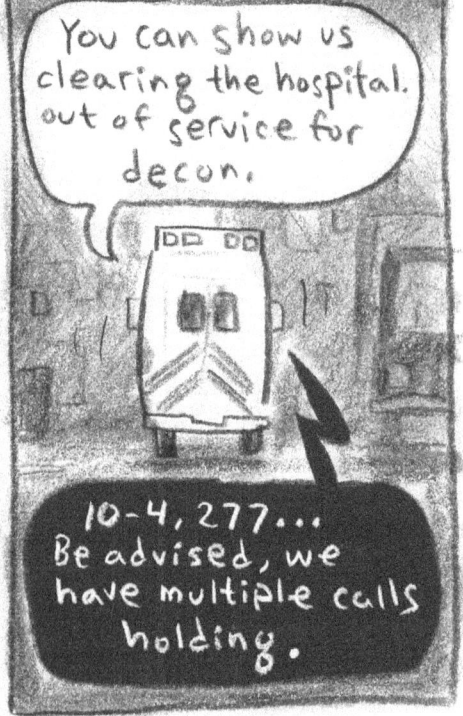

"You can show us clearing the hospital. Out of service for decon."

"10-4, 277... Be advised, we have multiple calls holding."

Decon-ing a truck was a colossal pain in the ass.

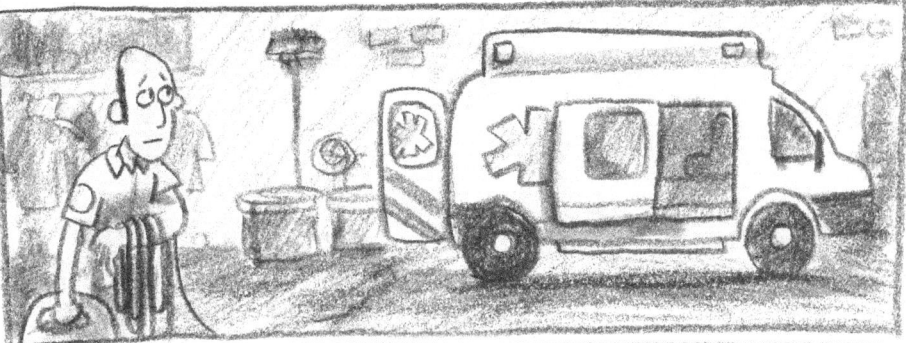

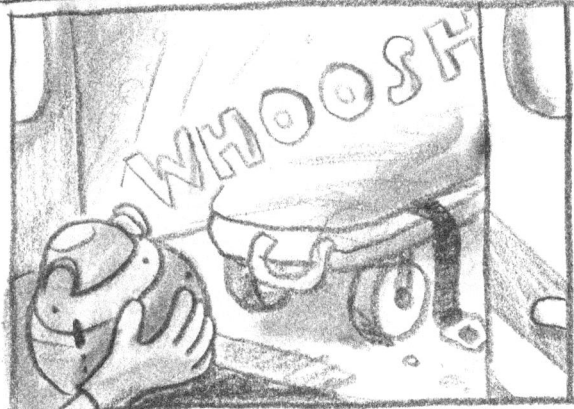

We used a fogging machine to marinate the patient compartment with some chemical called Lemocide.

I wonder what the long-term effect of that will be. Anyway, it was nice to catch a "break" for 20 minutes.

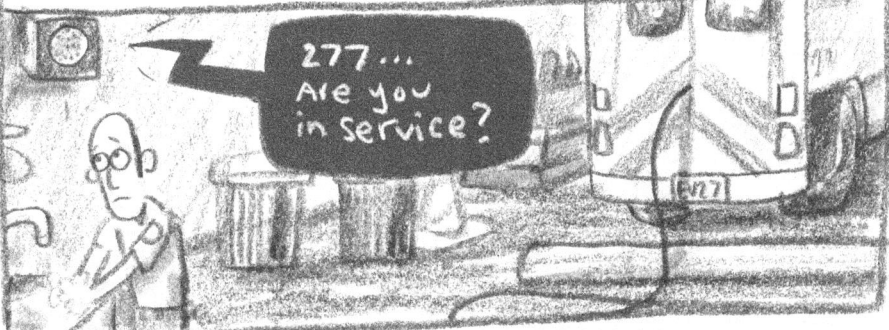

277... Are you in service?

The volume of calls had dropped — but you wouldn't know it.

"277 back in."

All the gearing up and decon-ing made calls take longer.

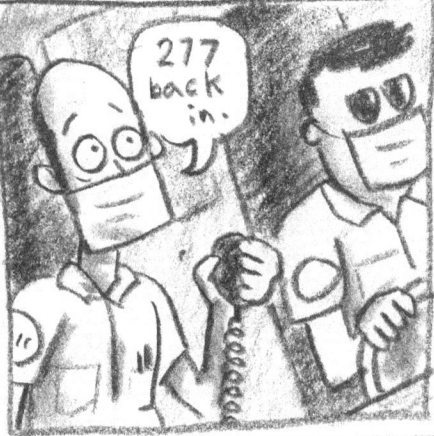

277: Respond to 14 Harper Road for adult male, difficulty breathing with altered mental status.

EEE WOOOO

'77 responding

And even if there were fewer calls — most calls were high acuity.

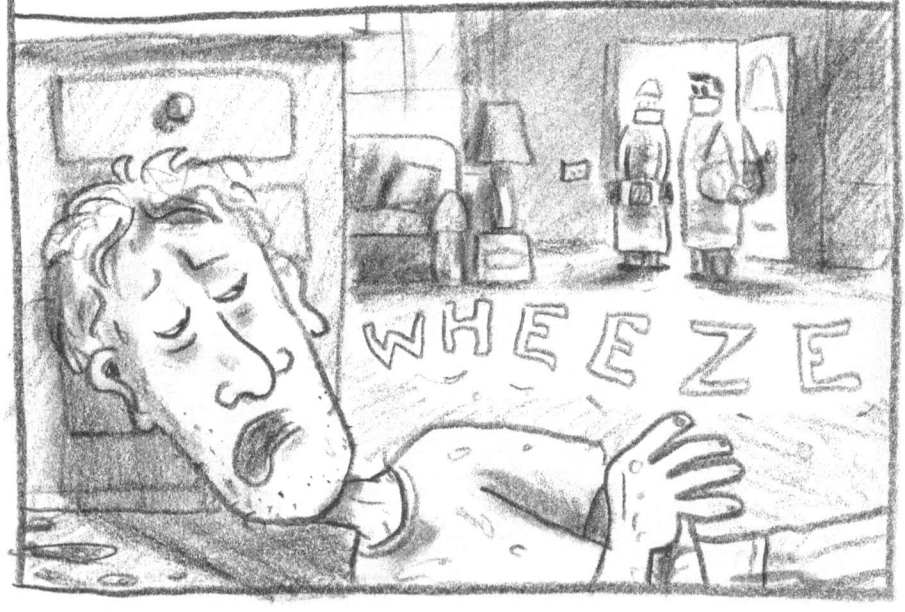

WHEEZE

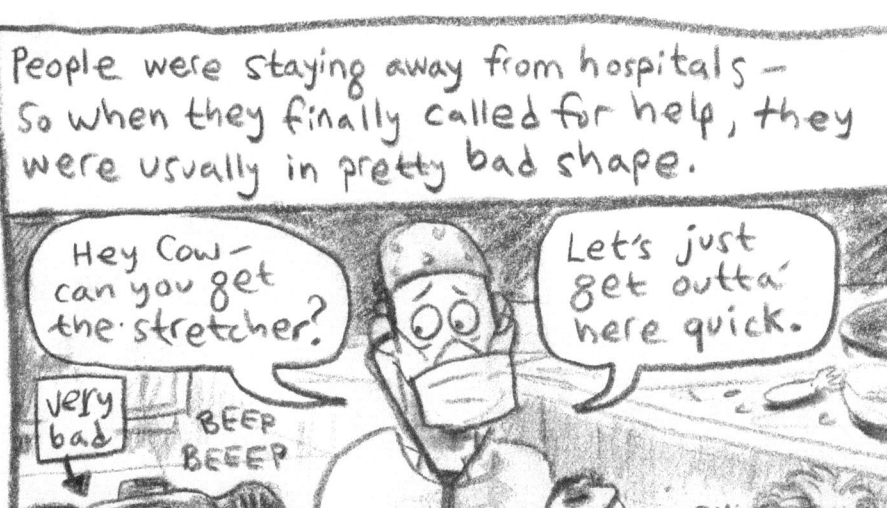

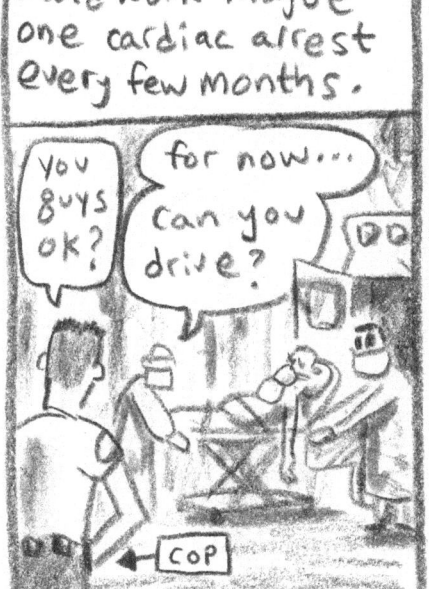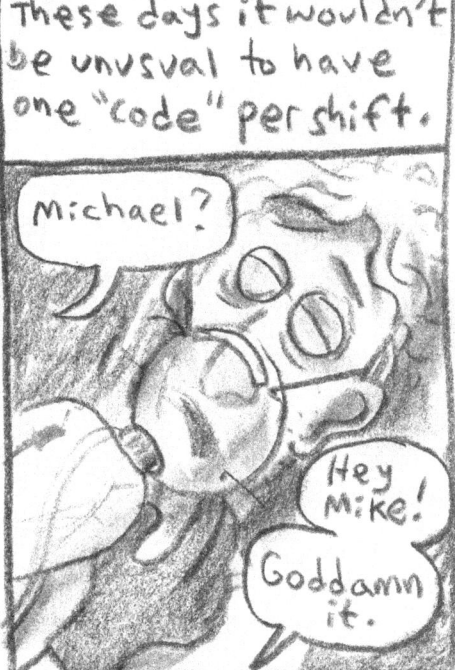

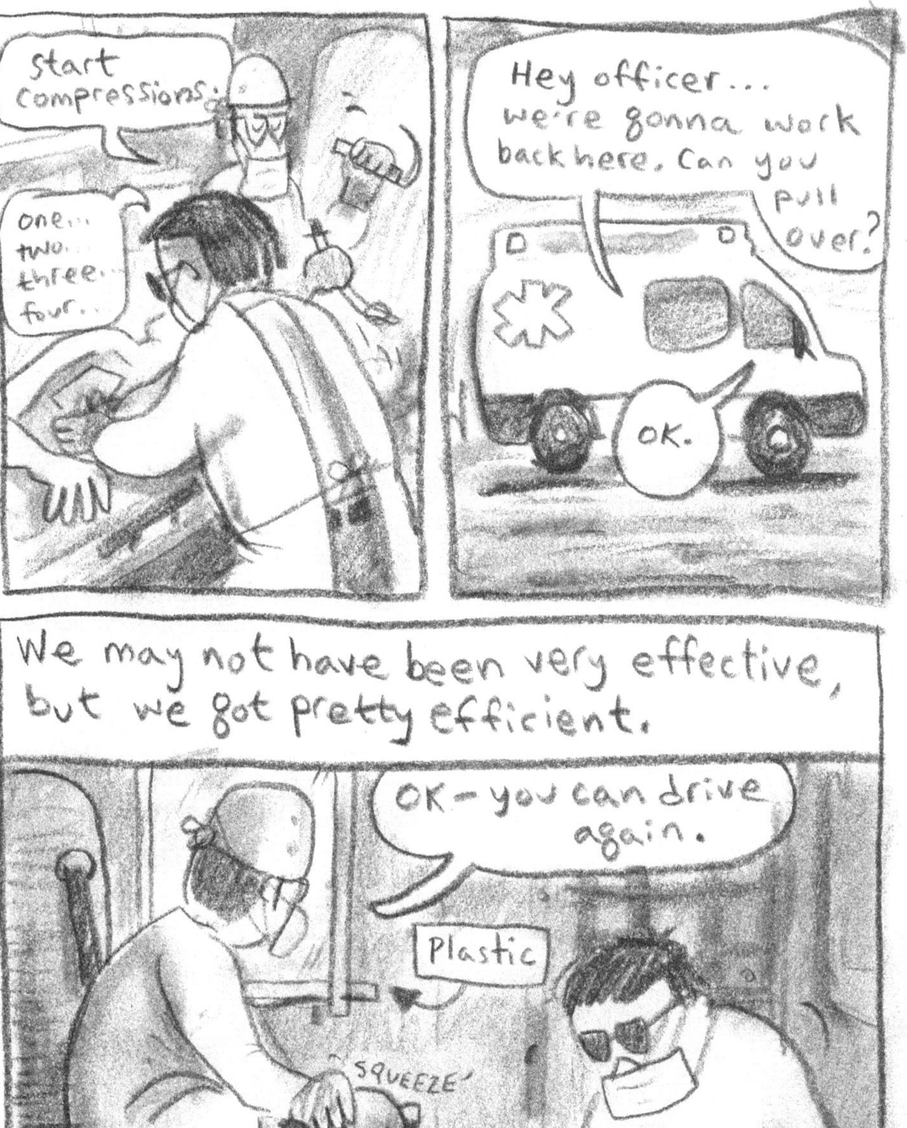

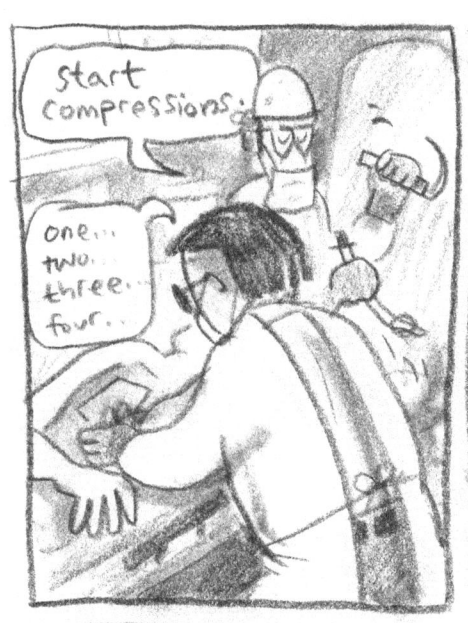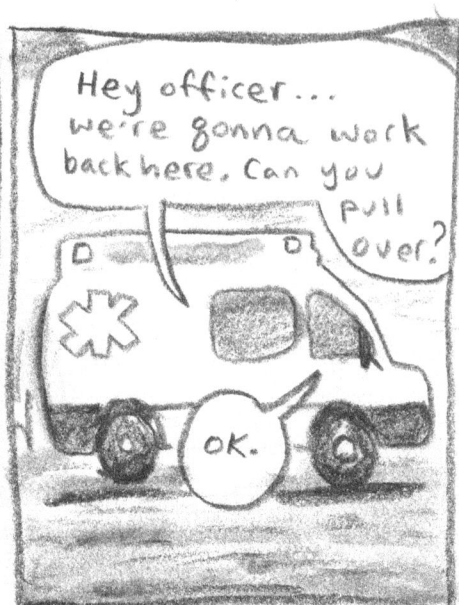

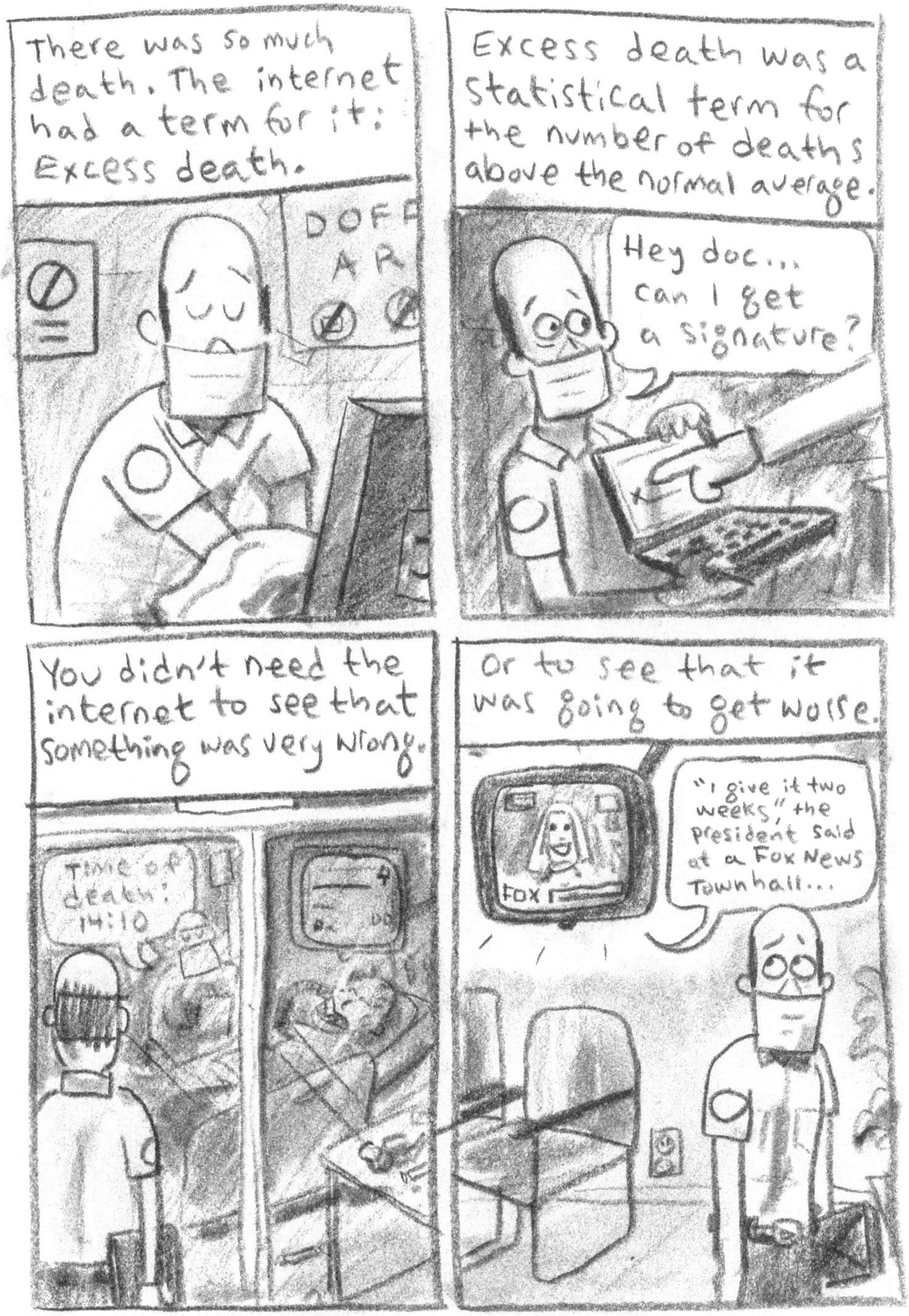

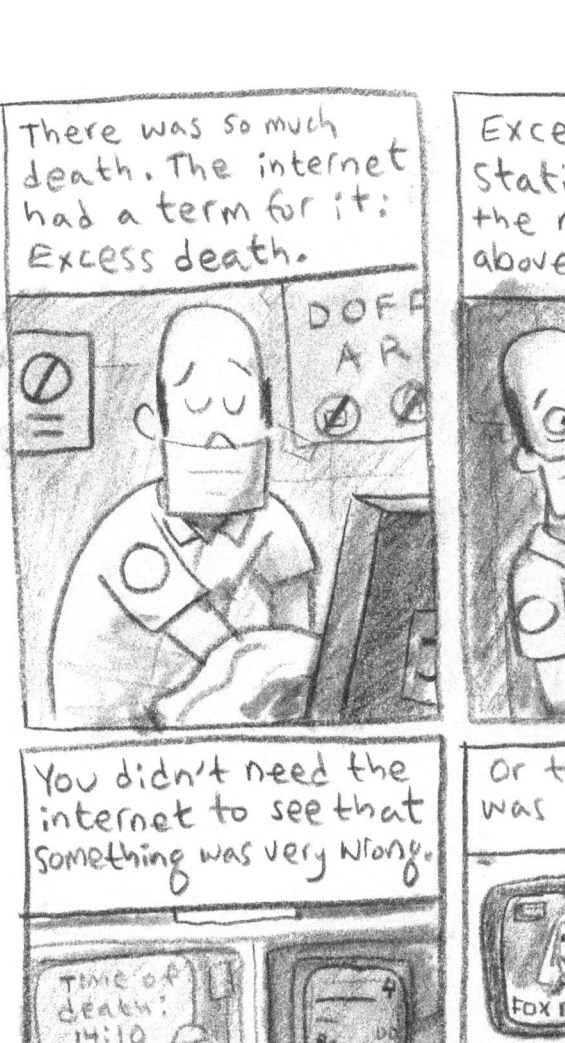

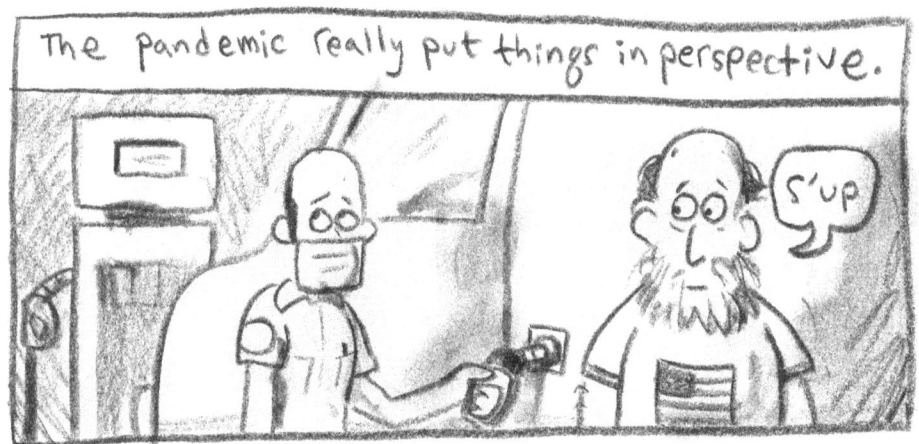

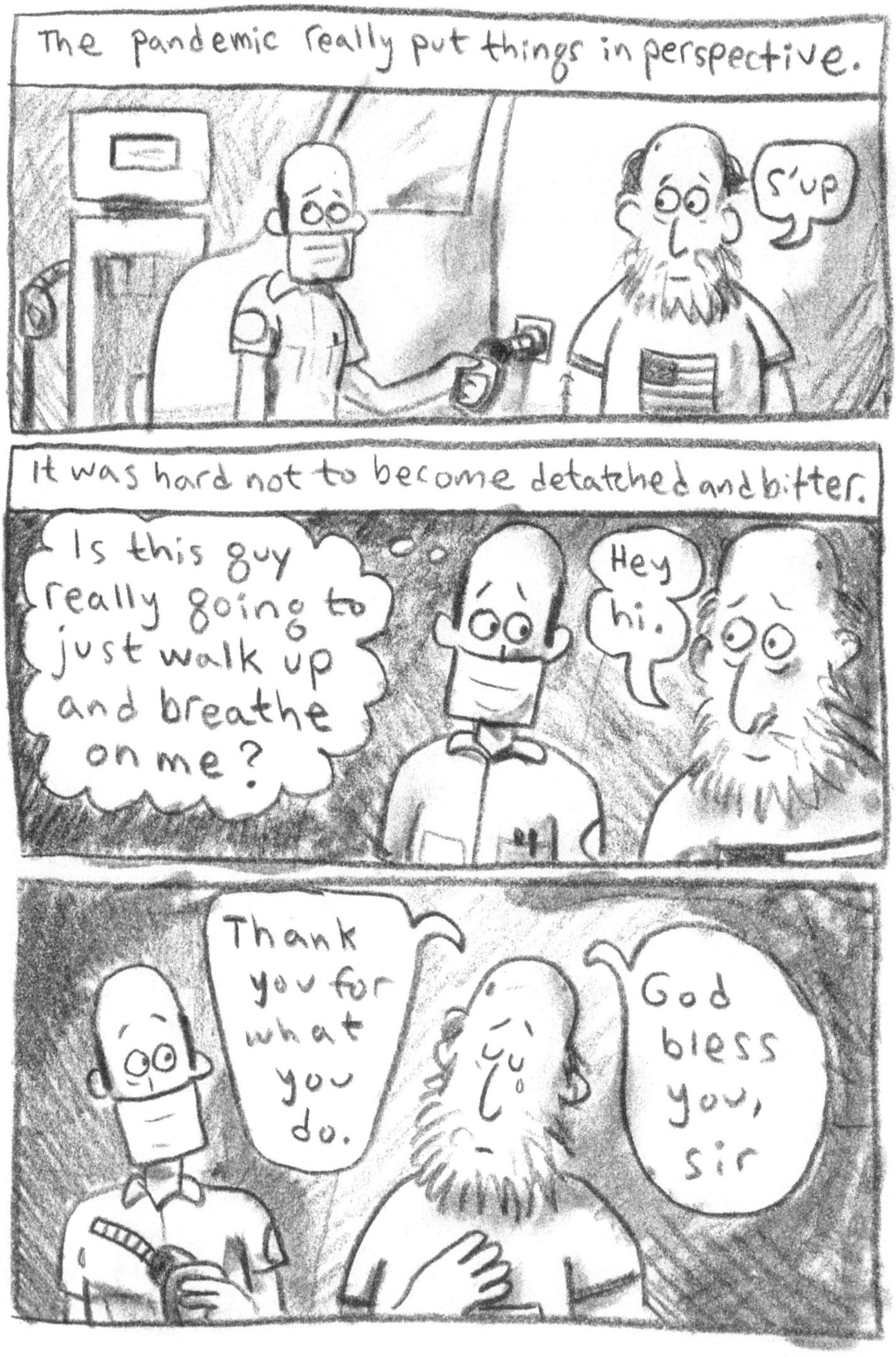

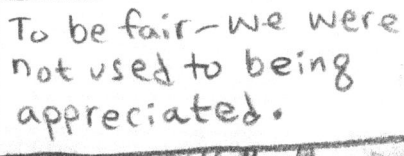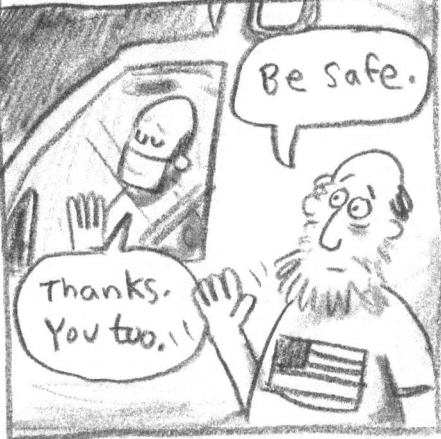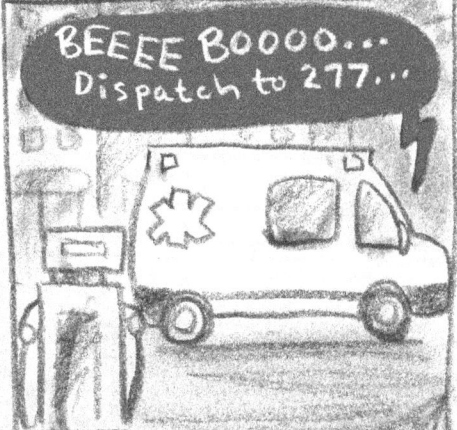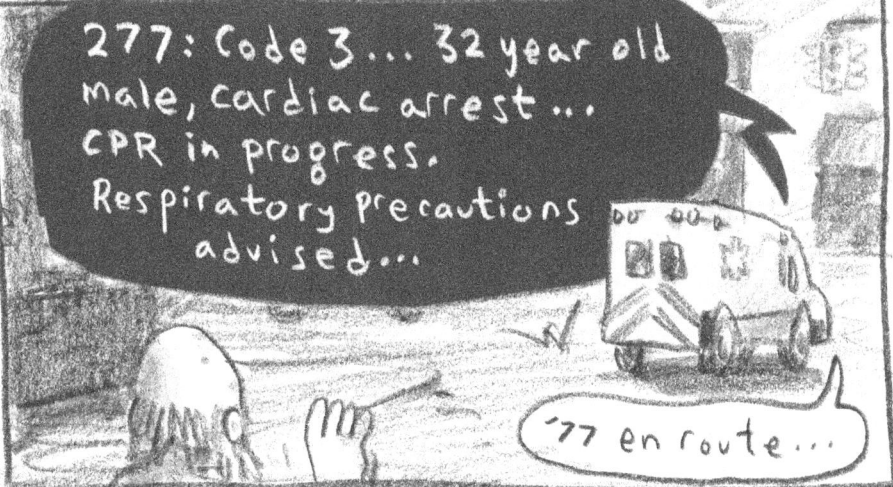

Anatomy of an Overdose

One type of call we saw a lot more of during the pandemic was overdoses.

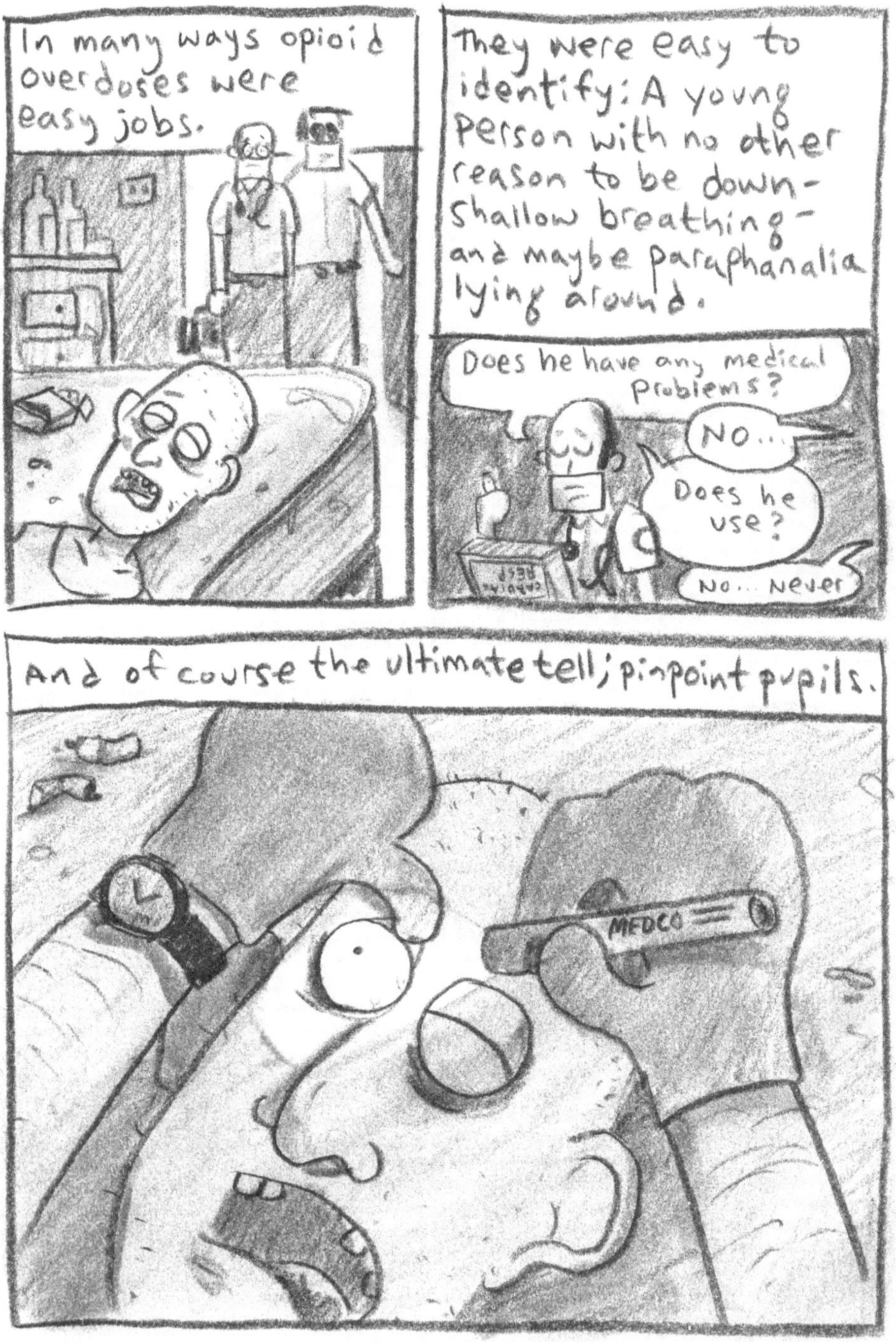

In many ways opioid overdoses were easy jobs.

They were easy to identify: A young person with no other reason to be down- shallow breathing- and maybe paraphanalia lying around.

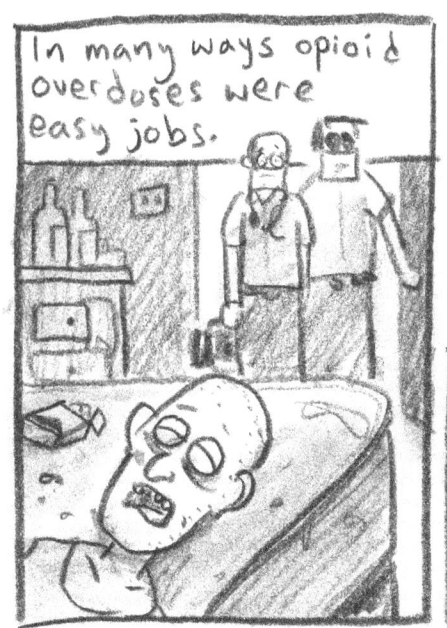

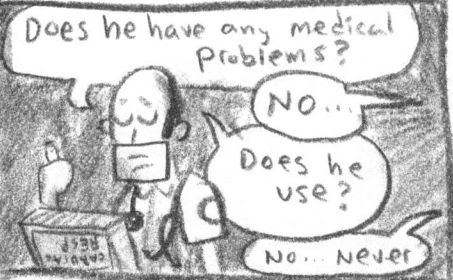

"Does he have any medical problems?"

"NO..."

"Does he use?"

"No... Never"

And of course the ultimate tell; pinpoint pupils.

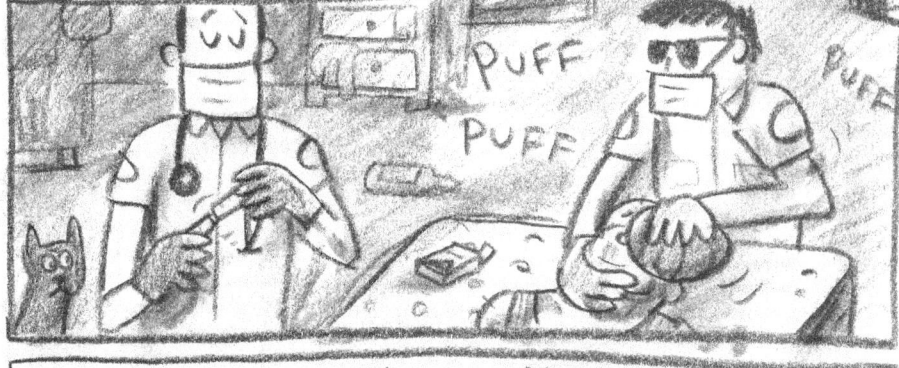

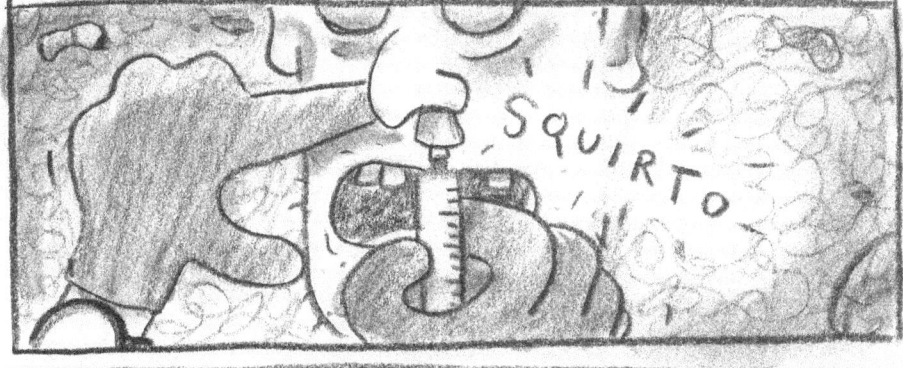

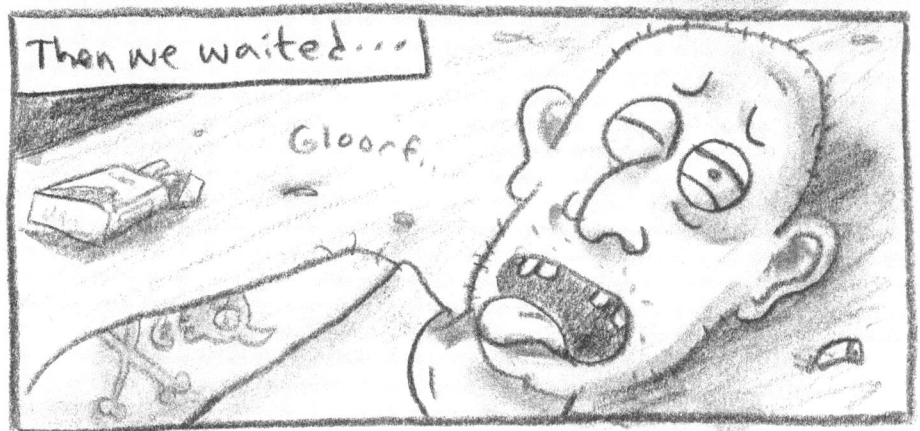

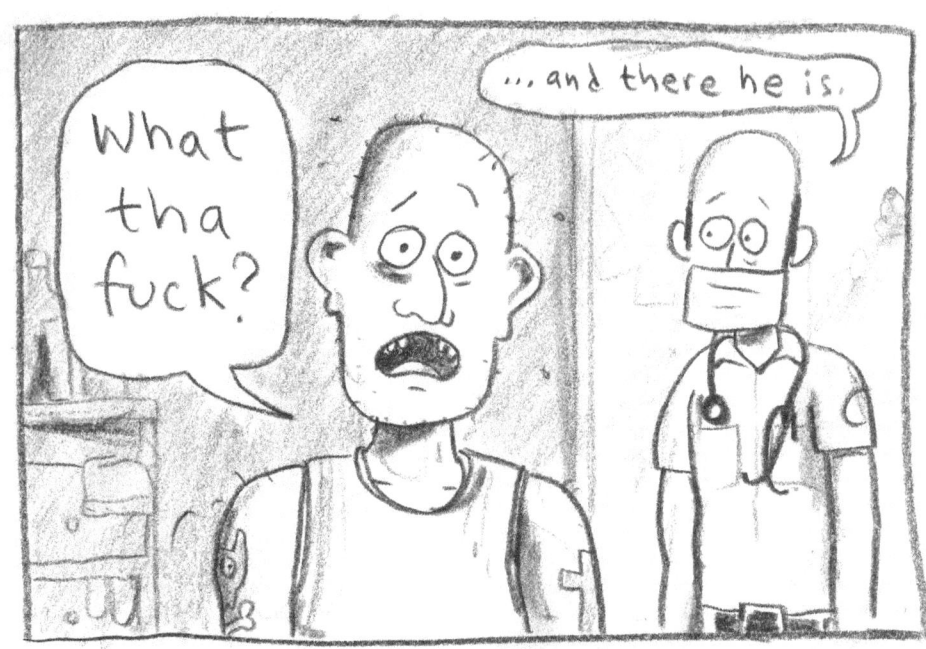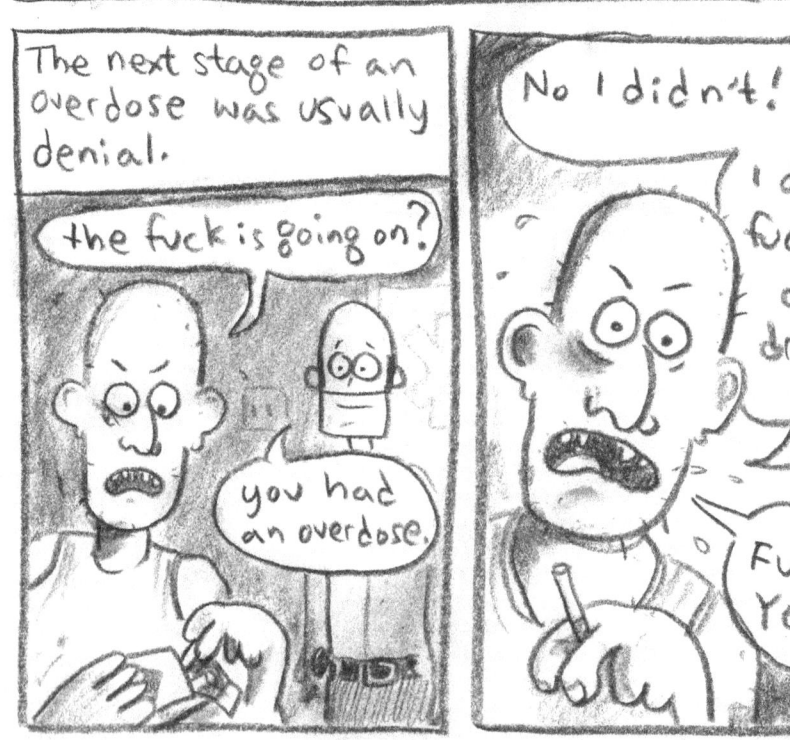

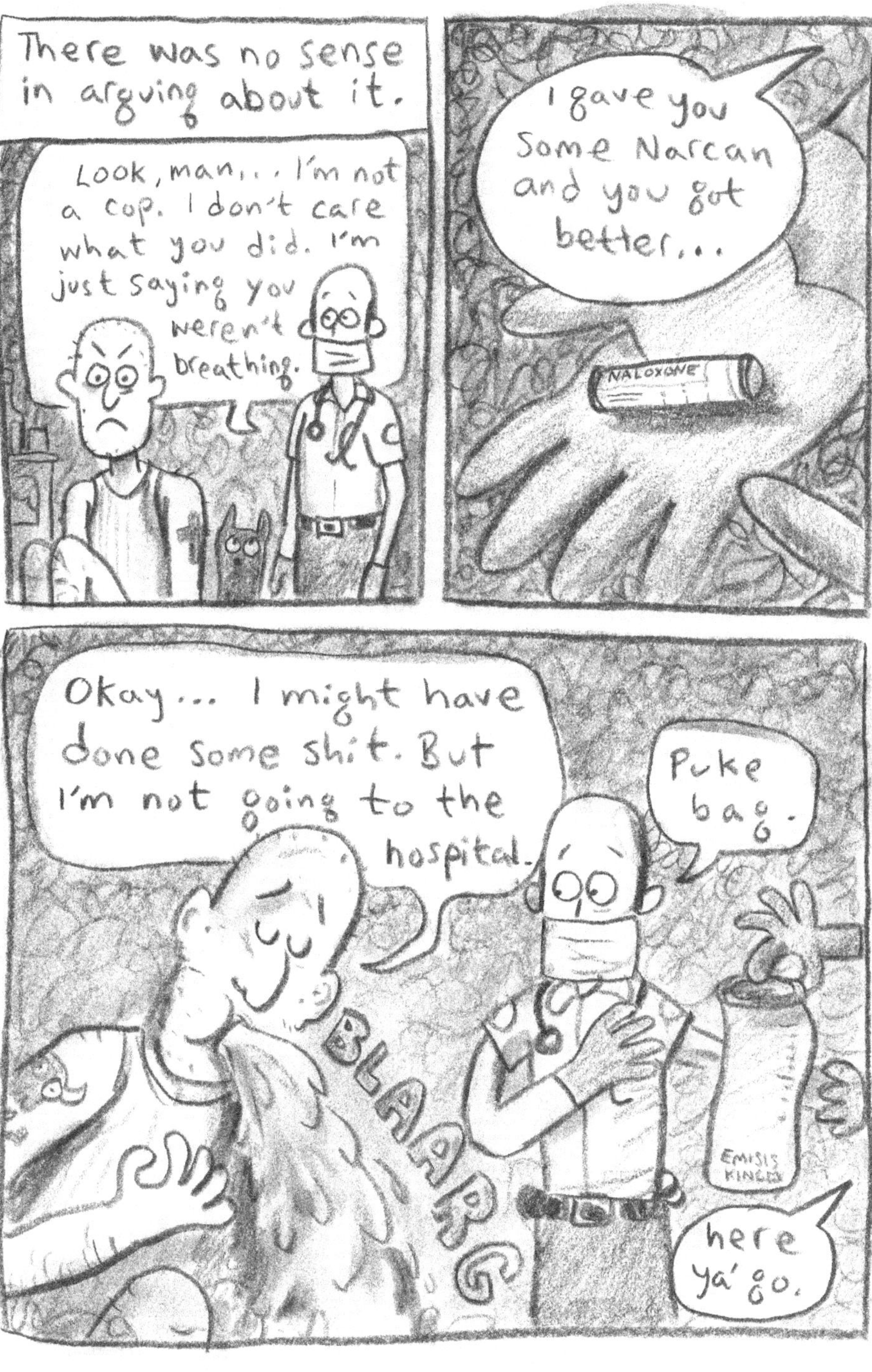

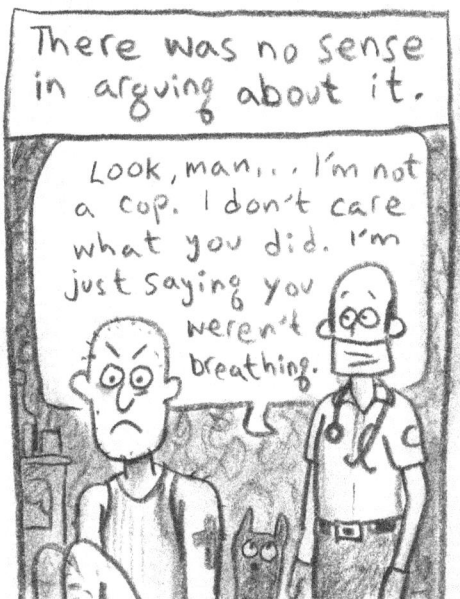
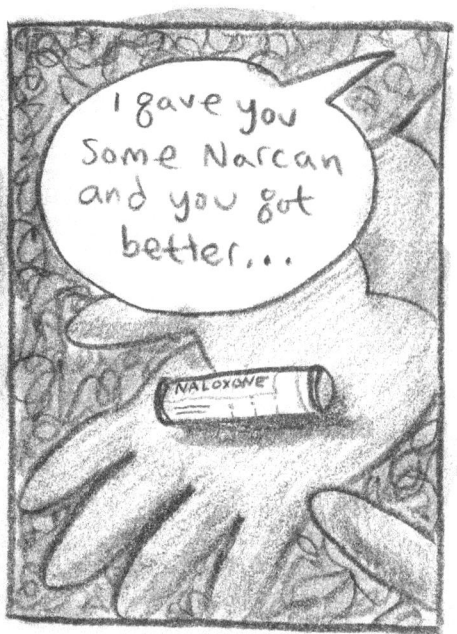

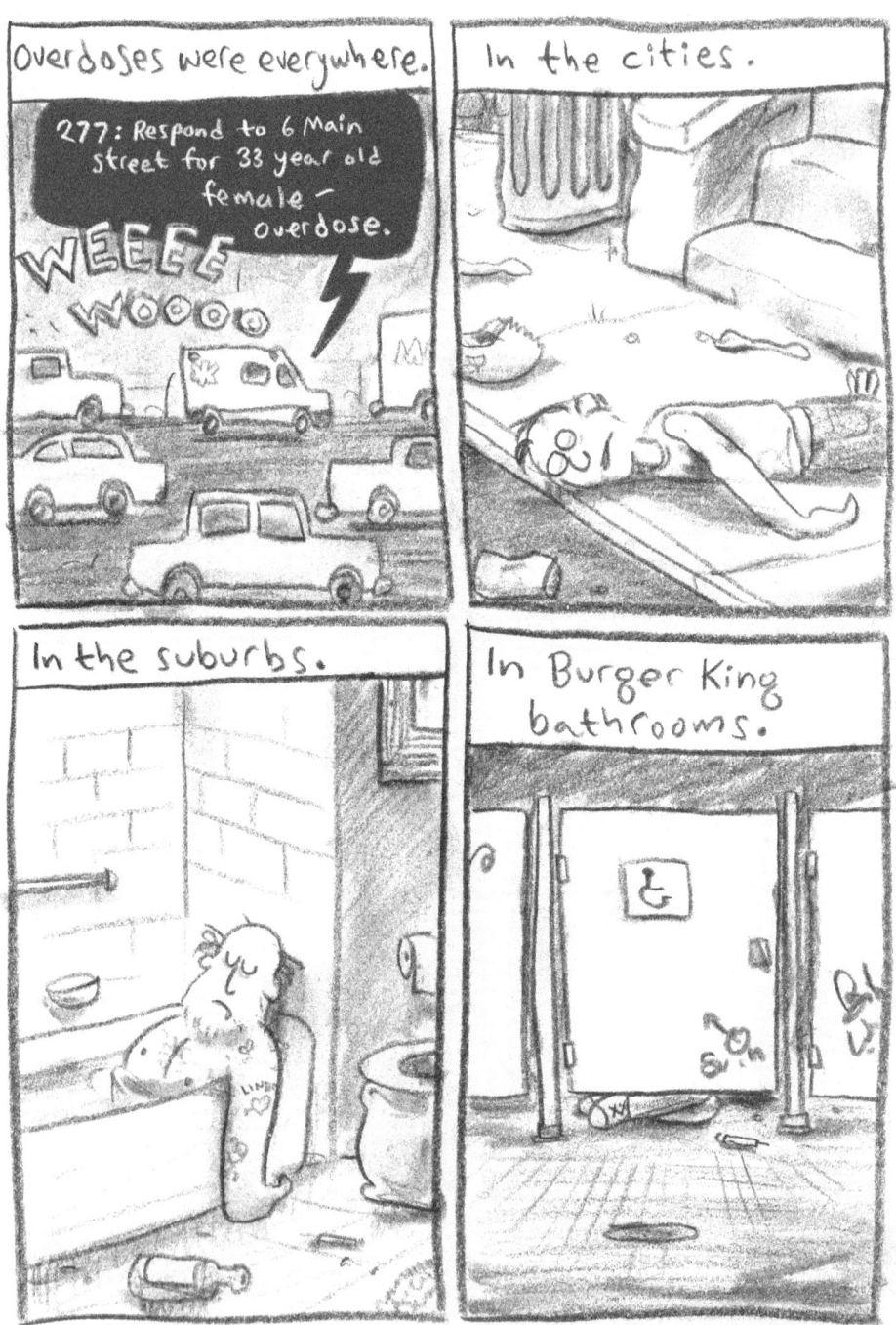

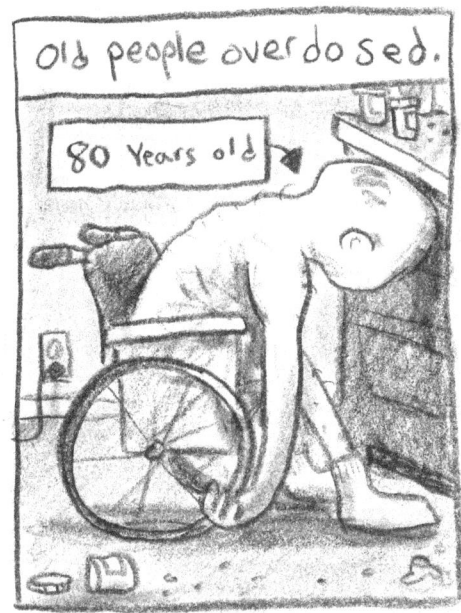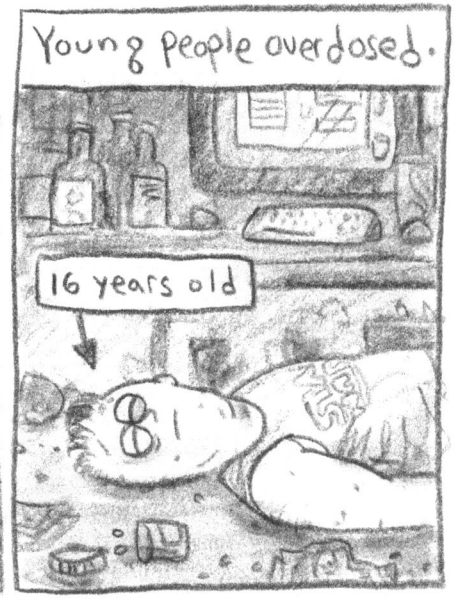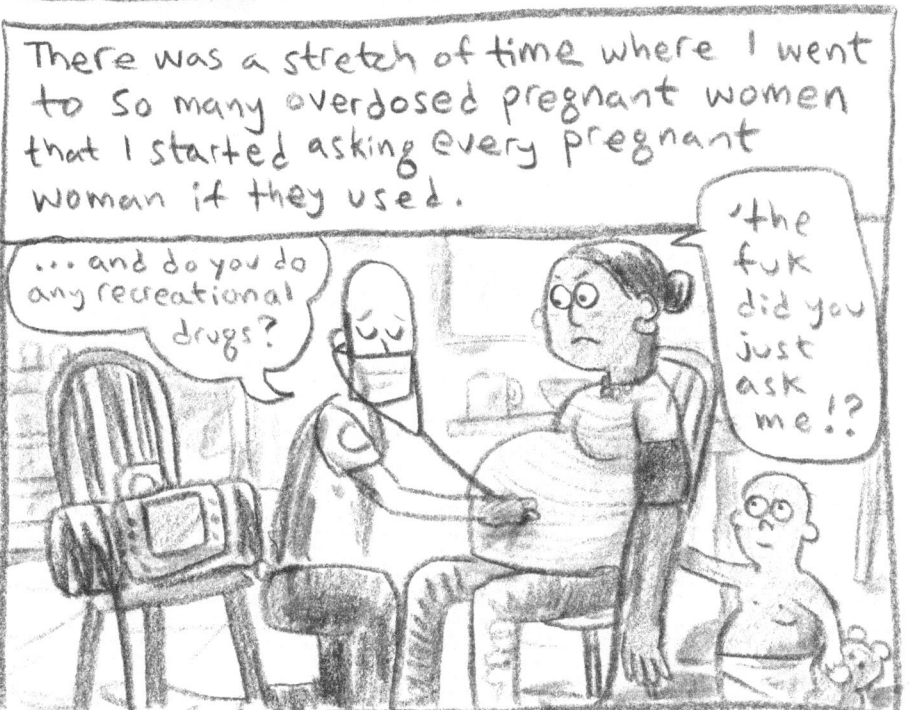

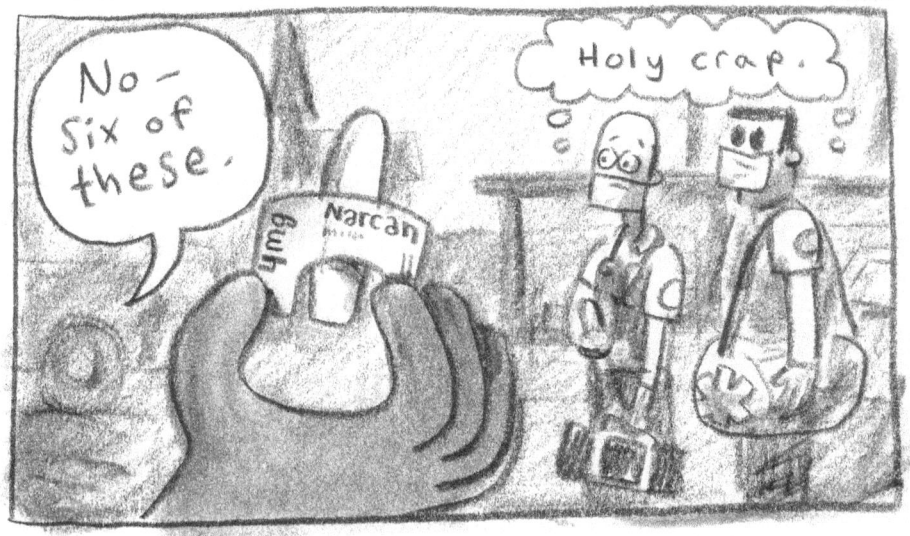

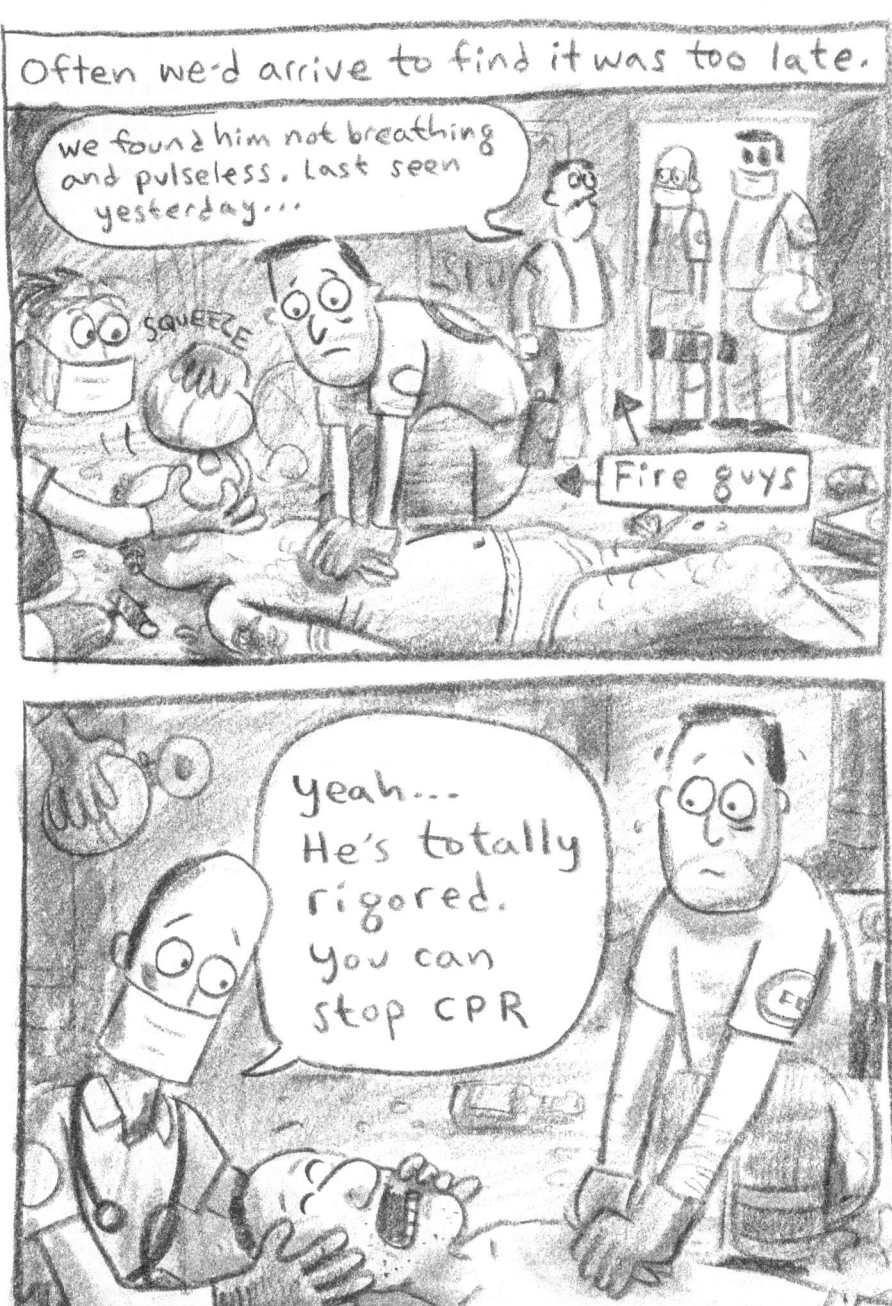

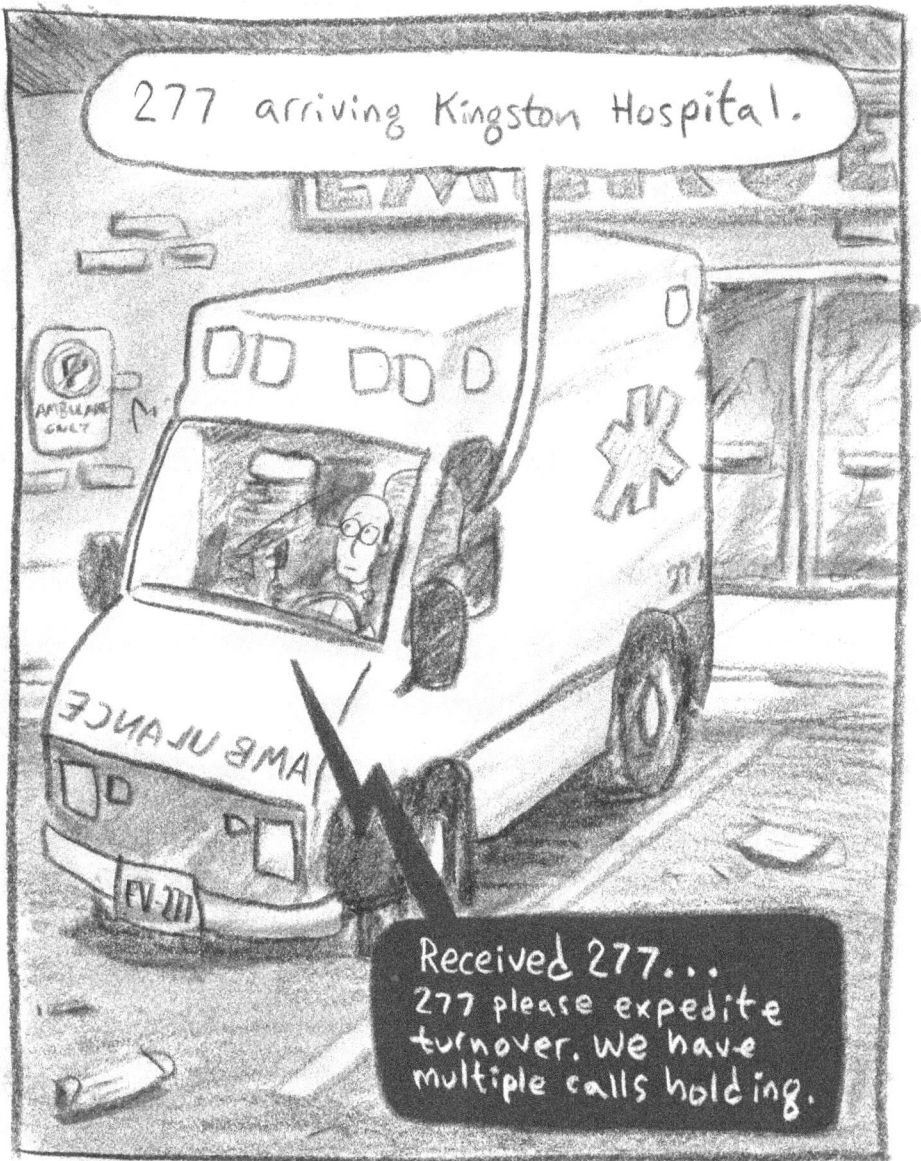

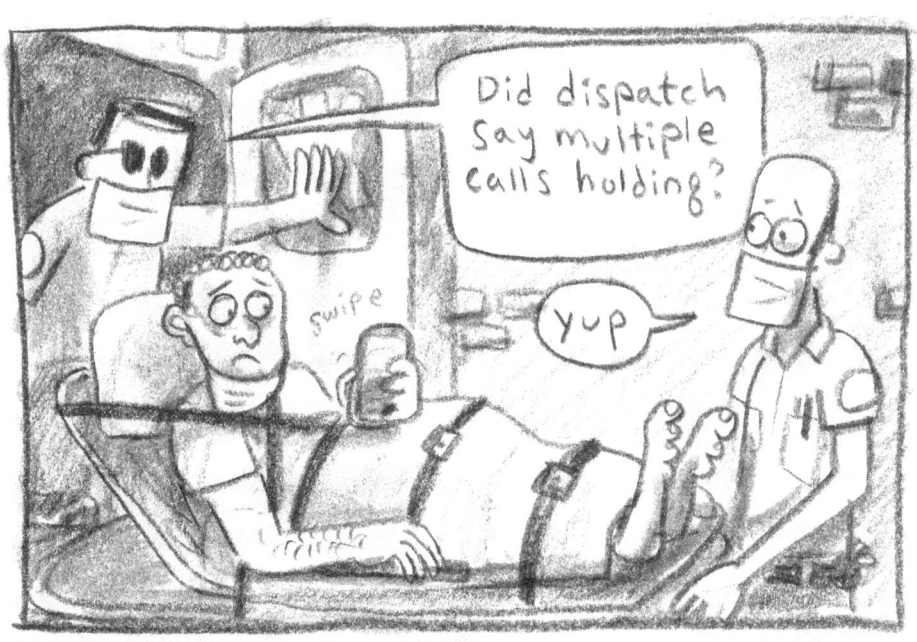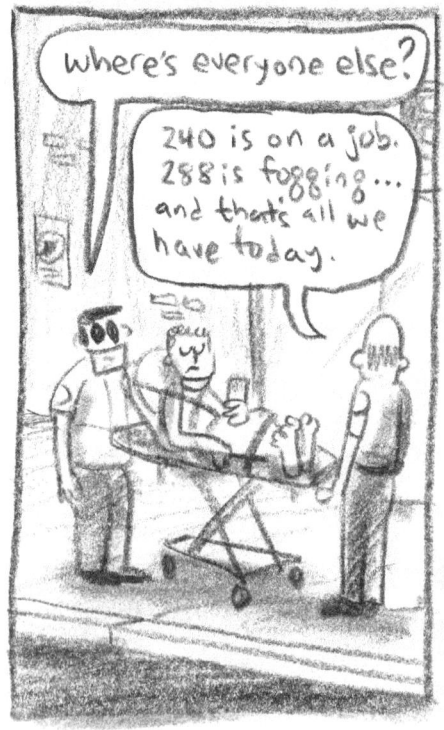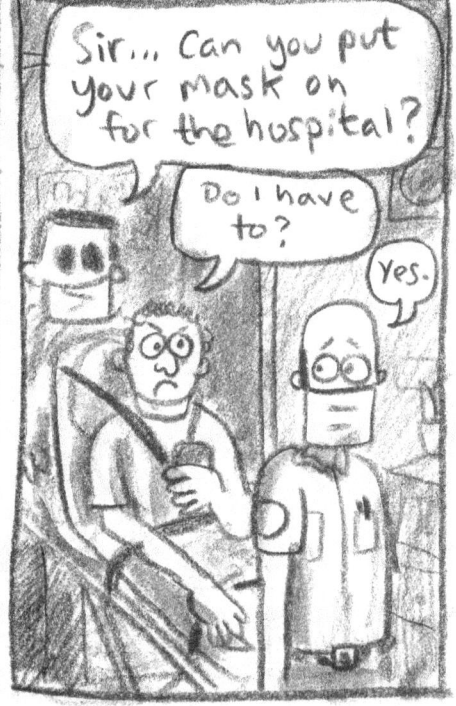

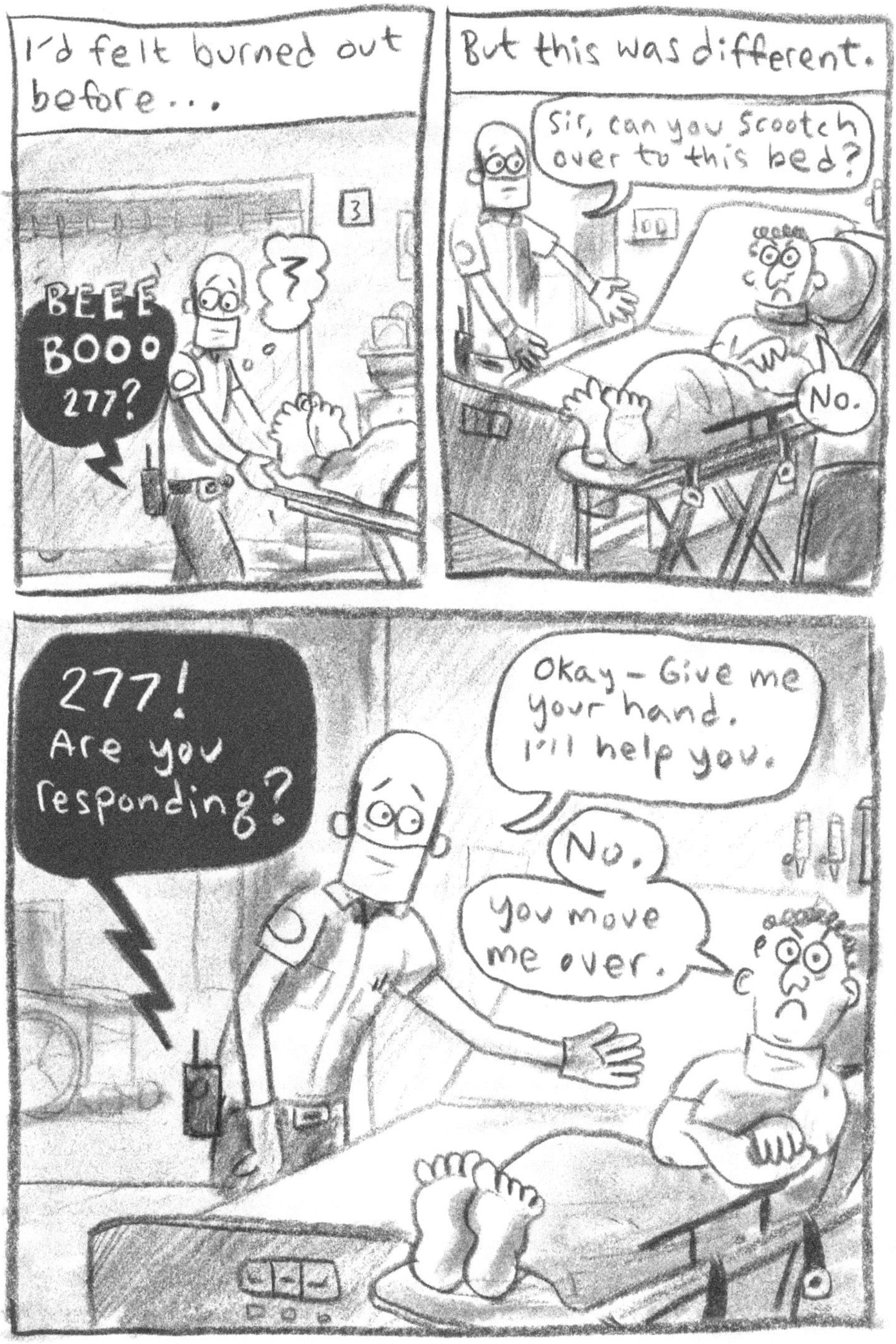

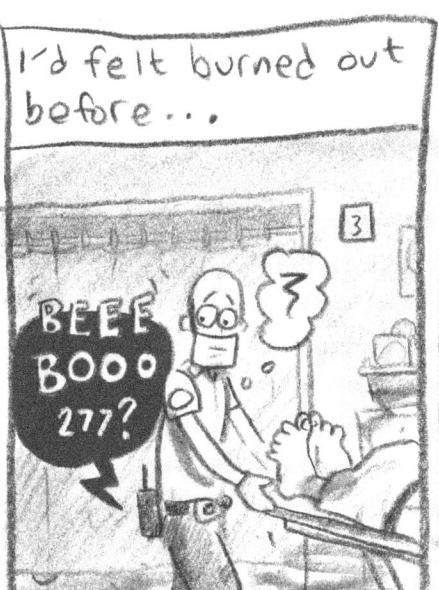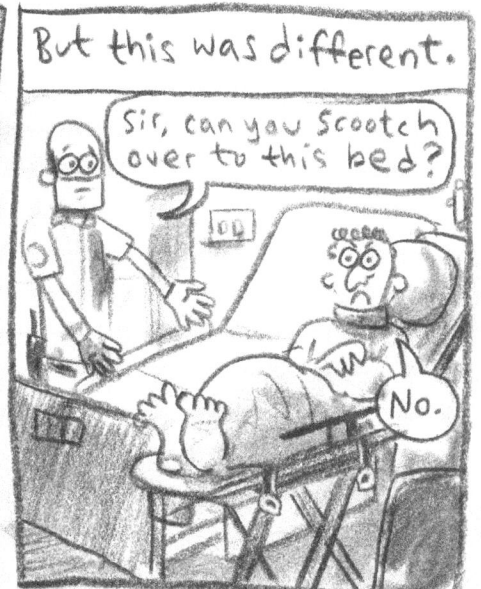

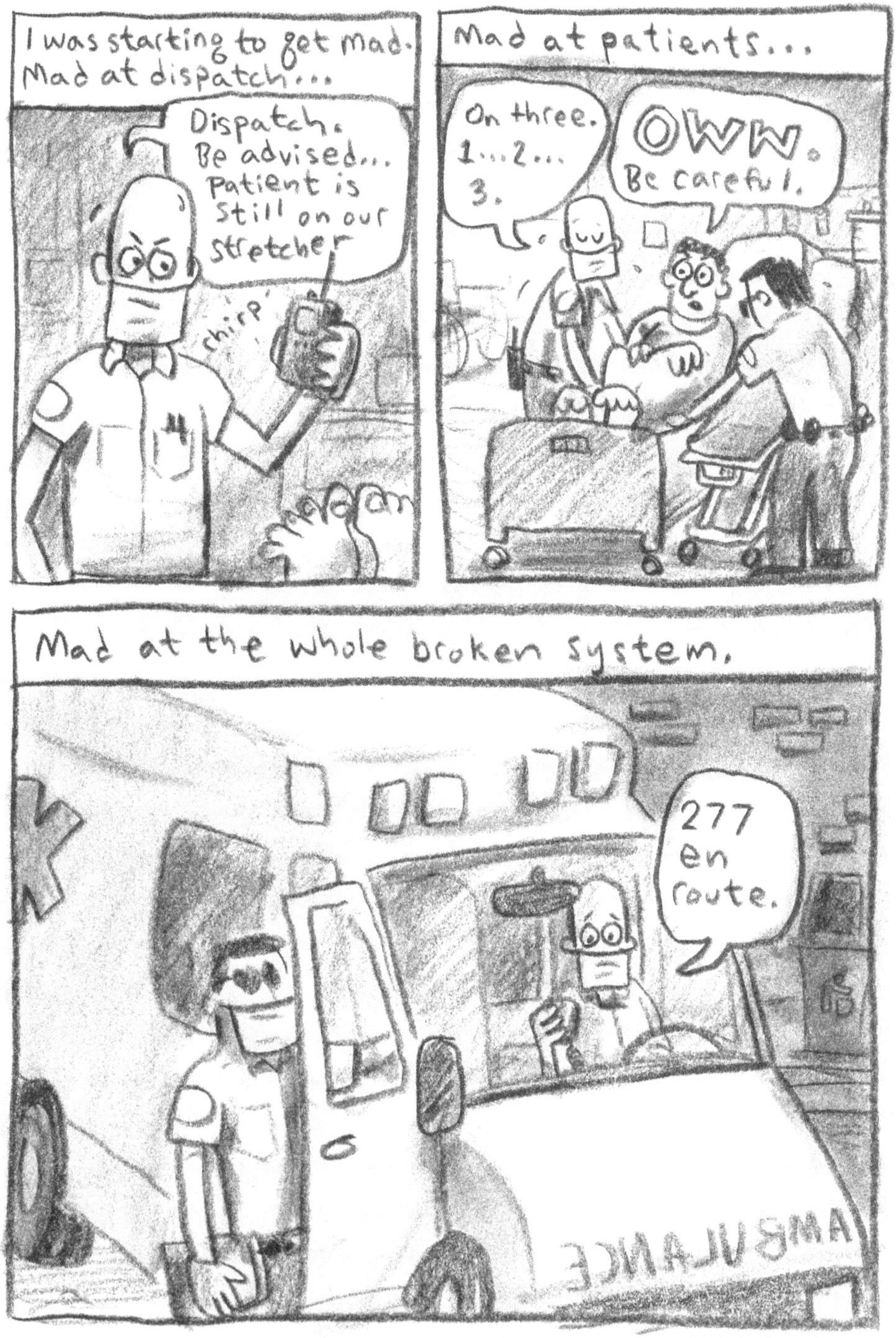

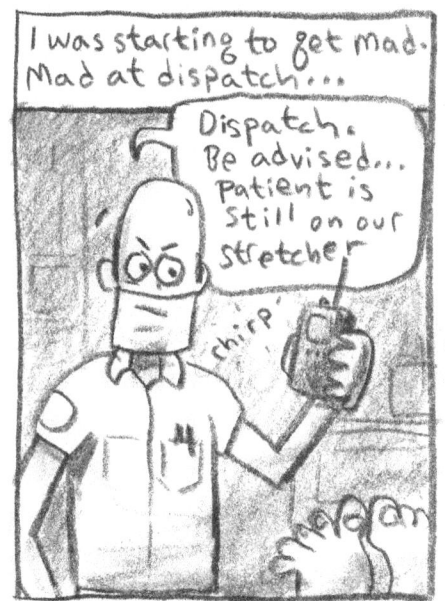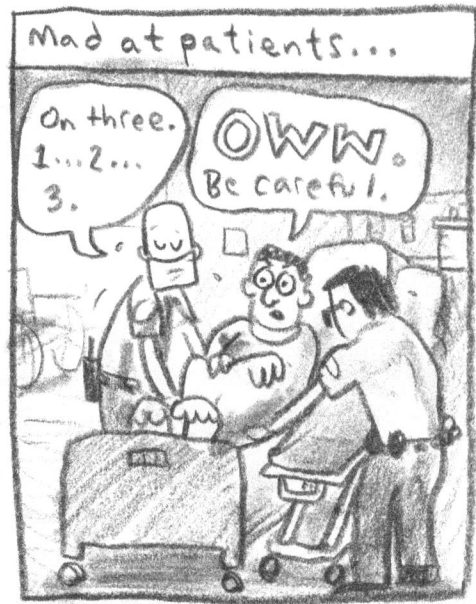

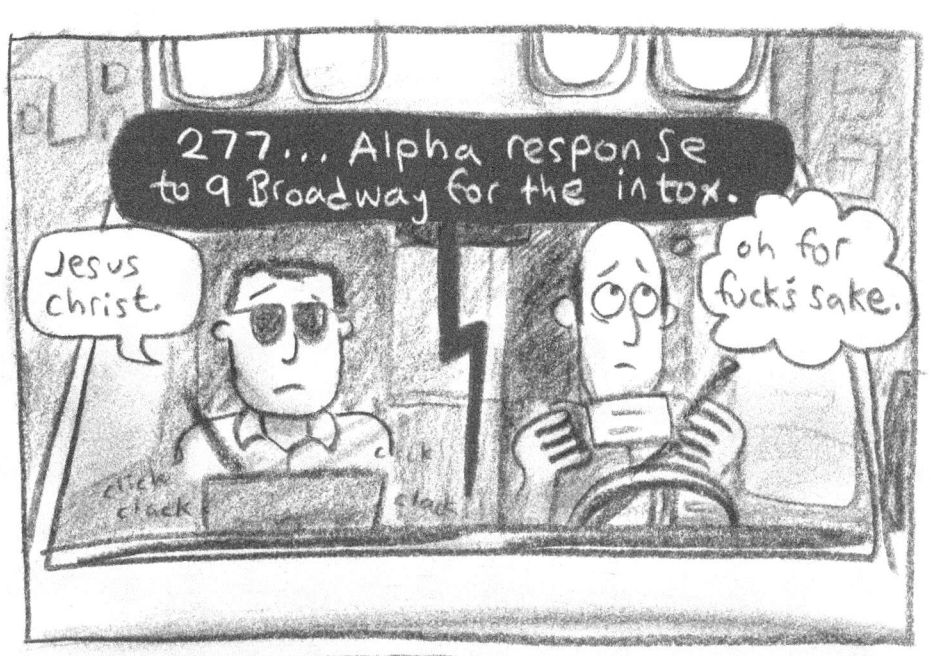

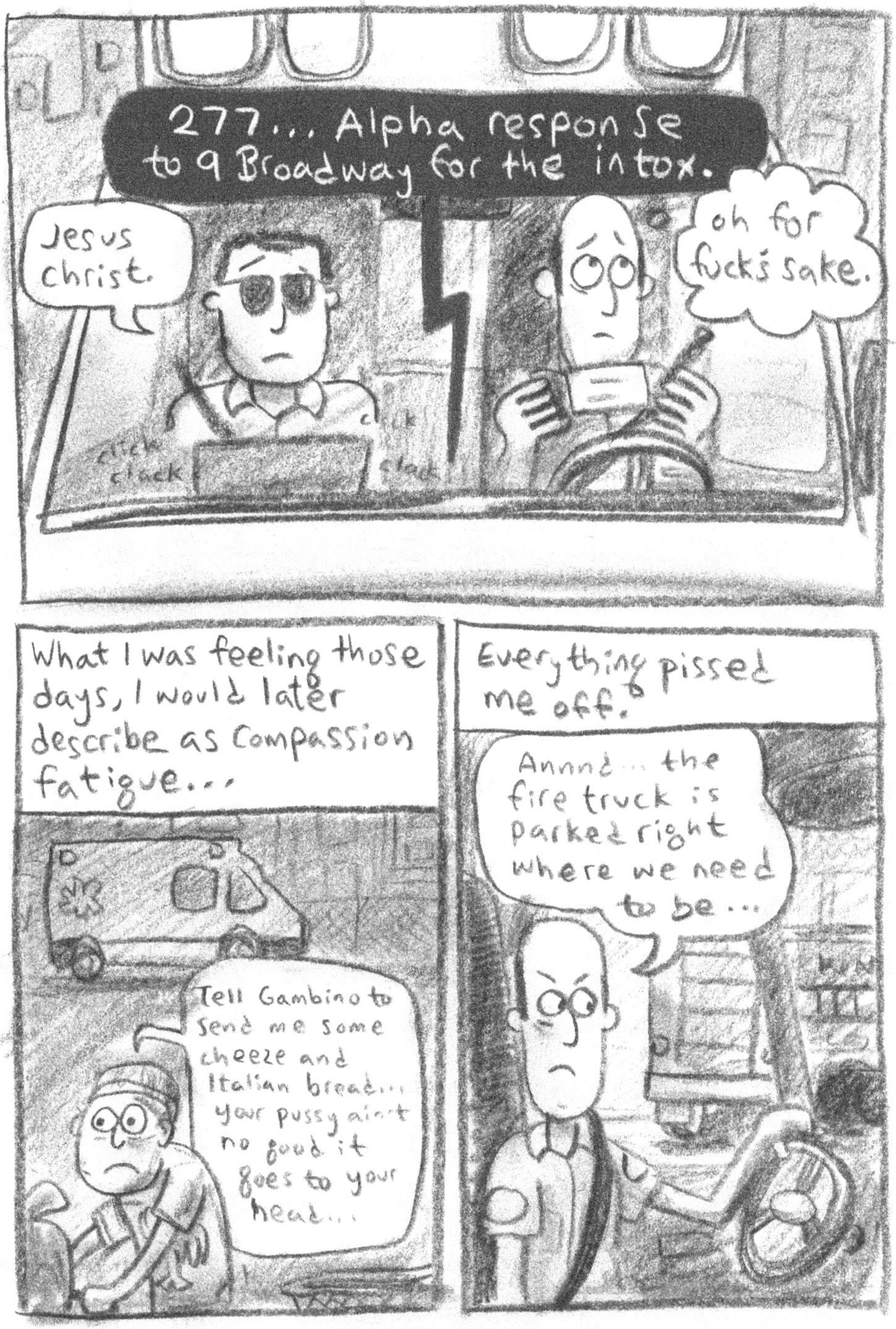

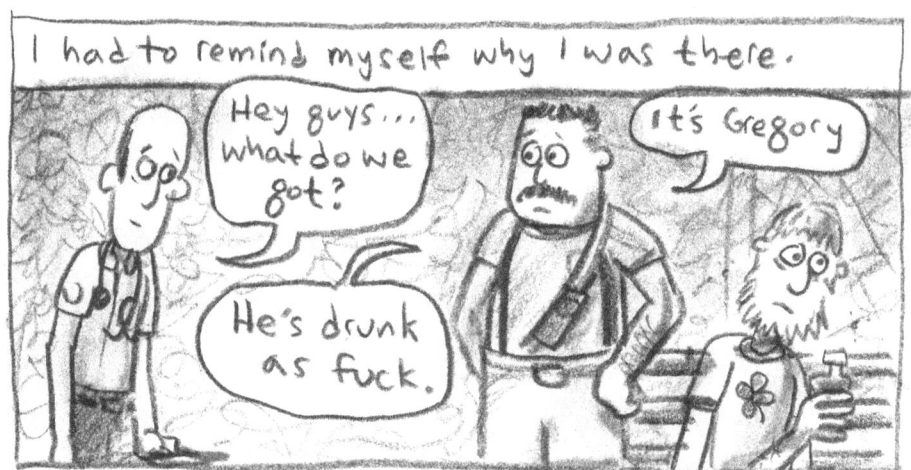

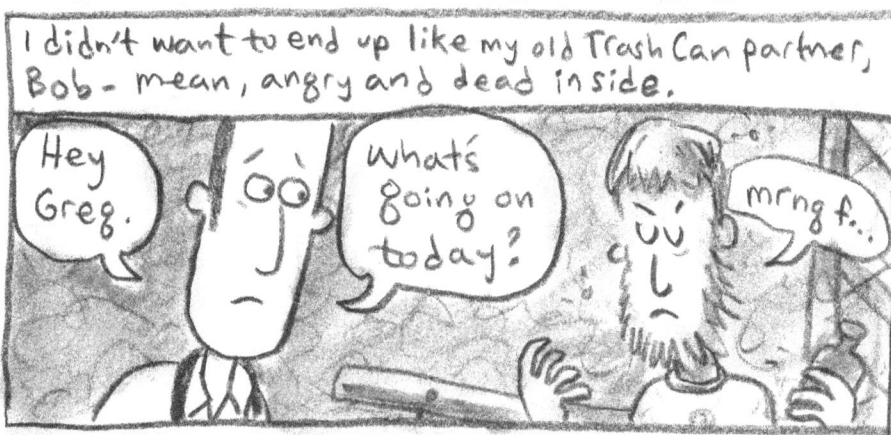

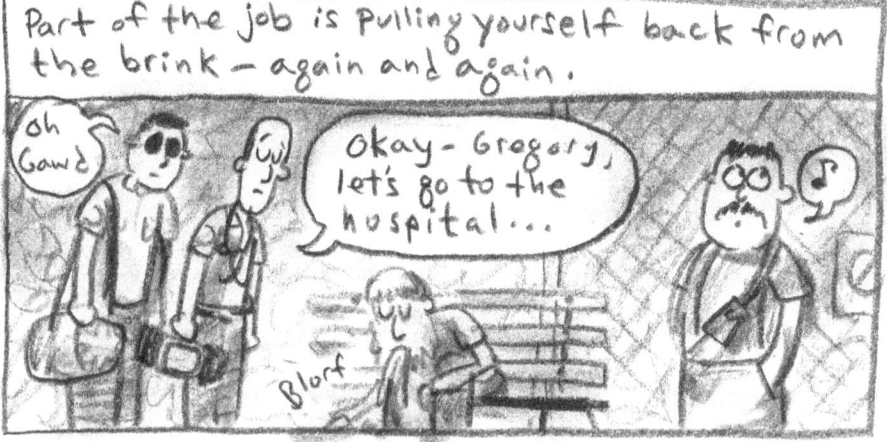

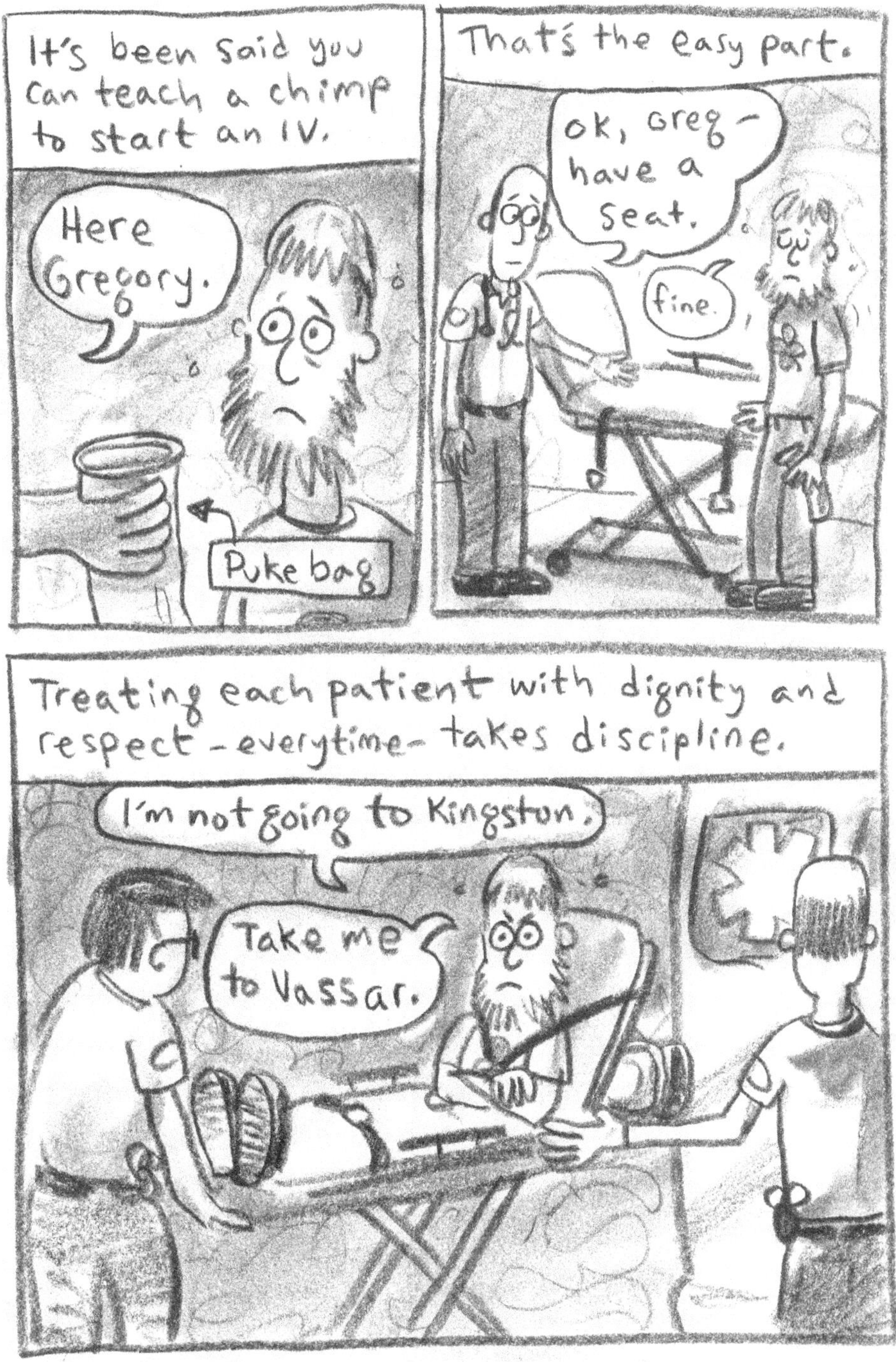

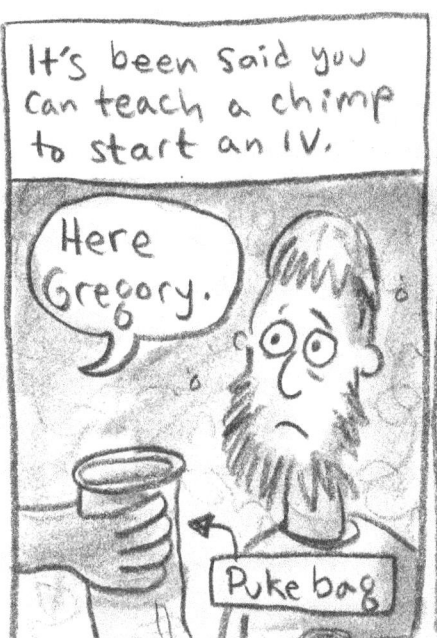
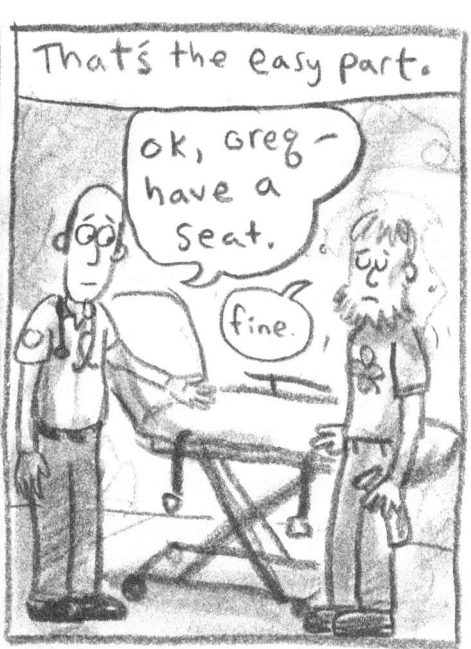

A Little Blip

One of the best things about EMS is the variety of calls. No two jobs were the same.

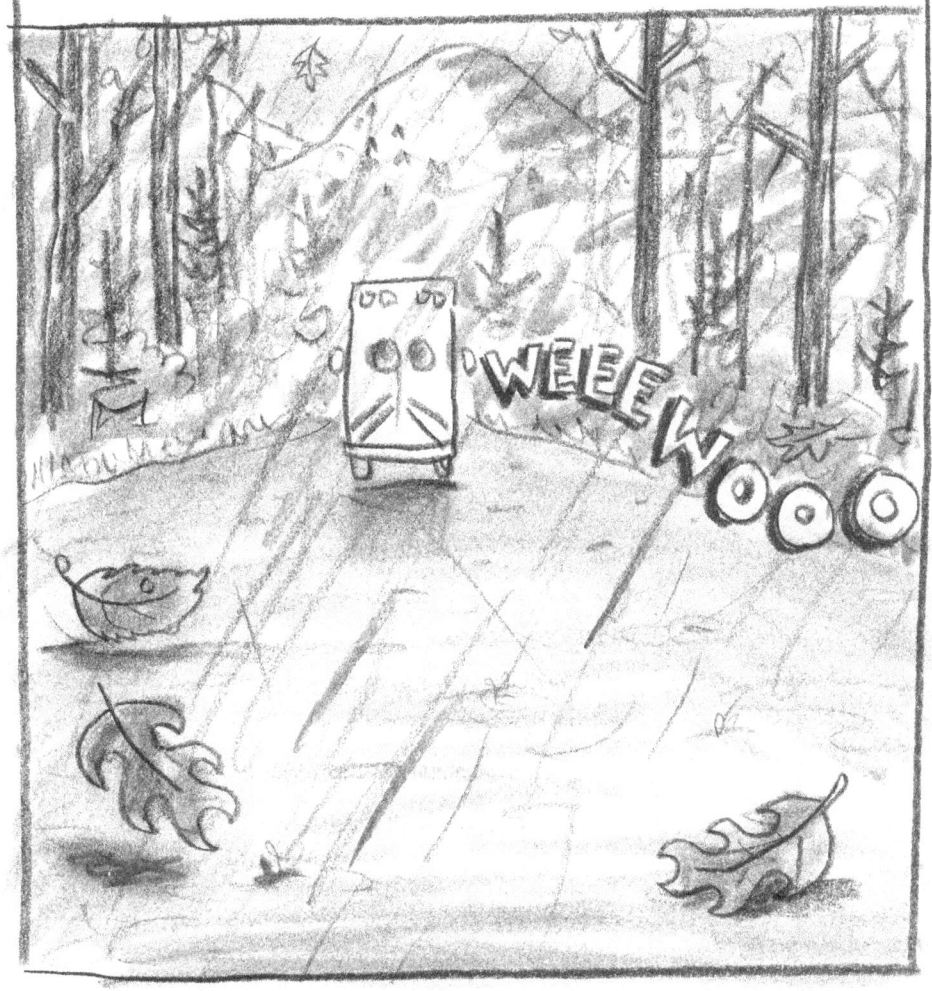

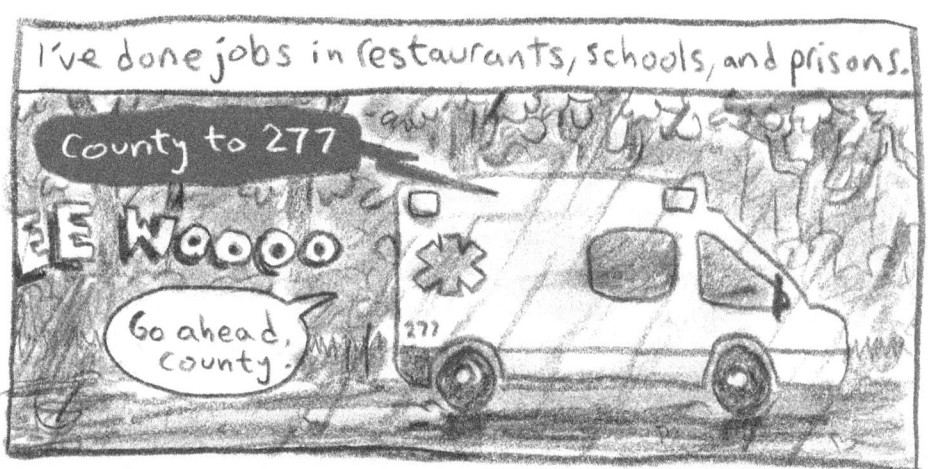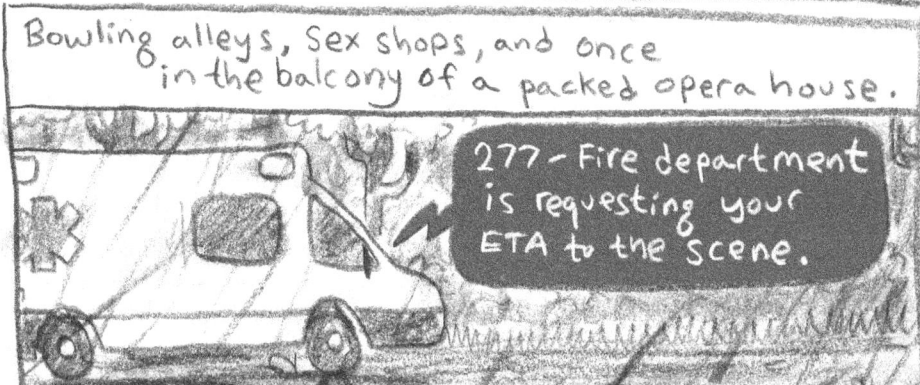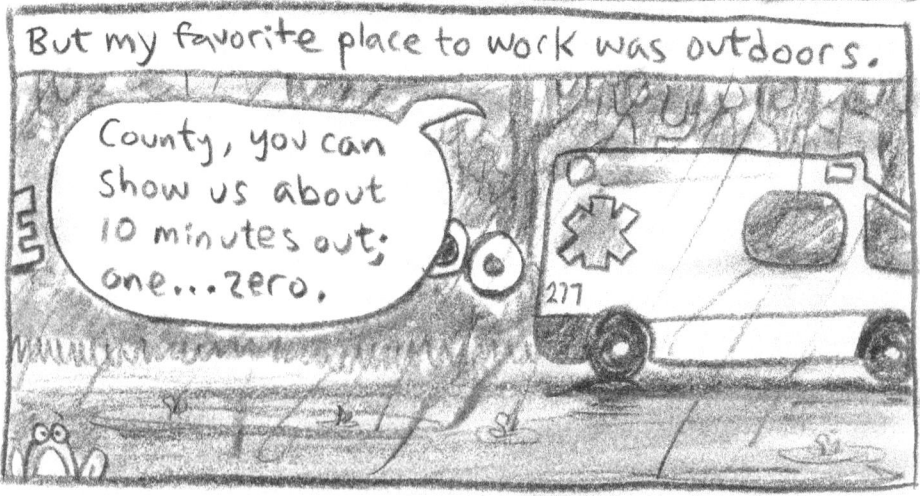

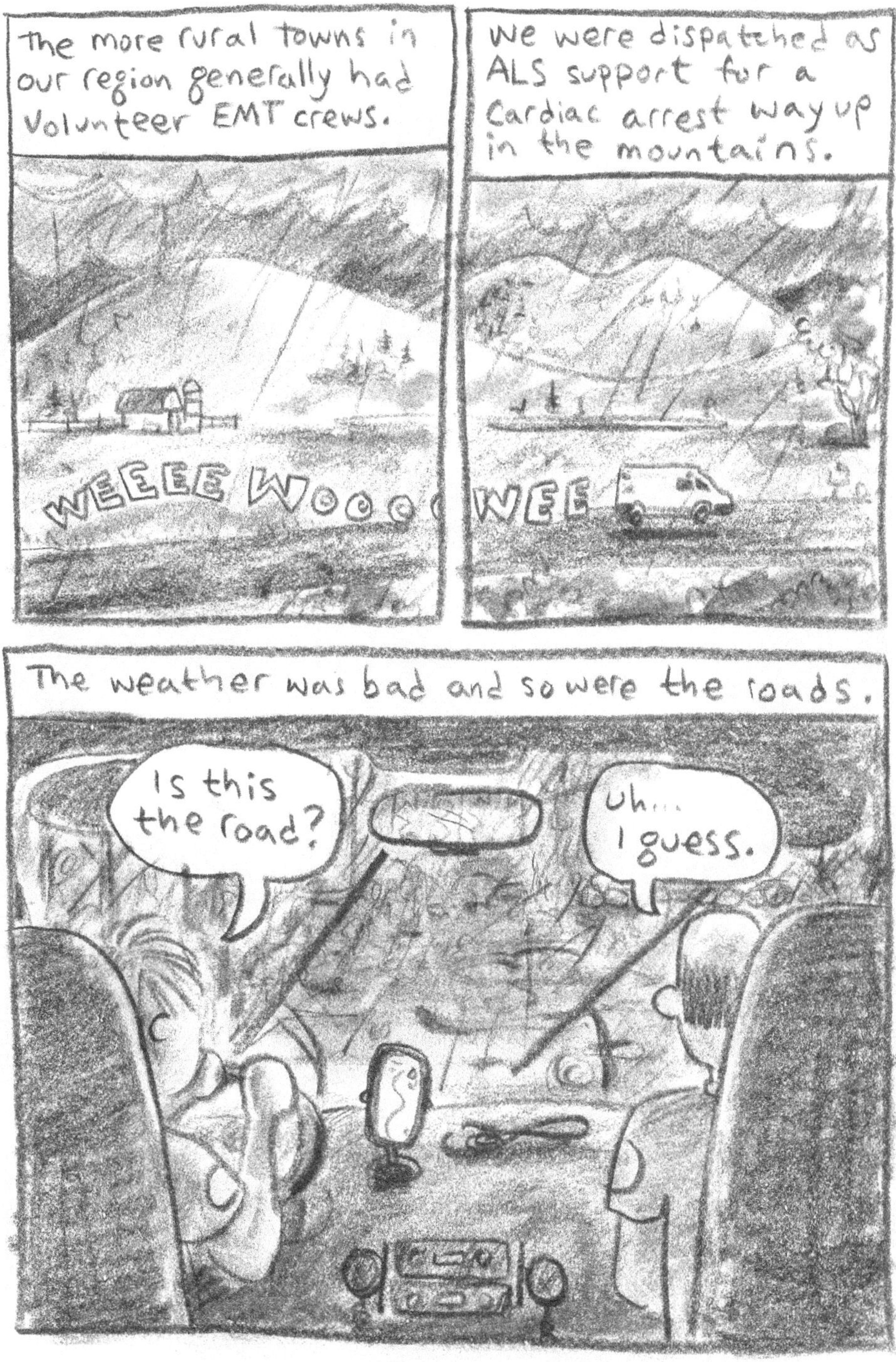

The more rural towns in our region generally had volunteer EMT crews.

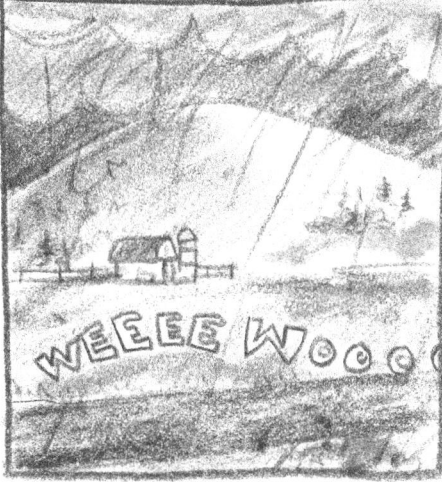

WEEEE WOOO

We were dispatched as ALS support for a cardiac arrest way up in the mountains.

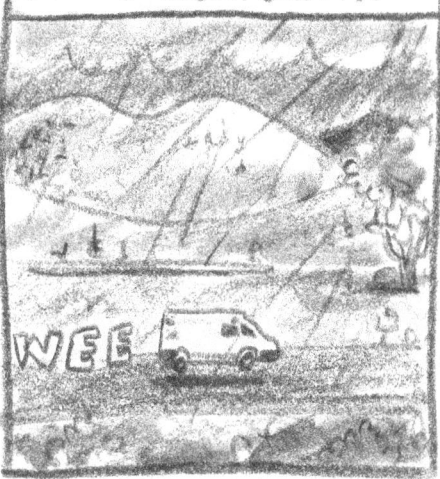

WEE

The weather was bad and so were the roads.

"Is this the road?"

"Uh.... I guess."

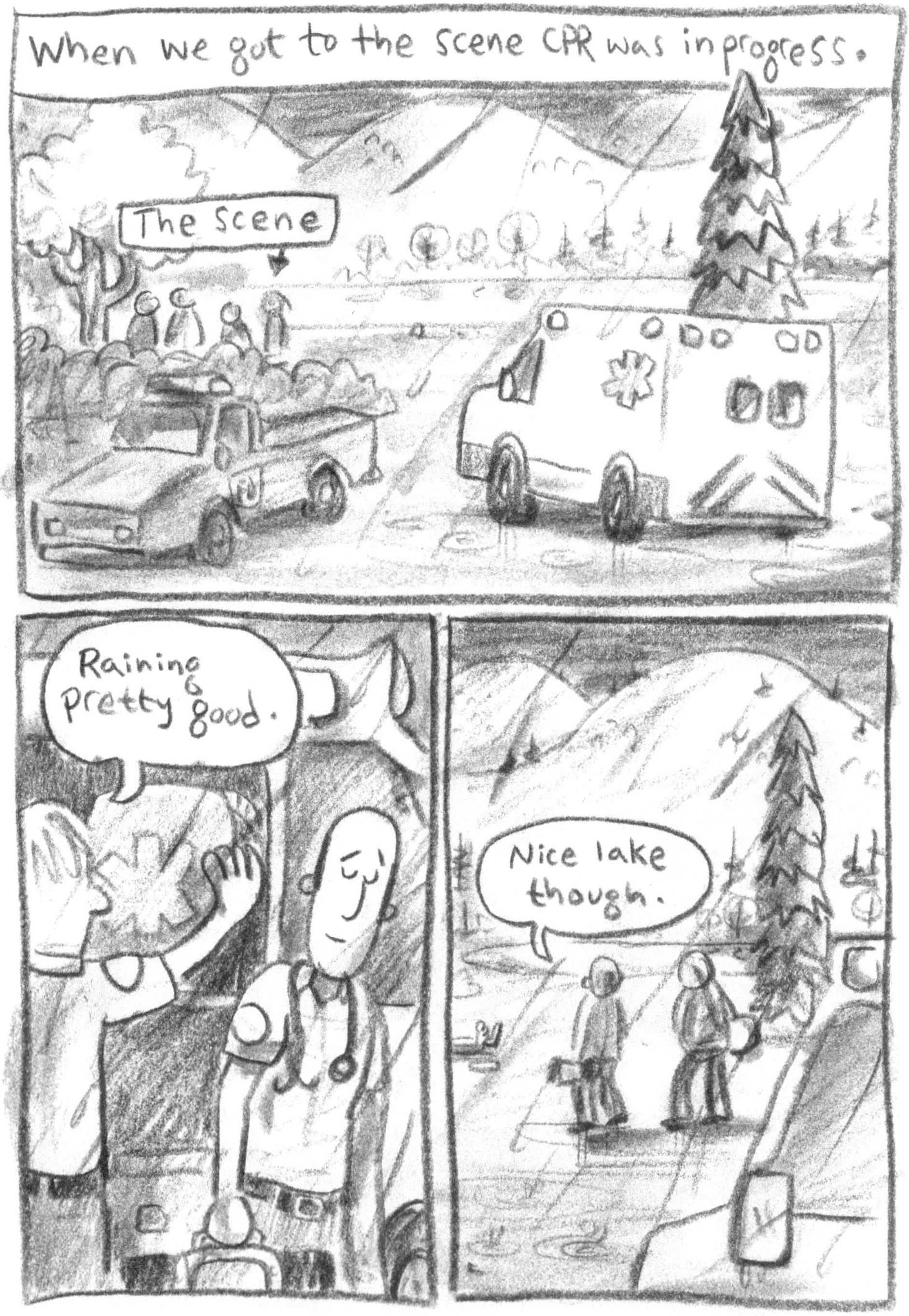

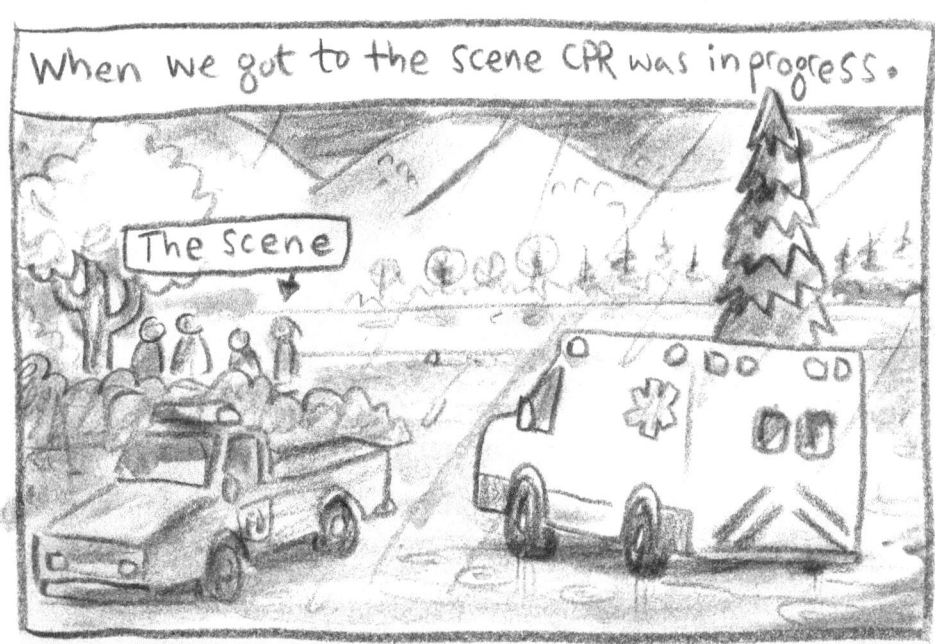

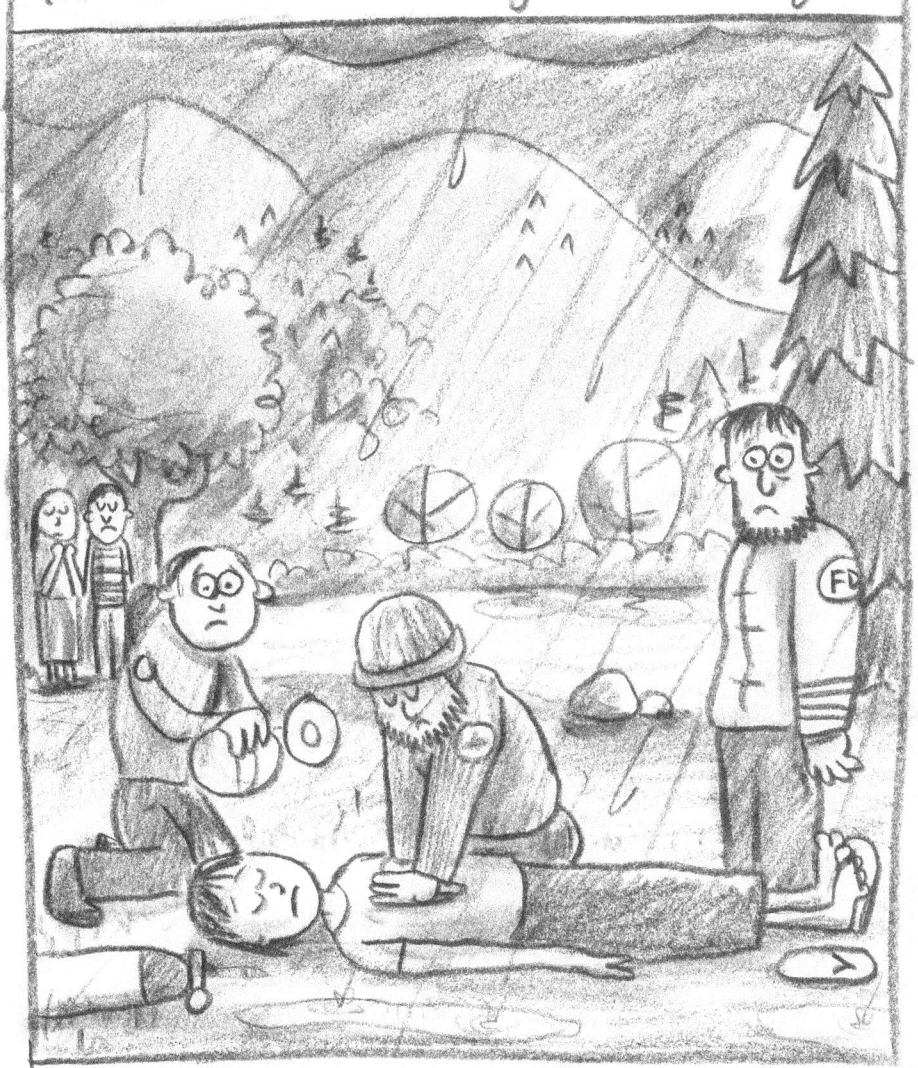

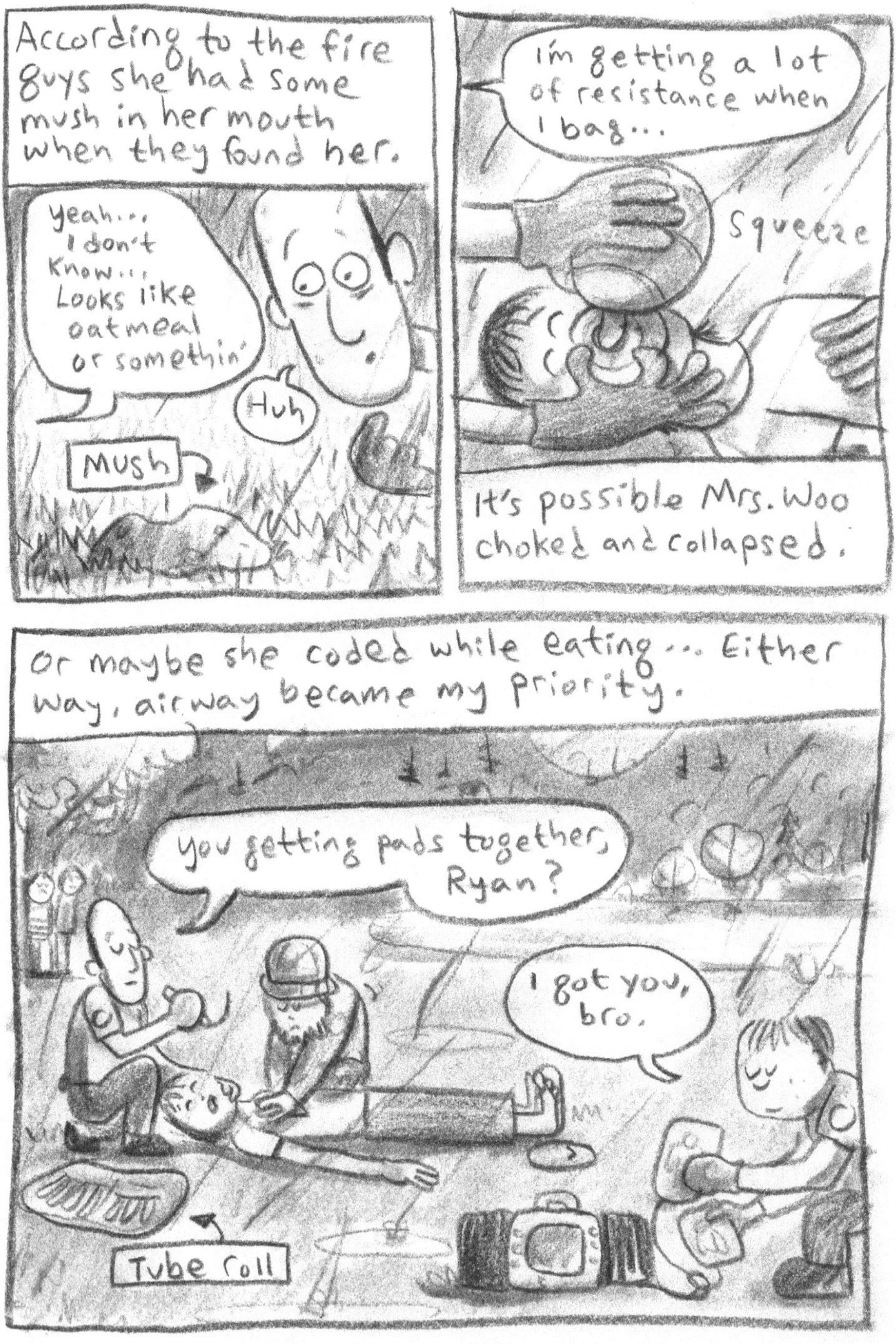

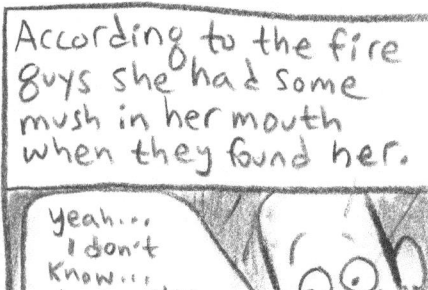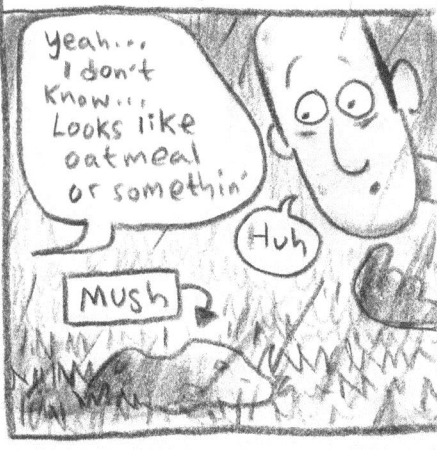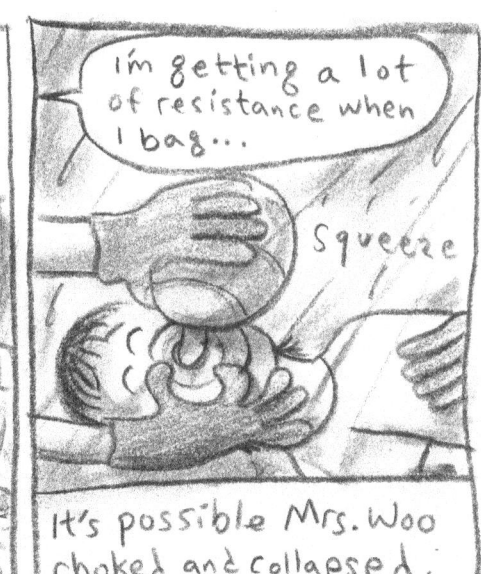

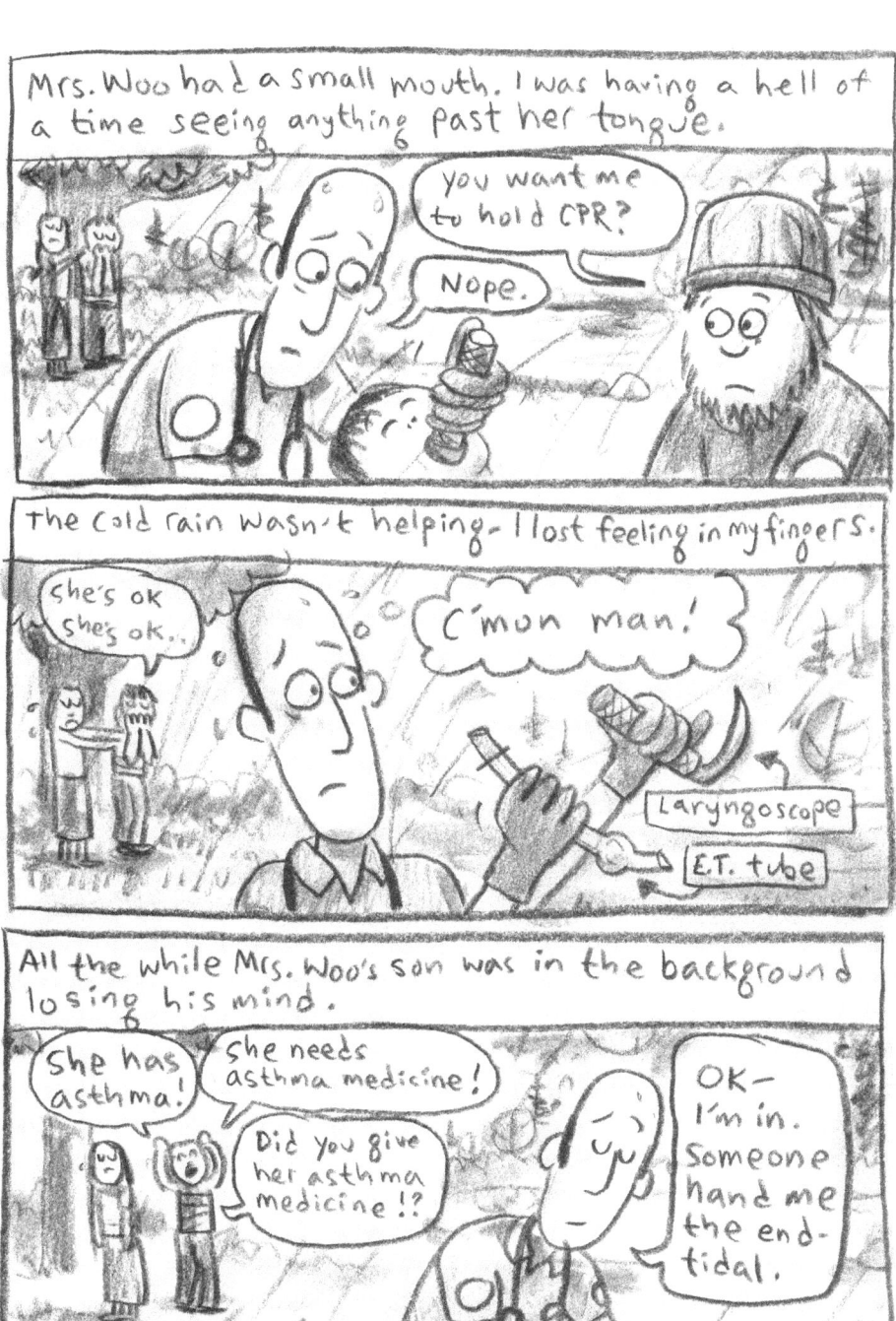

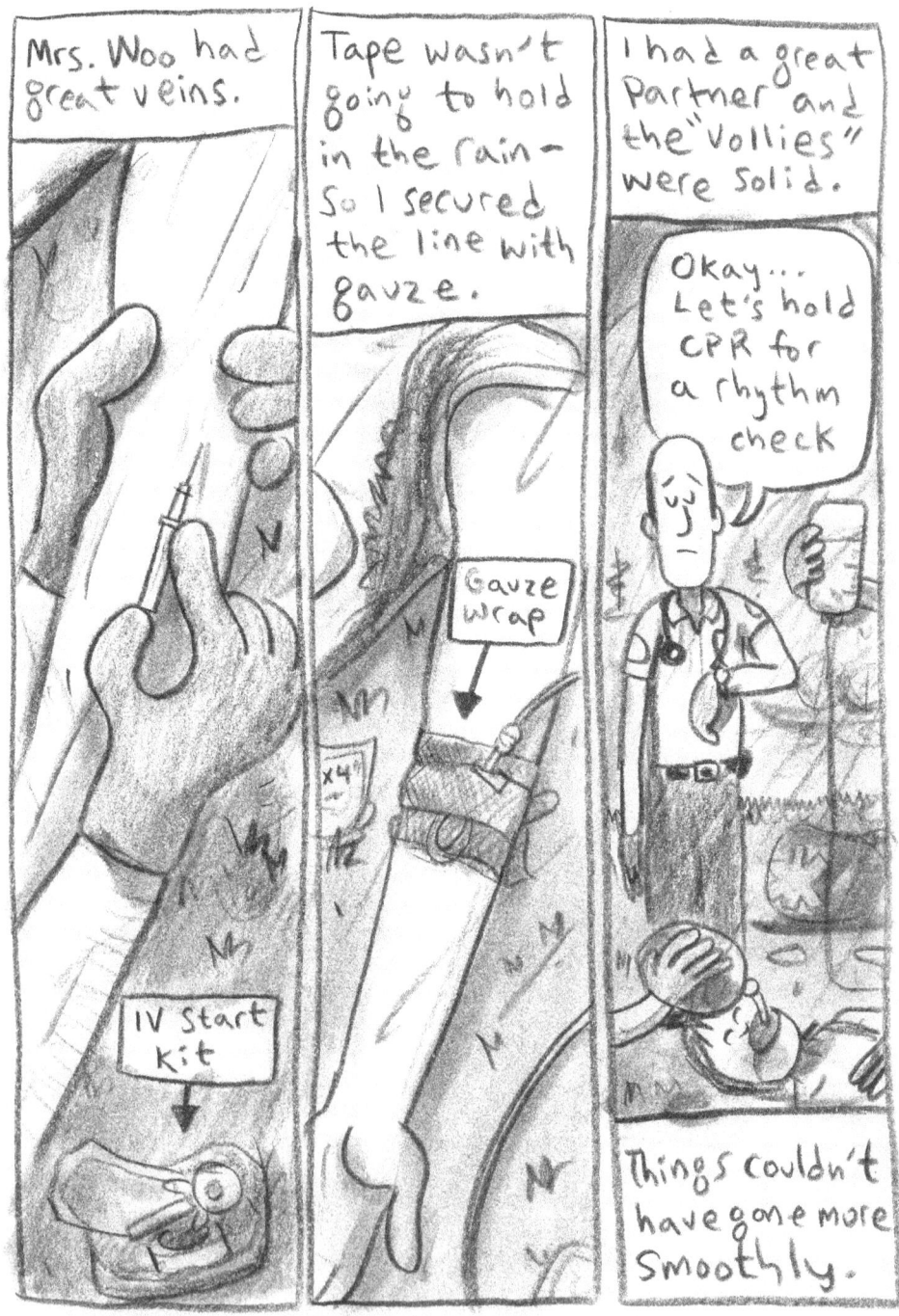

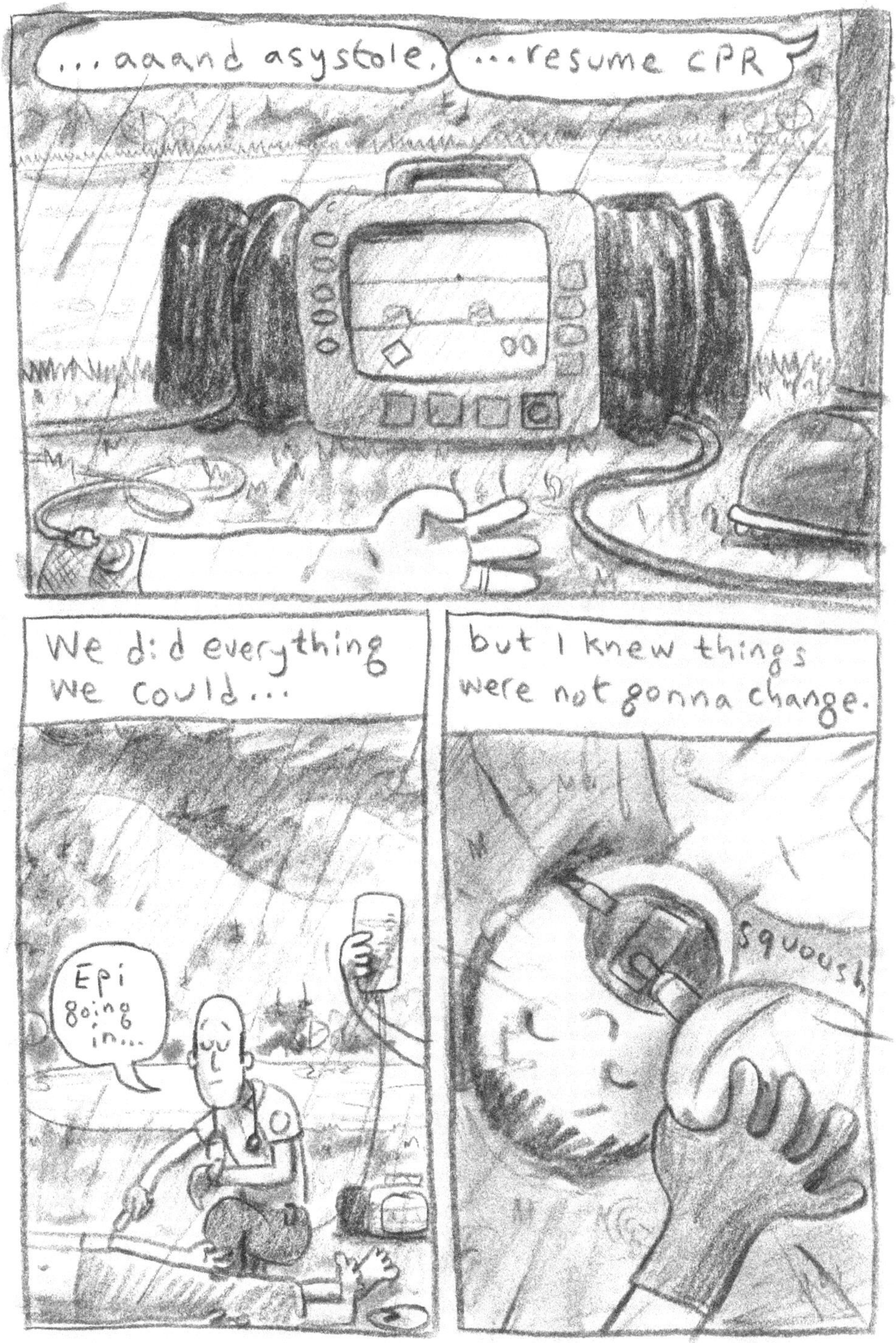

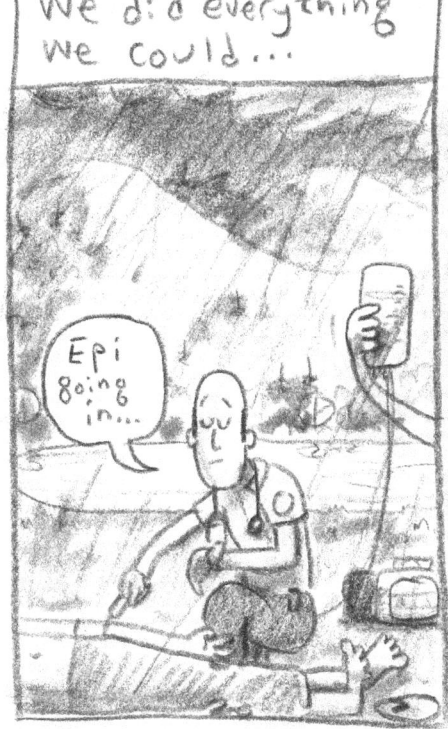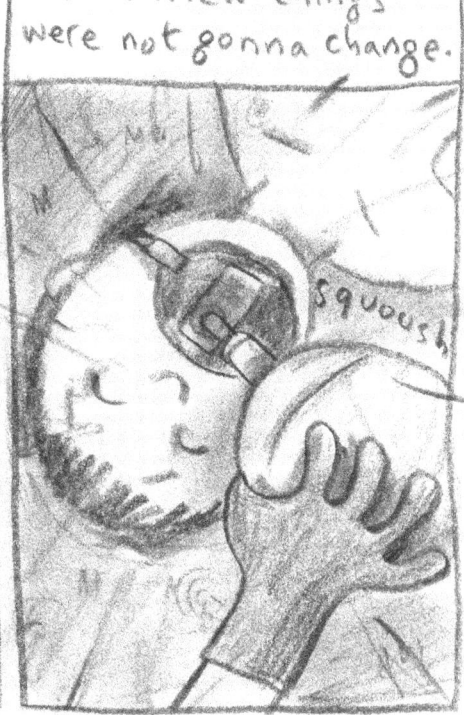

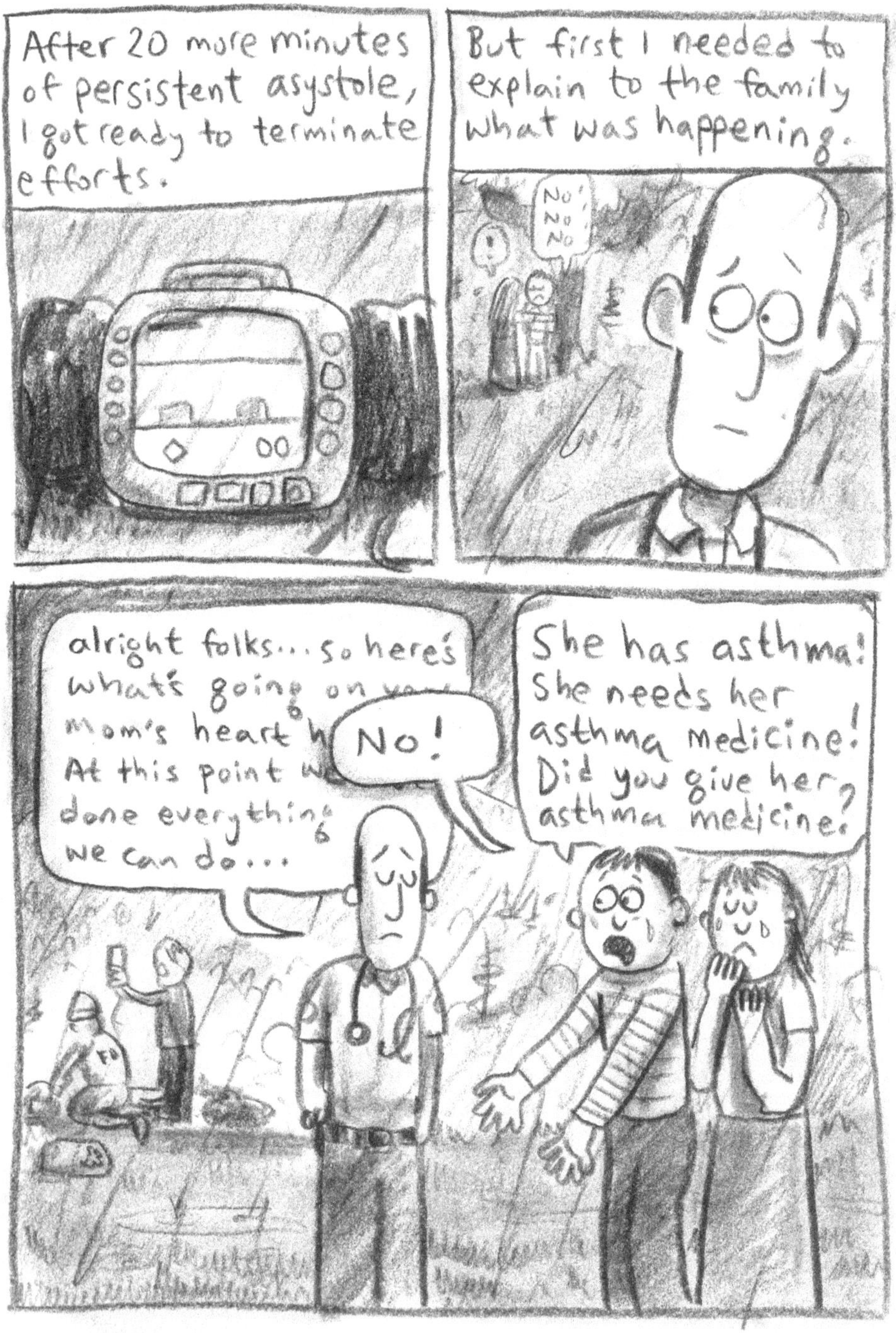

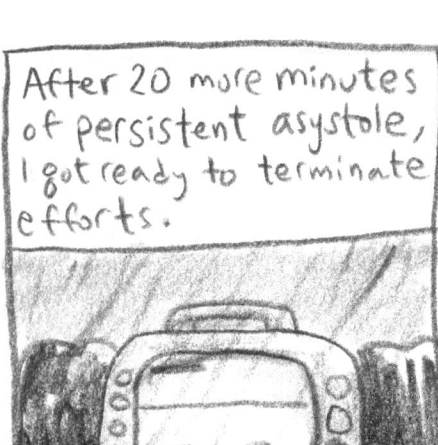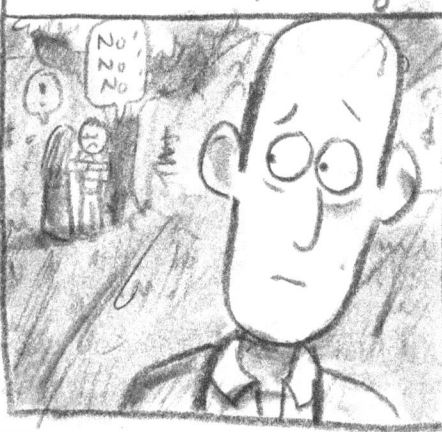

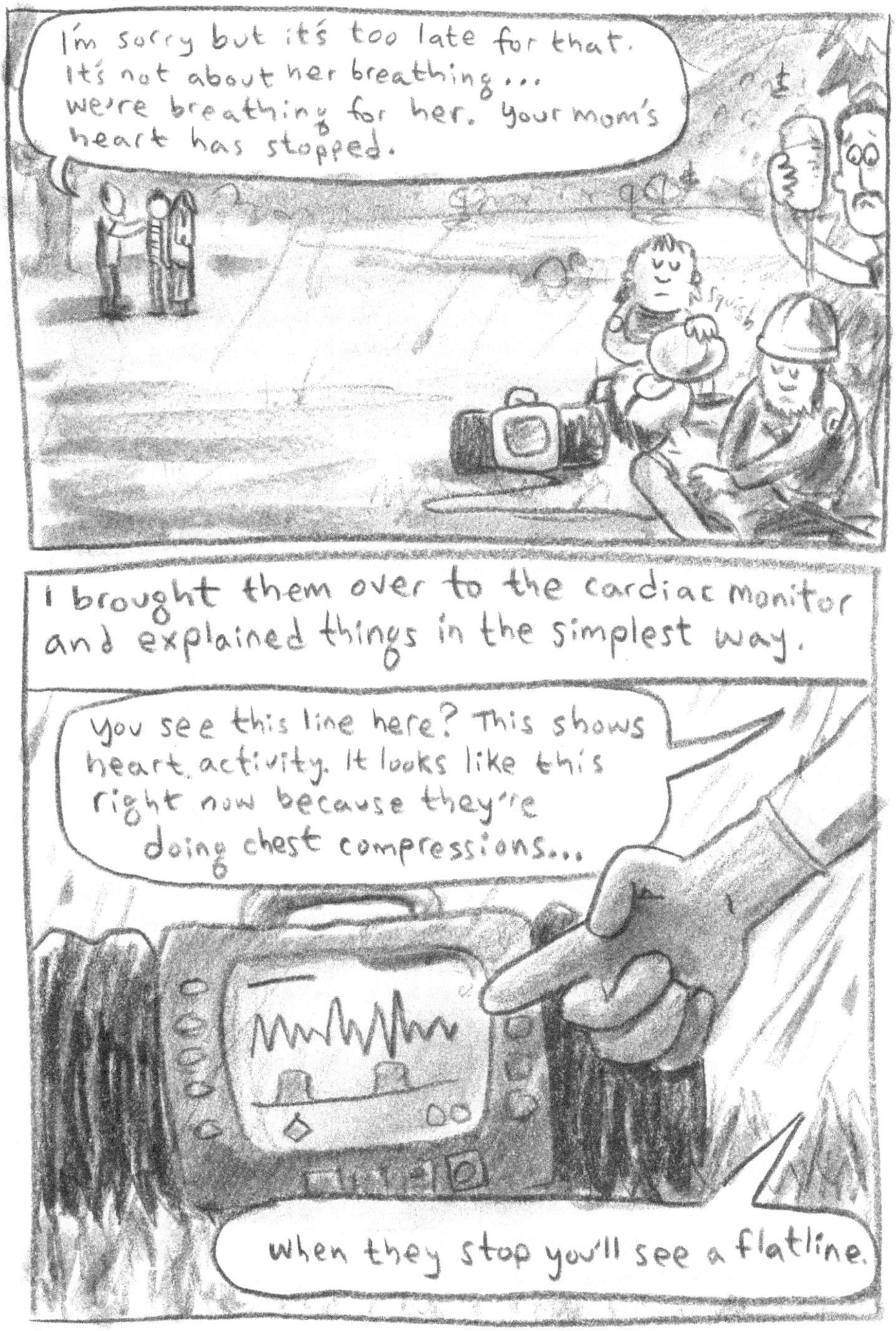

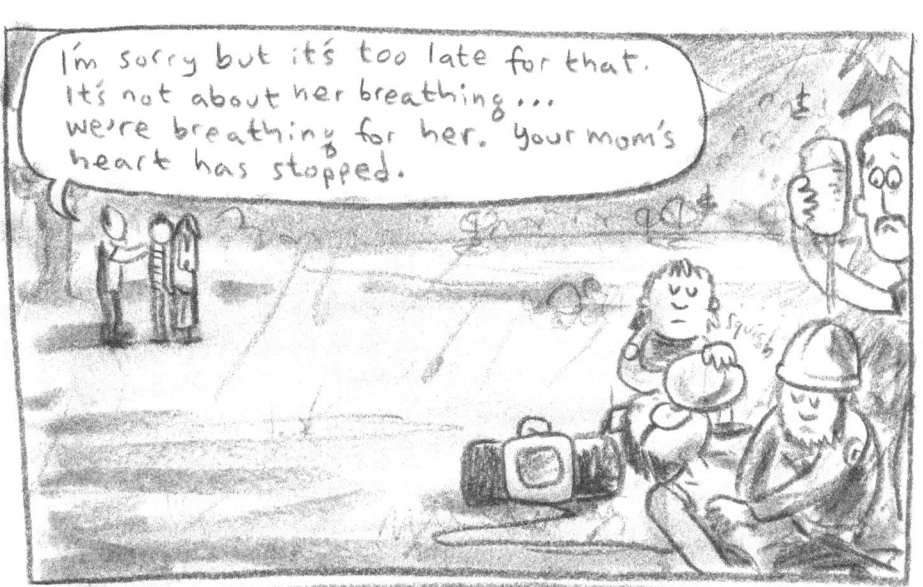

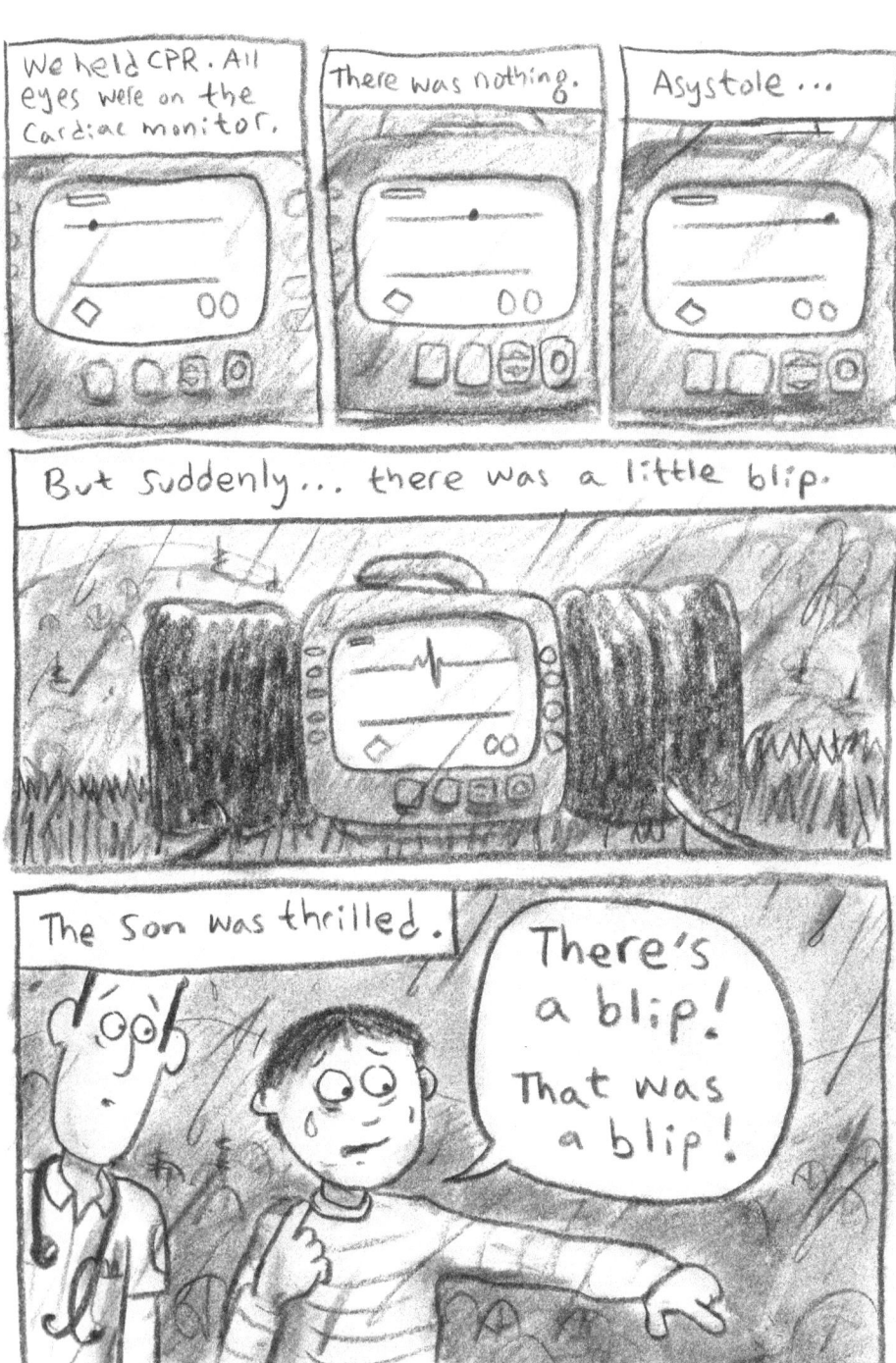

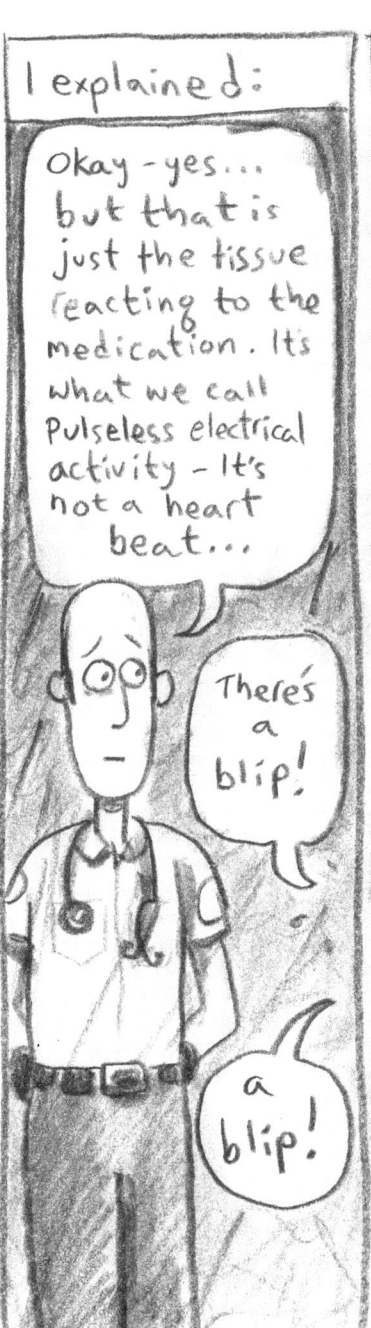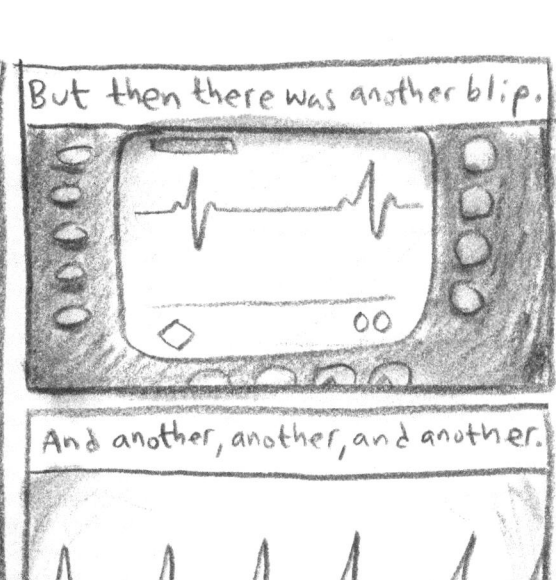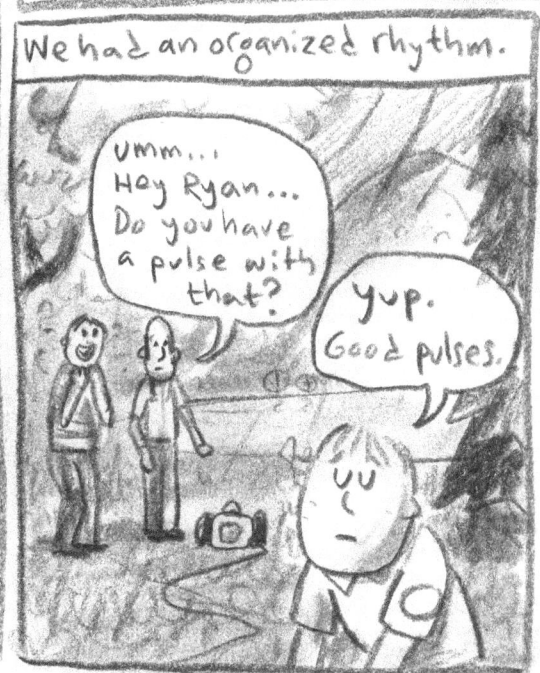

We loaded Mrs. Woo into the volunteer's ambulance and raced towards the hospital.

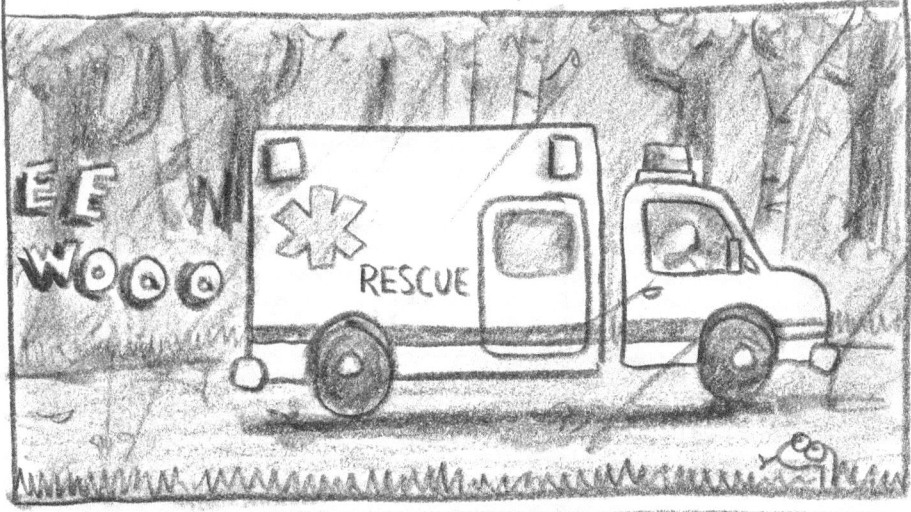

It was a long ride. I advised the hospital we were coming. Mrs. Woo's vitals were great. There wasn't much else to do so I started another IV.

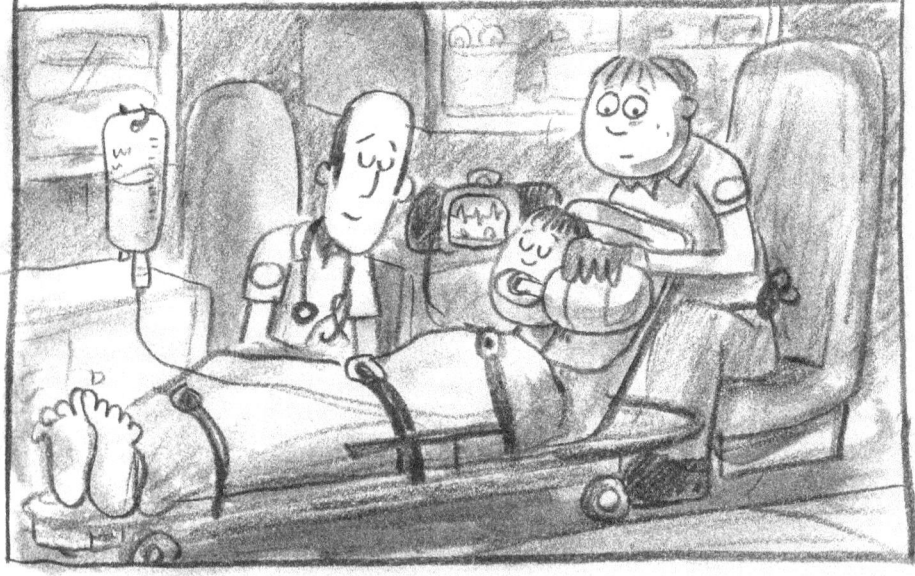

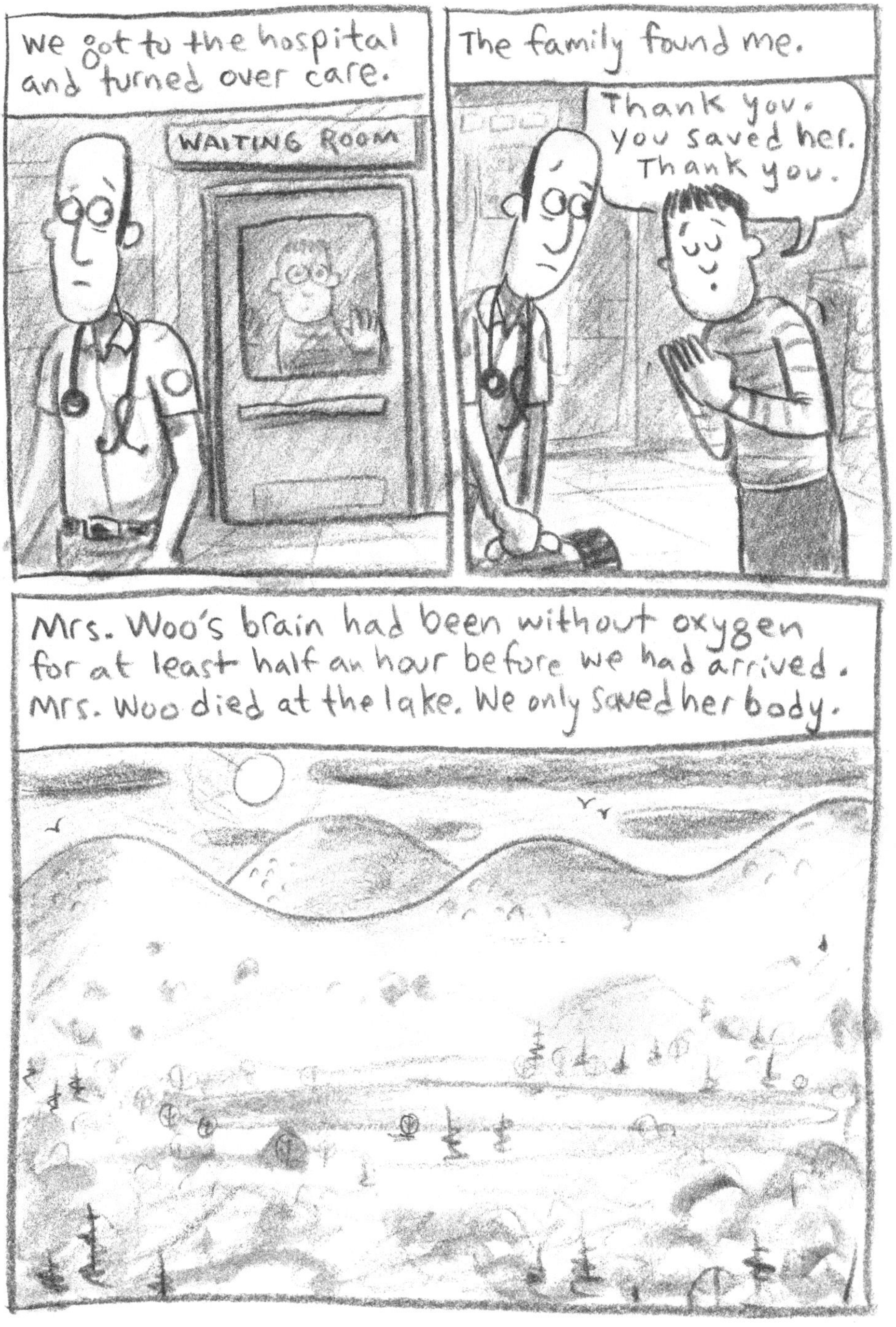

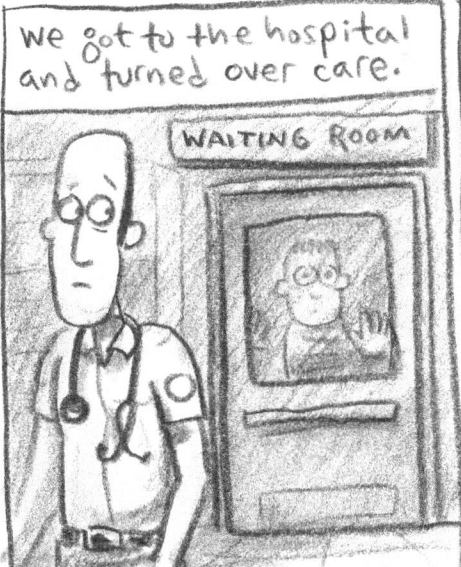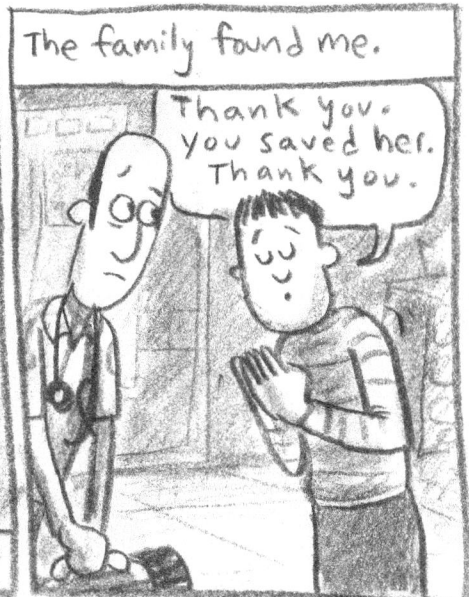

Another Time

I could not even guess how many cardiac arrests I've attended over the past ten years. Maybe a hundred. Maybe hundreds.

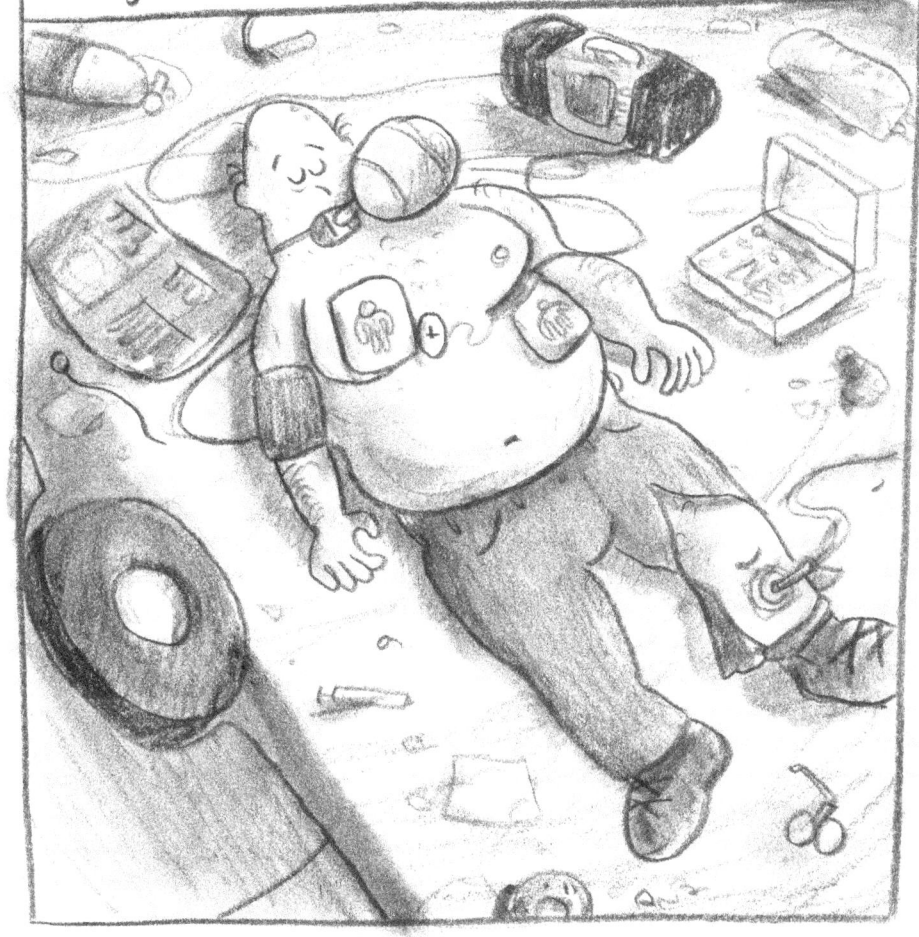

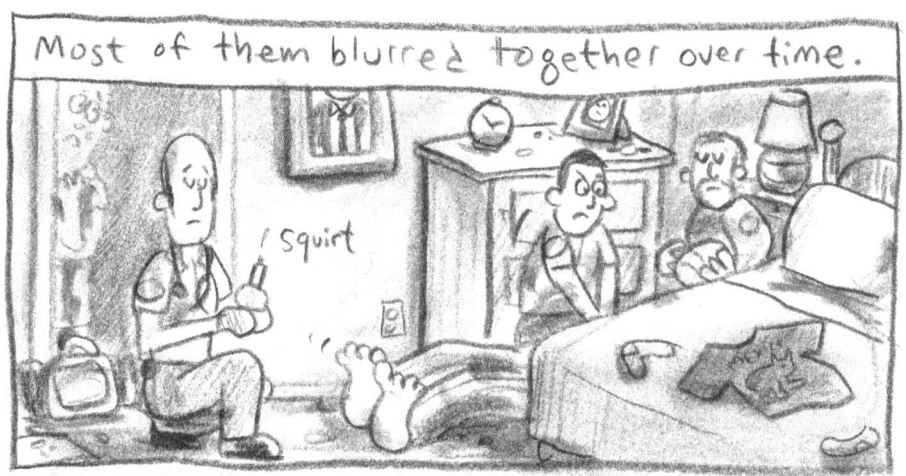

Most of them blurred together over time.

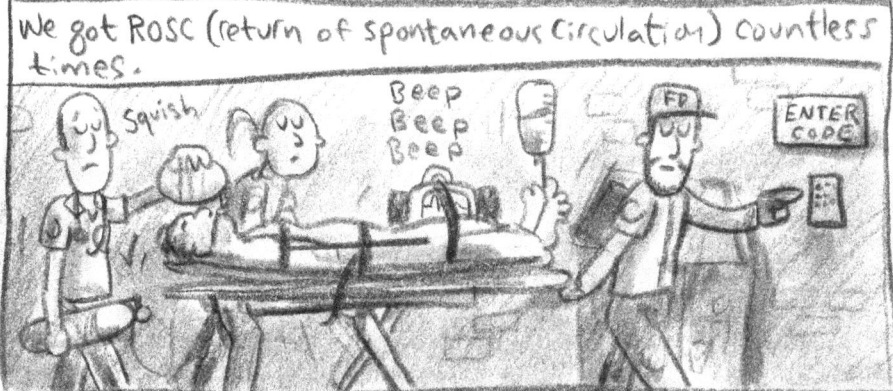

We got ROSC (return of spontaneous circulation) countless times.

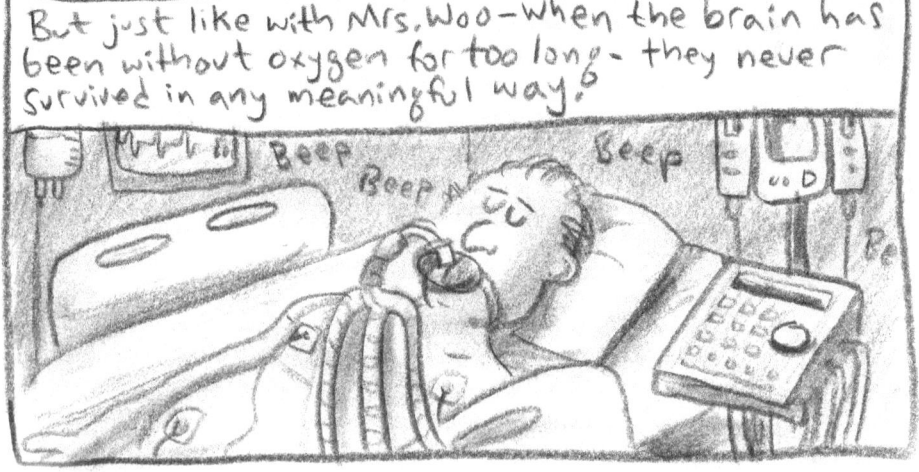

But just like with Mrs. Woo — when the brain has been without oxygen for too long — they never survived in any meaningful way.

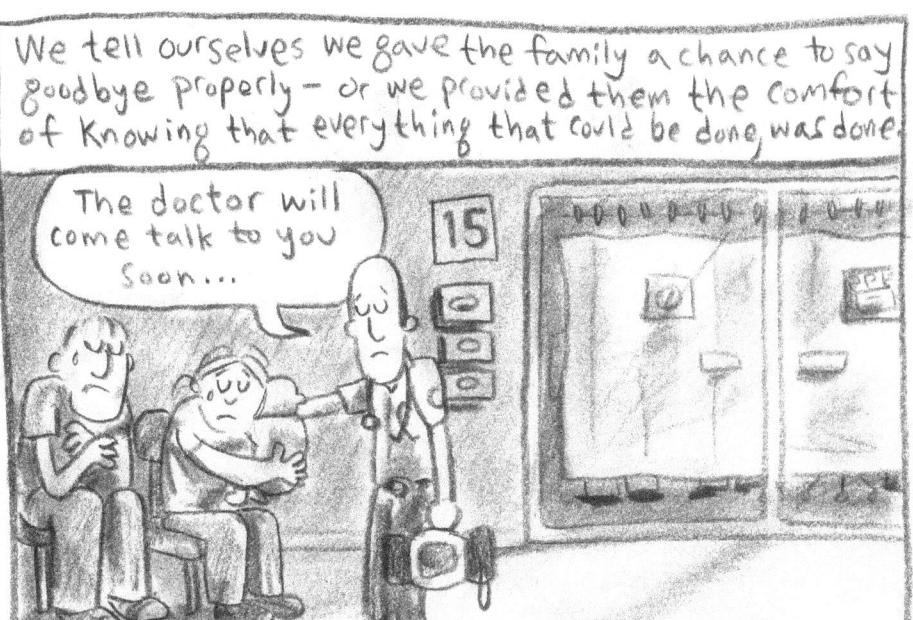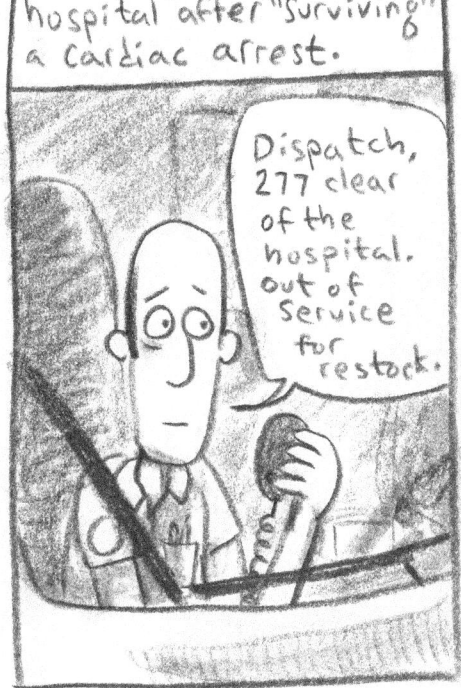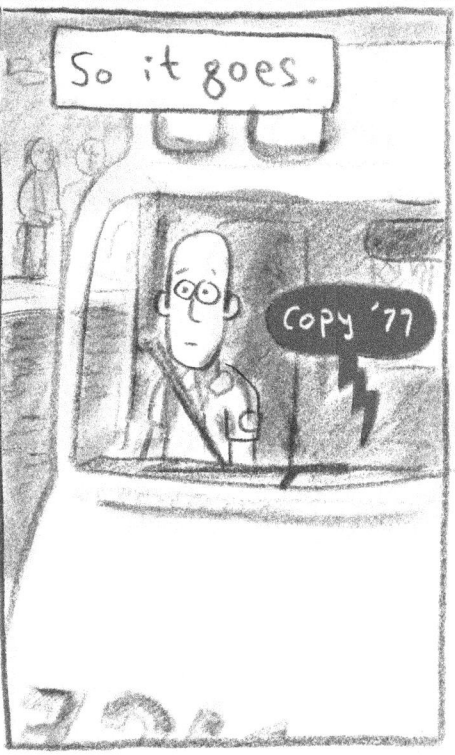

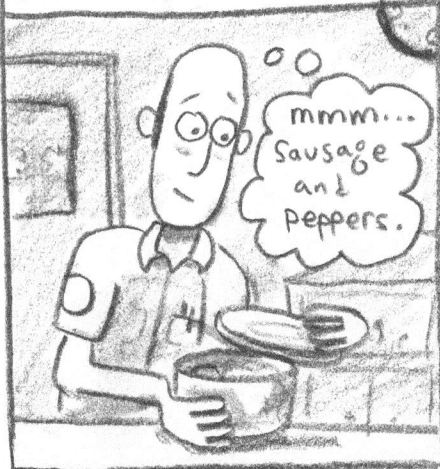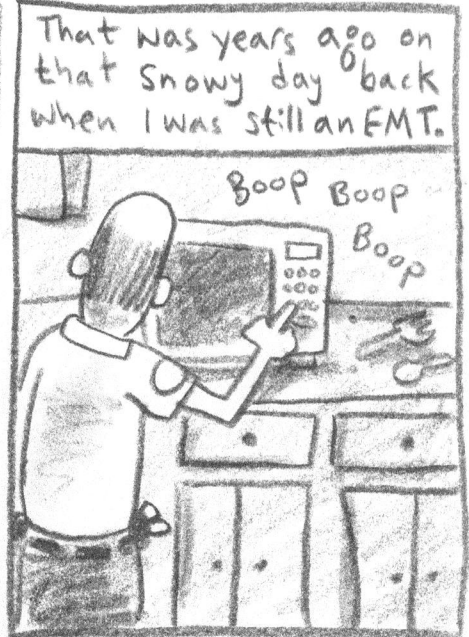

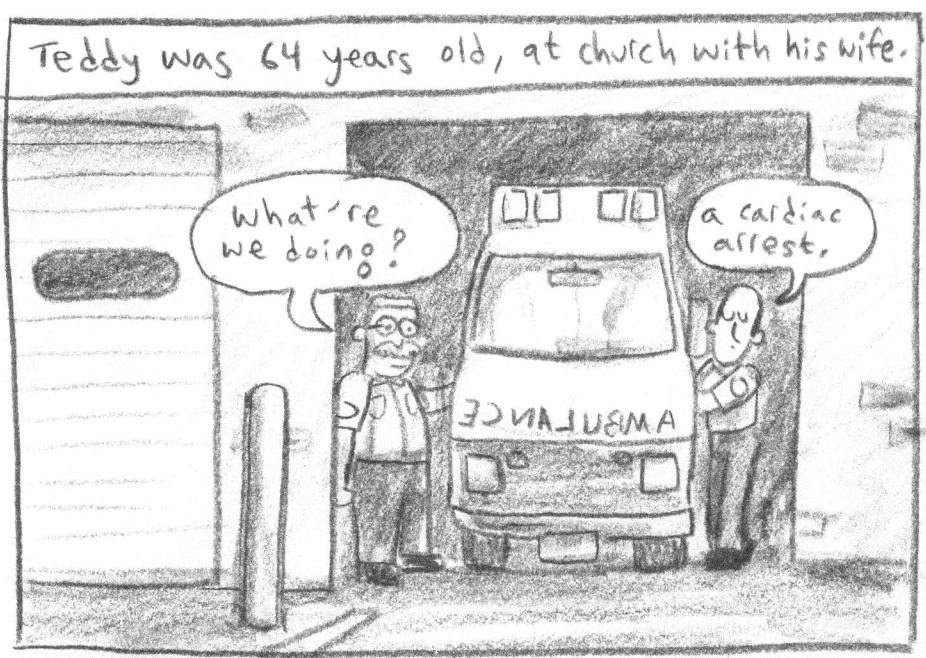

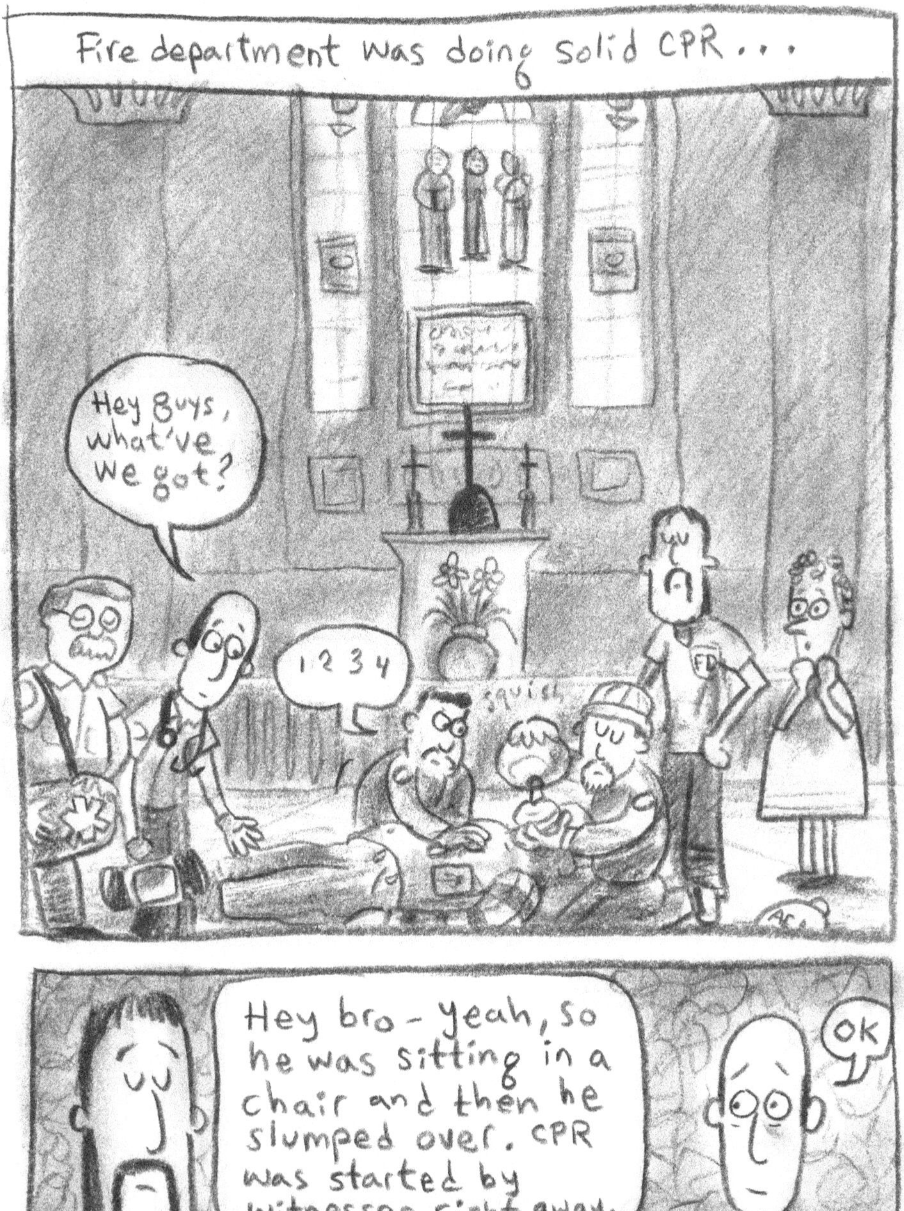

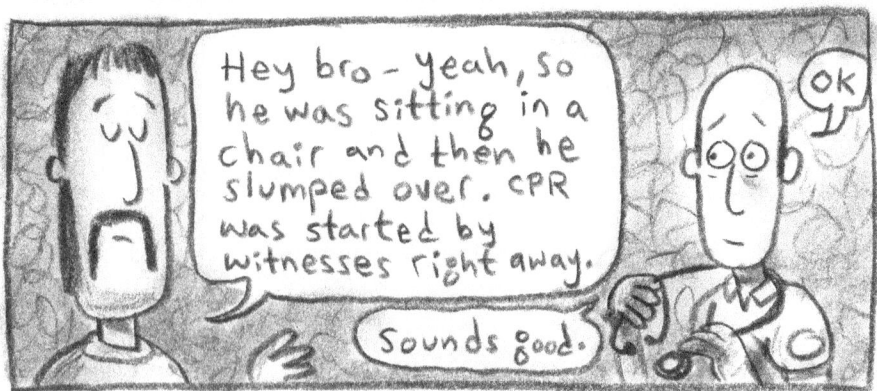

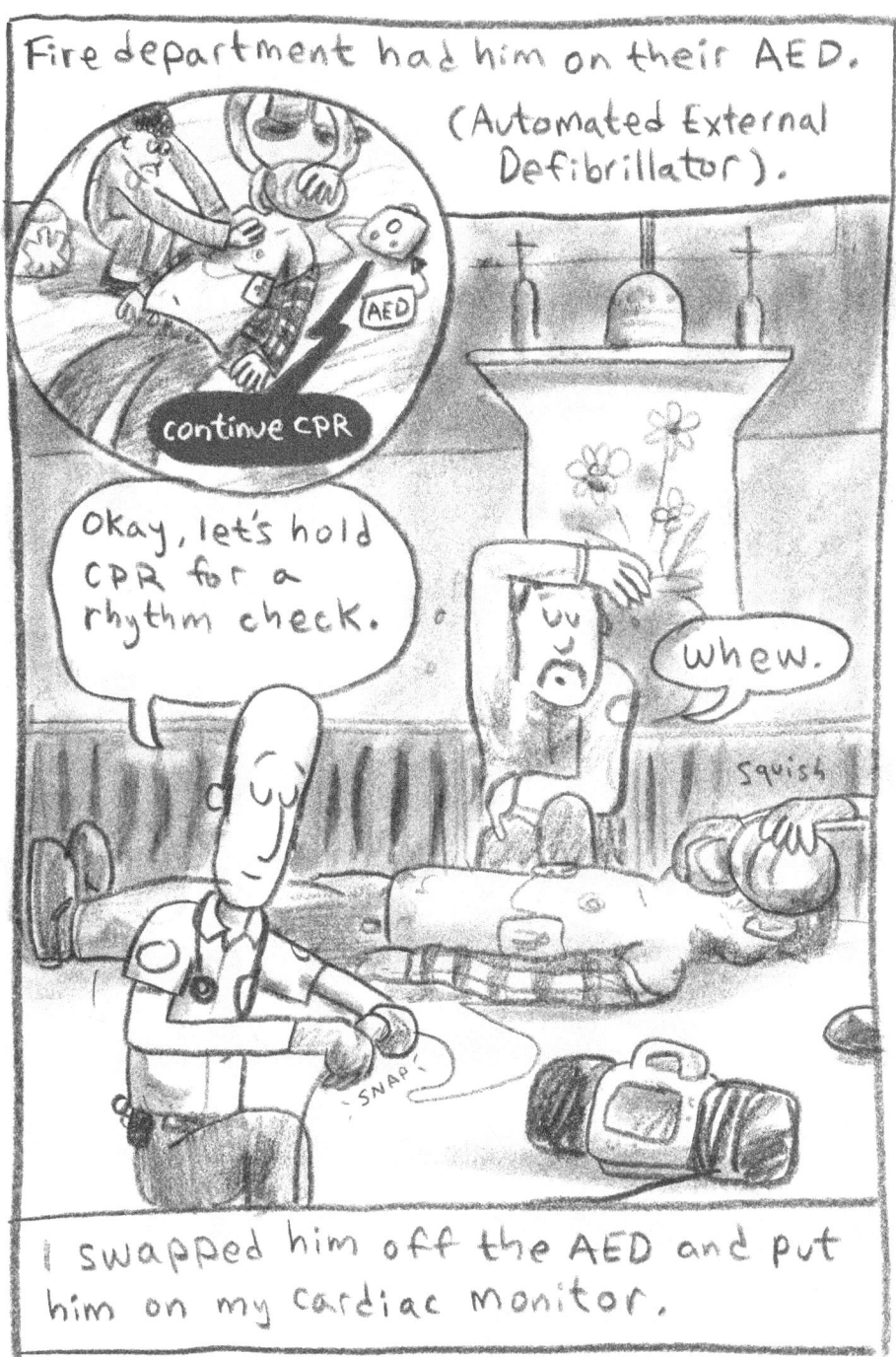

The rhythm was unmistakable.

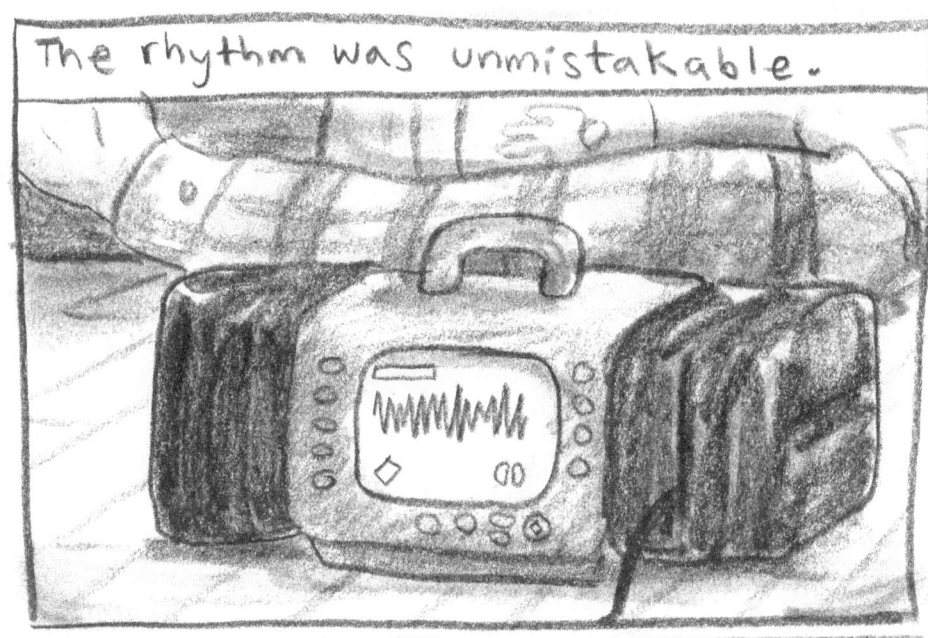

Teddy was in V-fib. Ventricular fibrillation. One of only two shockable rhythms.

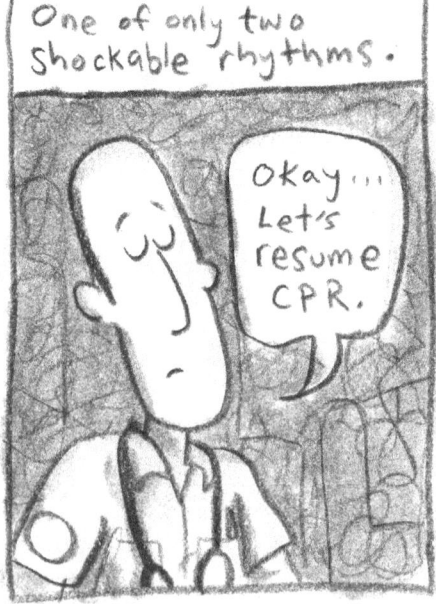

"Okay... Let's resume CPR."

It took a second for my brain to catch up.

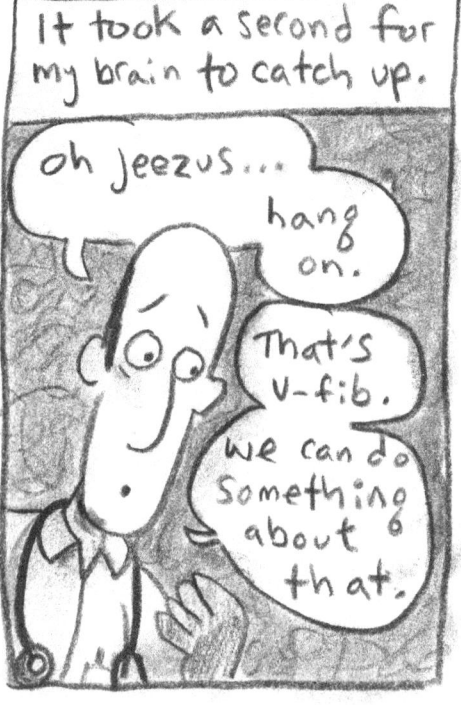

"Oh jeezus... hang on."

"That's V-fib. We can do something about that."

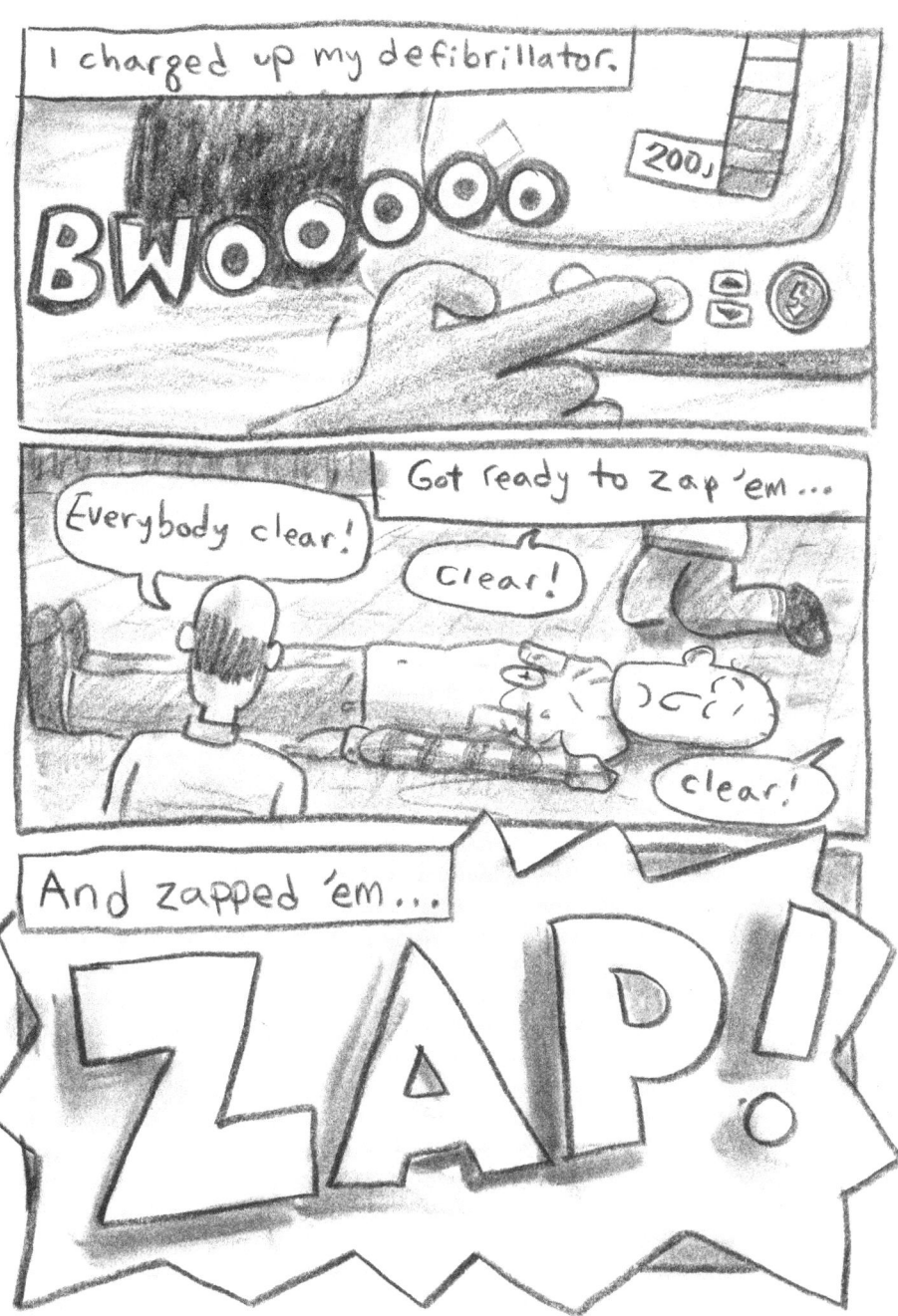

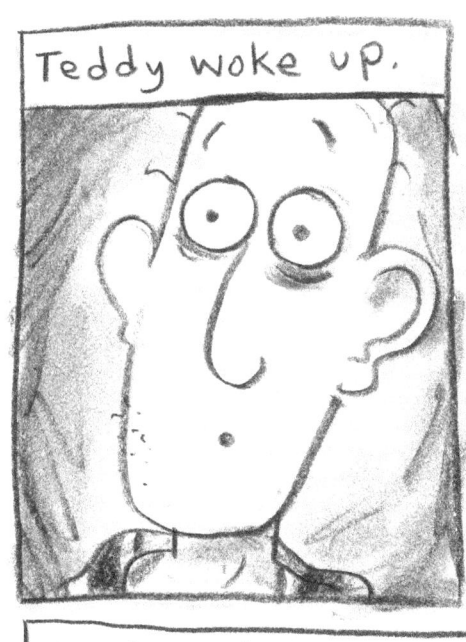
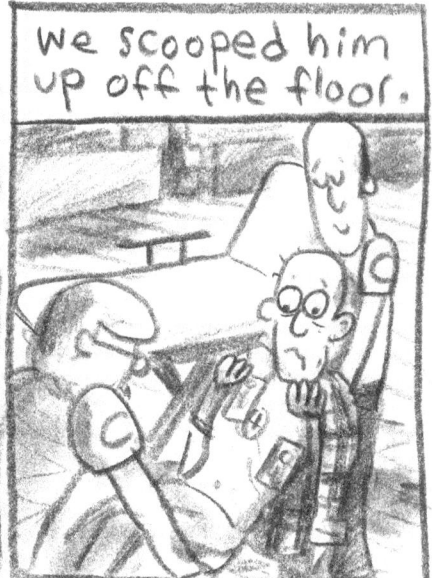
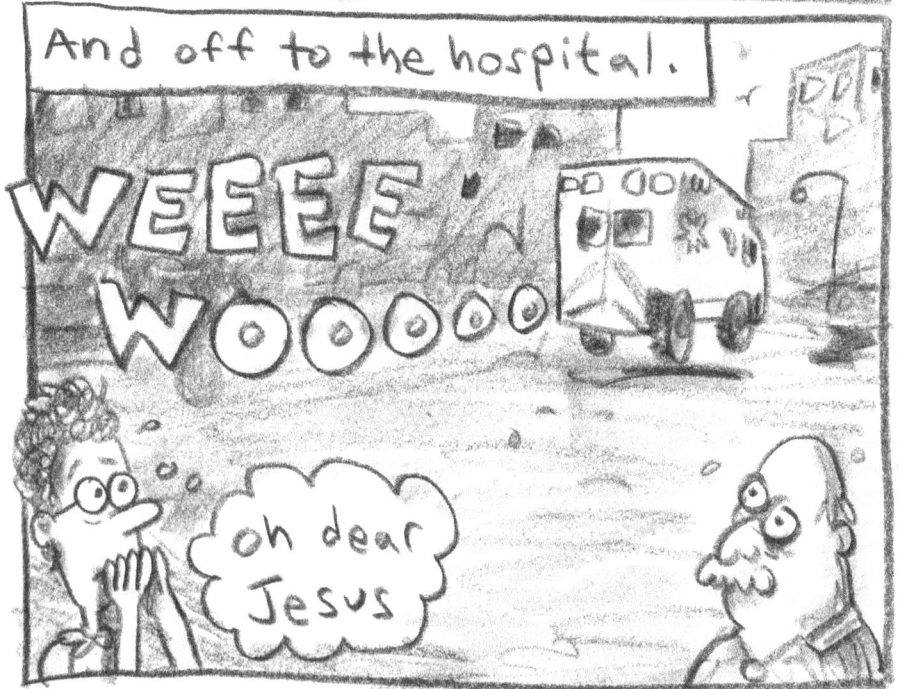

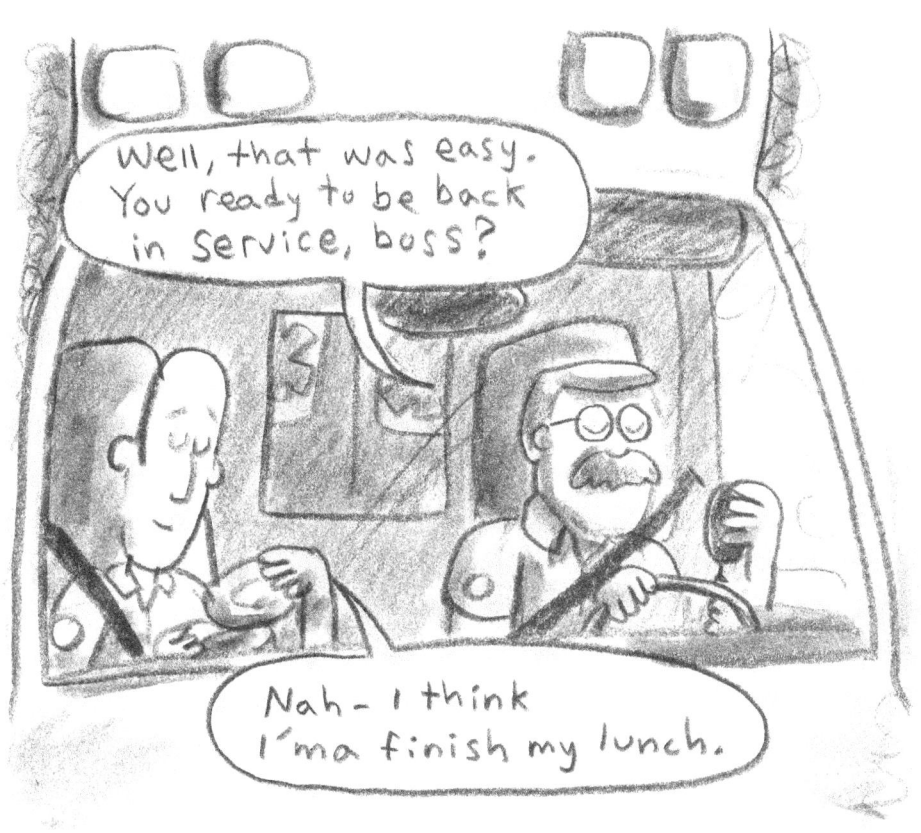

When we dropped Teddy off at the hospital, he was alert and oriented. His vitals were great. He was surprised to hear that he had just died.

424030

Afterword

It's been a few years since I made the pages you just read. A lot has happened. A lot has changed.

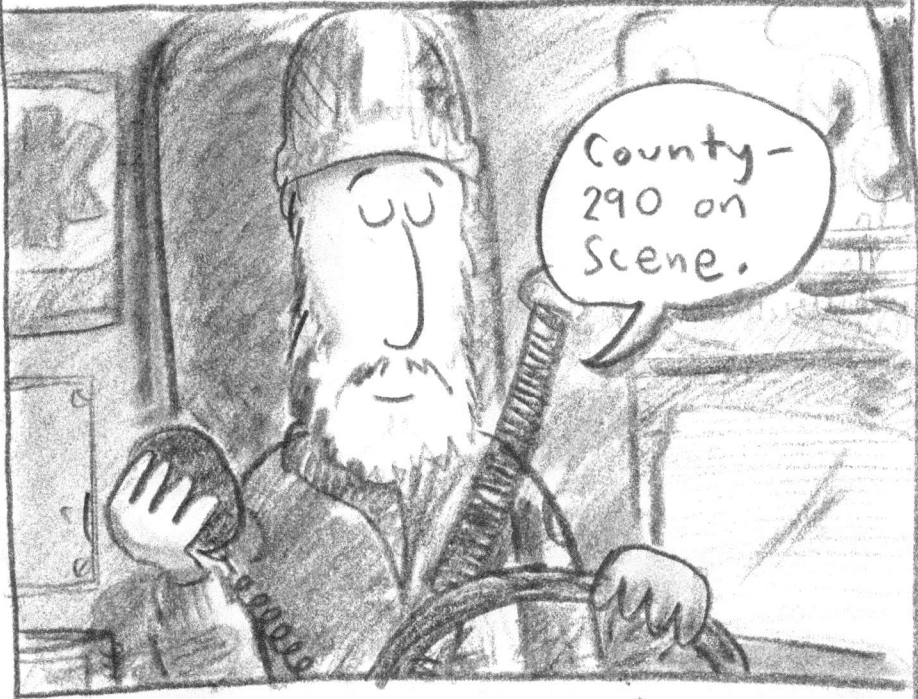

County-290 on scene.

Mobile Life got bought out by a bigger company. I was able to grow my beard back - my beard had become white.

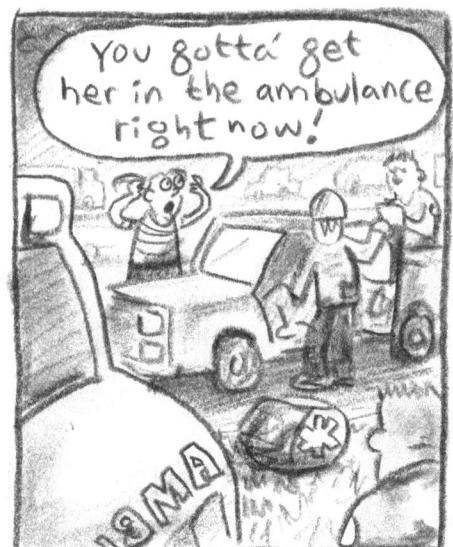
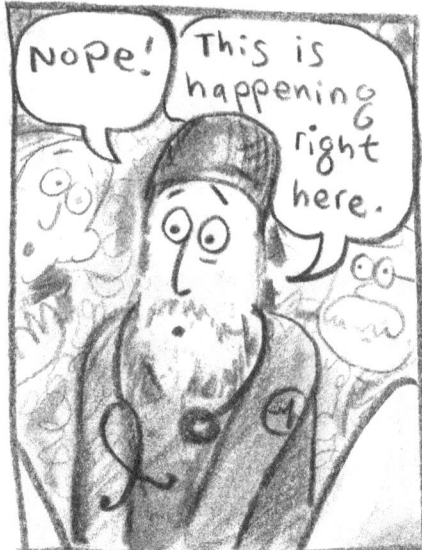
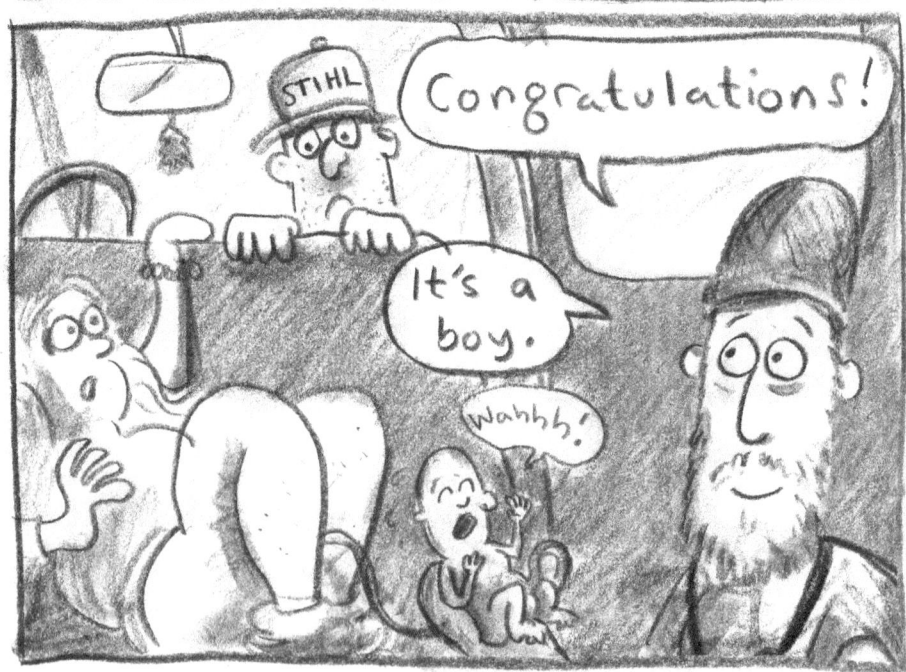

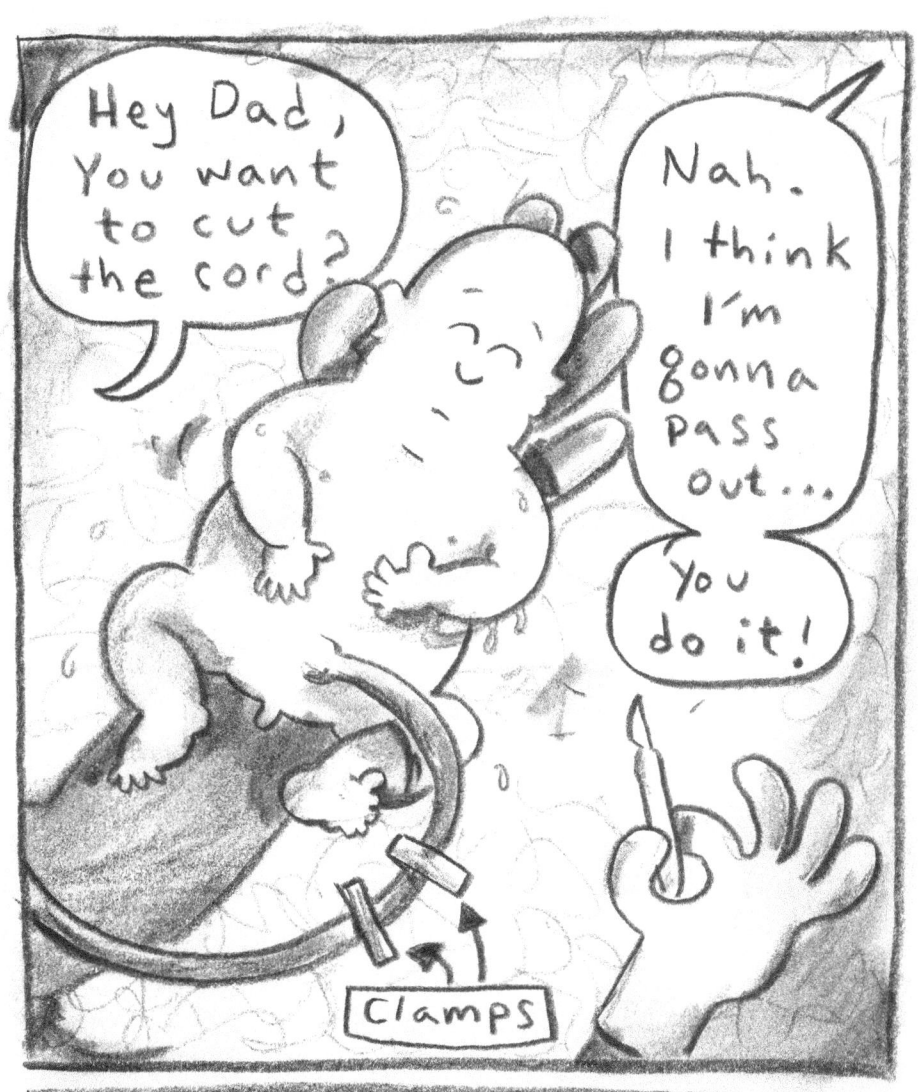

Eventually, I moved on to a smaller agency — a local rescue. So far, so good...

About the Author: Dave Horowitz is an artist and a paramedic. He lives and works in New York's Hudson Valley. He has also written and illustrated numerous books for children, including *The Ugly Pumpkin, Emergency Monster Squad, Humpty Dumpty Climbs Again, Five Little Gefiltes,* and many more.

More at **horowitzdave.com**
horowitz.dave *on Instagram*

www.ingramcontent.com/pod-product-compliance
Lightning Source LLC
Chambersburg PA
CBHW052128030426
42337CB00028B/5072